PSYCHOLOGY AND PERFORMING ARTS

PSYCHOLOGY AND PERFORMING ARTS

EDITED BY

GLENN D. WILSON

SWETS & ZEITLINGER B.V. AMSTERDAM / LISSE PUBLISHERS

SWETS & ZEITLINGER INC. BERWYN, PA

Library of Congress Cataloging-in-Publication Data

Psychology and performing arts / edited by Glenn D. Wilson.
p. cm.
"Compiled from the proceedings of the First International Conference on Psychology and Performing Arts held lat the Institute of Psychiatry, University of London in August 1990"--Pref.
Includes bibliographical references.
ISBN 9026511191
1. Performing arts--Psychological aspects--Congresses. 2. Performing arts--Therapeutic use--Congresses. I. Wilson, Glenn D. (Glenn Daniel) II. International Conference on Psychology and Performing Arts (1st : 1990 : University of London)
PN1590.P76P78 1991
791'.01'9--dc20 91-9691
CIP

CIP-Gegevens Koninklijke Bibliotheek, Den Haag

Psychology and performing arts / ed. by Glenn D. Wilson. - Amsterdam [etc.] : Swets & Zeitlinger
Proceedings of the First International Conference on Psychology and Performing Arts, held at the Institute of Psychiatry, University of London in August 1990. - Met lit. opg.
ISBN 90-265-1119-1
NUGI 711/925
Trefw.: uitvoerende kunst ; psychologie

Cover photograph by Kors van Bennekom - Hollandse Hoogte
Cover design by Rob Molthoff
Cover printed in the Netherlands by Casparie IJsselstein
Printed in the Netherlands

ISBN 90-265-1119-1
NUGI 711/925

Contents

Preface

This book is compiled from the proceedings of the First International Conference on Psychology and Performing Arts held at the Institute of Psychiatry, University of London in August 1990.

The aim of the conference was to bring together academics, clinicians and performers from around the world who shared an interest in the interface between psychology and the performing arts, including stage, music and dance, as well as more specialized types of performance such as mime, acrobatics, conjuring and puppetry. The conference was well-attended, with speakers coming from the United States, Canada and The Netherlands as well as Britain. Most found it very rewarding and the quality of the presentations can be judged by the selection reprinted here.

Two major questions were addressed: (1) What have psychology, psychiatry and other social sciences got to offer performers in overcoming difficulties and optimizing their art? (2) What does the theatrical process and experience have to tell us about human nature? The central presumption throughout the conference was that scientists and performers each have something to contribute to the other. A third major topic concerned the therapeutic applications of music, drama, dance and movement.

Glen Bryan, Alison Chumbley, Sharon Dawe and Andrew Worthington provided valuable assistance in the running of the conference. I am especially grateful to my co-organize r Shirley Chumbley, who handled the business arrangements for the conference.

Glenn Wilson
November, 1990

PART I
The Acting Process

Performance and possesion: The actor and our inner demons

Brian Bates

Department of Psychology, University of Sussex

The psychology of performance is a new approach to understanding the nature of human functioning by turning our attention to people who spend significant portions of their lives trying to understand and portray insights into ourselves: actors. In an ongoing research programme at the University of Sussex I and my colleagues are investigating the potential for psychology of using the work and experiences of the actor as a paradigm for understanding aspects of inner and interpersonal dynamics (Bates, 1986). This research, in which the indigenous psychology of the actor is explored as a source of knowledge for the development of psychology in general, complements the work of others (e.g. Wilson, 1985) who are applying the insights of scientific psychology to understanding the ways in which performers work.

This chapter considers certain experiences of actors which imply a new understanding of the concept of 'possession'. As part of this research the actors Charlton Heston, Liv Ullmann and Anthony Sher were interviewed, and material from those interviews, and others published elsewhere with these actors, are used as a basis for the analysis.

Possession was a powerful experience which lay at the centre of the actor's way in traditional societies. The actor became possessed by the spirits, gods, deities, of the 'other world', manifestations of external and universal forces incarnated in performance as 'spirit personalities' (LaBarre, 1972). Today, we associate possession with superstitions, primitive cultures and modern medical opinion considers possession states to be psychopathological.

Psychiatrists, dealing today with people distressed by involuntary possession (now called hysteria or dissociation), and seeing possession in an exclusively clinical environment, have reinforced the taboo of the state in Western societies. And psychiatric discourse represents the behaviour of a possessed person as '...gross non-reality ideation, abnormal perceptual experiences, (and) profound emotional upheavals' which constitute a 'schizoid' state - regarded as a serious pathological condition (Lewis, 1971). In other words, stripped of its scientific-sounding but assumption-ridden bias, this is saying that possession is a mental state involving highly imaginative ideas, unusual perceptual experiences and strong emotion - which is what actors experience in almost every performance.

Of course, our image of possession is of a person totally out of control, dominated by some psychic force more powerful than himself. But the common image of a zombie-like body, inhabited and controlled by an external agency, is misleading. While we often assume that the possessing force completely obliterates consciousness and will, even in traditional societies when actors 'become' the spirits and are 'possessed' by them, they do not lose contact with the requirements of the performance they are giving.

For example, one traditional shamanic actor says of a possession experience: 'I was obliged almost without ceasing to utter cries, weep, sing, dance and roll upon the ground where I went into horrible contortions; I was forced to jerk my head and feet in all directions, howl like a bear ... (but) I am never absent, I always know what I am doing or saying' (Cole, 1975 p. 42).

The traditional actor's state of possession is a powerful phenomenon, which alters the actor's behaviour and experience to that of the 'spirit'; but it is nevertheless a performance. It is a controlled possession. The traditional actor has a double consciousness; one part is possessed, the other observes and controls.

In contrast with the traditional actor's experience, contemporary actors' partial 'possessions' no longer involve spirits or deities but, rather, dramatic characters, imaginary people. And the character somehow asserts a presence which the actor finds difficult to exclude from his own life. Of course, most of us have been involved at some time with tasks or projects that have stayed with us, occupied our thoughts even while we are not working on them, 'haunted' us. But for an actor, when the project is an imaginary person who is occupying mental, emotional and physical space within him, the presence offers intriguing glimpses into the construction of the self. Especially when the character takes over in performance, briefly but decisively.

Charlton Heston had an attack of panic on stage in London. But who panicked? Heston or the character? As part of my research into the psychology of performance, I interviewed Charlton Heston in some depth about a recent experience on stage which illustrates the process of possession during performance.

He was playing the role of Commander Queeg in his London production of *The Caine Mutiny Court Martial*. The play concerns the court martial of Queeg, who is accused of bad captaincy and also of pilfering from his ship's supplies. He, on the other hand, alleges mutiny, because subordinate officers took over the command of his ship when they felt he was heading it for destruction in a storm. The proceedings lead to Queeg's breakdown in court; a performance for which Charlton Heston won critical acclaim from London theatre reviewers.

There is an intense moment in the cross-examination when the lawyer (played by Ben Cross), defending the subordinate officer, traps Commander Queeg in a lie. Queeg, with a darting movement of Heston's eyes, shows that he is trapped. Panic. And the emotion of the scene surprised Heston.

He explained to me what happened, 'Ben Cross and I had been using more and more that moment when he looks at me and says, "Commander, there are many points of dissimilarity between you and the testimony of other witnesses. If you like I'll ask for a five minute recess so that you can put your thoughts as best as you can." He's using more and more a moment of real sympathy, because he does hate the fact that he is going to have to destroy Queeg's career to defend his client.'

Heston entered this moment in the play carrying with him the feelings of Commander Queeg. He explained that as Queeg he didn't feel sorry for himself. He felt persecuted. He also felt just in his cause; he was one man against a whole ship of mutineers. He did his best. He served for years without making one single mistake and he could prove it. His reputation had been spotless until then, and he would not have besmirched it by lies and distortions. But Heston points to the breaking point in Commander Queeg's emotional armour, 'It's all mixed with fear, because somewhere deep down he knows it isn't true.'

Charlton Heston lost control. 'That moment when Ben gives Queeg a chance to escape, the emotion builds up, and the last night it frightened me, as Queeg. To the point where there was, in my judgement, too much emotion. I couldn't control it.' At the crucial moment in the scene the character took full possession and Heston realized that it was his own emotion being expressed. He had allowed the character Queeg to possess him.

In discussing this experience with me, Charlton Heston continually returned to the 'loss of control' when 'real' emotion took over from acted emotion. When an actor 'puts himself in the character or, to express it in terms of possession, allows the character to 'enter into himself', he feels the emotions *of that character*. How can this happen?

The actor uses his imagination to construct a vivid picture of what the situation would be like, and then reacts as if he were the character. He registers the emotions, and how they can be expressed to the audience, during the rehearsal, and then practices it until the emotion becomes automatic rather than a charge. It is distanced a little from the actor's own primary experiences of emotion, and becomes the emotion of the character.

Of course, in performance the actor must invest the character's emotion with spontaneity and vitality. He must prevent the 'fixing of emotion' in rehearsal from becoming too mechanical. The emotions of the character need to be fuelled by the juices of the actor's own emotion. Even with the actor's inner self observing and controlling, it is hardly surprising that there exists the risk of confusion. 'Fixed' emotion can suddenly merge with that of the actor, and the actor experiences emotion as himself. In other words, it was not Commander Queeg who panicked. It was Charlton Heston. And for one surprising and disturbing moment, Charlton Heston was suddenly and totally possessed by Commander Queeg.

But while it's possible to conceive of the actor's own emotion becoming fused with that of the character, we are still left with an unclear picture of where the character's emotion comes from. For although actors might act the emotion, we have all witnessed performances in which the quality of the emotion was undeniably real.

In the film *Face to Face* Liv Ullmann depicts a psychiatrist breaking down. In one six-minute scene the character loses and gains and loses control of her emotions. Of her control, as the actress, over the emotional energy of this long, demanding and extremely intense scene, Liv Ullmann told me in an interview, 'I like to think I'm in control all the time, that it's not the character doing it. But it's a mixture.' She explains that, 'There are two ways of crying: one is that you allow your character to cry; but the other is that you get so moved by yourself that you cry. And then you are in deep trouble because you are into self-involvement.'

She emphasizes the importance of being a channel, 'Actually the fun of acting is to use your openness in such a way that the character can come through you. And if the character needs to cry, it's the character and not you feeling all over the place. It's a kind of openness that allows you to stand beside and watch, like having an instrument so tuned that whatever you choose to play on it will come out right. The moment you feel too much private anger or private anguish you aren't in tune anymore' (Ullmann, 1977, p. 96).

A further dimension is revealed when she reflects on a particular stage role. Acting in the play *The Chalk Circle*, Liv Ullmann is playing a character called Grusha. Revolution has come to the village where she lives in poverty. Everyone has fled the murder and fire that followed in the wake of war. While she herself was running away she found an infant abandoned by its mother. In playing the scene, Liv Ullmann describes an unexpected experience, 'Grusha is sitting beside the baby whose mother has abandoned it, and as she bends down to pick it up, a tear comes into her eye and rolls down her cheek. Suddenly the tear is there and it is a wonderful feeling. And I am surprised because I hadn't known she would weep at that moment.. But it is no longer myself caught in an emotion, not I that weep' (Ullmann, 1977, p 97).

So how can we understand such a process in which the actor contains a character's emotions? It sounds as if an 'alien being', in the form of a character, is literally using the body and mind of the actor in order to exist. Of this process Ullmann says, 'I see myself as a sieve. Everyone's feelings flow through me, but I am never able to retain them. In the evening I am put aside empty - only to be inundated the next day with new emotions' (Ullmann, 1977, p 96).

The opening and maintenance of these emotional 'streams' are like an exercising of one's psychic being. But although Liv Ullmann describes herself as a kind of empty vessel through which emotions flow, she nevertheless recognizes something crucially important for our understanding of the way in which 'possession' works, namely that the character and herself are one and the same person.

The character within Liv Ullmann is experiencing its own emotions, but they are derived from Liv's own emotional 'reservoir'. The possessing character, personality, being, is allowed a stream or channel of space into the 'backlog' of the actor's experience, going right through the layers from deep unconscious to surface persona. Sometimes, Liv does not know where the emotions come from; sometimes, the possessing character surprises her.

But the observations of Liv Ullmann and other actors make clear that when the possessing character becomes too powerful, it dips into other areas of the actor's psyche, and begins to take over control.

Possesion Reconsidered

Who are the dramatic characters, the beings that possess modern actors like succubi, using parts of their emotions, and yet leading an independent existence as the 'Mask' seen by the audience? To answer that question we need to look afresh at the nature of possession.

Psychotherapist Rollo May advocates a redefinition of 'demonic possession' (May, 1970). He suggests that the 'demon' be defined as any natural function in the individual that has the power of taking over the whole person. 'Demonic possession' is, then, the takeover of part or all of the personality by one of these powerful functions. He maintains that we all have 'demons' within us, aspects of ourselves that we have not allowed freedom, and that have remained lost, ignored, or hidden - and there are lessons to be drawn from Rollo May's suggestion, because we are 'possessed' every day of our lives.

Everyday Possesion

Most of us are aware that significant portions of each day are spent in 'daydreams', fantasies, and a kind of reverie in which we talk to ourselves. This inner talk is essentially identical to the way we might talk to someone else, except that the words are not spoken out aloud. This self-talk even has the structure of an inner conversation, evidenced by the curious mixture of pronouns, names and modes of address employed. Often an inner voice says 'I' ('I'd better hurry up'), but also from time to time says 'You' ('You're going to be late again'). Sometimes one part of the inner self even offers a statement, directive or question, and another aspect responds with an answer (Caughey, 1984).

Of course, it can be argued that this internal dialogue is simply the way we voice ideas in our minds, and that it differs from the 'split self' experienced by the possessed person who, while perhaps aware of what is happening, is nevertheless in a trance. But the basic characteristic of a trance state is that the mind is fully, or almost fully engaged by an activity that excludes it from awareness of 'external reality' as we usually conceive of it. In other words, a person in a trance has lost their mind, but only in the sense that the mind has been relieved of moment-to-moment checks against the social environment that is the hallmark of the state we would recognize as 'normal waking consciousness'.

Individuals, alone in a room, or driving a car, or doing anything that isolates them from social intercourse, enter a state akin to trance, in which they float away on a sea of internal reverie. When someone knocks on the door, we 'come back to ourselves', to social reality. In fact, it is clear that significant portions of our waking lives are spent in mild trance states, in which we carry on an internal dialogue with a presence which resides inside us. But the 'character' possessing us does it in private and silently, while the character played by the actor possesses in public, and is expressed externally.

Actors create imaginary characters within themselves and deal with them in the same way we deal with the imaginary self that lives inside us. But we often forget that our inner self, with which we converse and argue, is an imaginary construction, a trick of the mind which allows us to negotiate with our life experience in the form of an inner character.

The actor constructs a new inner character; the imaginary person he is to play. And in so doing, he calls upon the various depths of his inner experience in new ways. Whether the actor tries to work from within that experience to build a character, or creates first an idea of the character and allows his emotional resources to respond to it, either way the actor is activating his inner experience around a new focus. Creating characters keeps life experience moving, flowing and flexible.

Antony Sher, in his book *Year of the King* (Sher, 1985) chronicles his preparation of the role of Richard III, and one reviewer summed up vividly the picture he paints, 'Sher must himself become the freaks or friends he imagines, permitting them house-room inside him.... Though he begins to assemble the character authologically, from mimicry of others and from trying on a battery of prosthetic disguises, as he goes on he sheds the assumed personae, the false noses and lank wigs, admitting that Richard is himself: he uses his own voice, his own hair, his own body, his own personality. For the coronation, he appeared naked: what is acting, after all, but self denudation?' (p. 25).

It is interesting that possession is expressed as self-denudation. The allowing of creatures within oneself is the same process as revealing oneself. The theatre director Peter Brook says that 'Actors are mediumistic: the ideas suddenly envelop the whole in an act of possession.... the actors are penetrated by themselves' (Conrad, 1985). So actors possess themselves.

When an actor is partially 'possessed', either by a character that takes over during the performance, or maintains a presence in the mind afterwards, he is essentially experiencing, confronting, digesting aspects of his inner self. Aspects that might never be realized if the only inner self available through which experience could be expressed was the usual inner self with which we converse silently.

Creating a character which calls upon so much of the hidden, repressed, inner experience of the actor that the character possesses the actor, is less common but not unusual. In these cases actors sense something of themselves in their performances which lead them to feel possessed. That 'something' was once held in awe by members of traditional societies. It is the level of human experience which is deeply embedded in all of us. It is the secret of self-possession.

In a sense, to be influenced by hidden, unknown aspects of ourselves is a sort of possession. The ghosts of our life experiences lead us this way and that without our conscious knowledge. For most of us, who do not enter into depth psychotherapy, the deep waters of our unconscious run undisturbed by even a dipping toe of consciousness. Our only clues to the hidden parts of ourselves are the fragmented images of dreams, and the frequently inexplicable nature of the strength of our emotional response to everyday events.

Developing a performance psychology, in which we begin to explore aspects of human functioning using the work of the actor *as a paradigm*, illustrates vividly some of the insights evolved by other paradigms but sheds new light on the *nature* of the processes involved. Psychology has as much to learn from actors as actors have to learn from psychology.

References

Bates, B.C. *The Way of the Actor.* London: Century Hutchinson 1986
Caughey, J.L. *Imaginary Social Worlds.* University of Nebraska Press 1984
Cole, D. *The Theatrical Event.* Middletown, Connecticut: Wesleyan University Press 1975
Conrad, P. 'An actor possessed.' *The Observer.* 23 June 1985
LaBarre, W *The Ghost Dance: Origins of Religion.* New York: Delta 1972
Lewis, I.M. *Ecstatic Religion: An Anthropological Study of Spirit Possession and Shamanism.* Baltimore: Penguin 1971
May, R. 'Psychotherapy and the Daimonic.' In J. Campbell (Ed.) *Myth, Dreams and Religion.* New York: Dutton 1970
Sher, A. *Year of the King.* London: Chatto and Windus, 1985
Ullmann, L. *Changing.* London: Weidenfeld and Nicolson, 1977
Wilson, G.D. *The Psychology of Performing Arts.* New York: St Martin's Press, 1985

Actor and mask as metaphors for psychological experience

Katharine Hitchcock and Brian Bates

Department of Psychology, University of Sussex

As part of an ongoing programme of research we are exploring the psychology of the performing artist as a central paradigm for understanding certain aspects of human functioning (Bates, 1986). In this chapter we outline several perspectives from which the actor's use of masks suggests insights into the experience of multiplicity and fragmentation.

The ideas that we each play roles: mother, father, wife, lover, children, and various other occupational and social roles, is familiar to almost everyone. In 1959, Erving Goffman made academic Shakespeare's earlier claim that "All the world's a stage" and the people in it are "merely players" by detailing the performative quality of human behaviour and in so doing demonstrated the value of a theatrical vocabulary for furthering sociological analysis (Goffman, 1959). More recently it has been shown that conflict between the demands of the several social roles we might simultaneously occupy and/or more personal belief and value systems, is a major feature in any so called "crisis of identity" (Breakwell, 1983). Even within the playing of one role, we find ourselves behaving in quite different and sometimes unexpected and contradictory ways.

Psychologically, the experience of multiplicity and fragmentation often presents as "voices in the head". Much of our time for example is spent talking to ourselves, about what we have done and said, imagining what we should have done and said and what we intend to do and say in the future. Along with other kinds of imaginings, recent studies have shown that about 2/3 of our waking life is spent in such reverie (Pope, 1985). Such voices, even if sometimes in direct and fierce competition with one another, are considered to form a part of our normal everyday consciousness. Our usual response however is to favour one voice over and above the others. We regard the many other voices as incursions, and as threatening to our familiar sense of ourselves.

If we listen to these voices, establishing their right to be heard, and come to recognize, as Jung did, our complexes as *persons*, we come to discover both their autonomy and their influence over us. In the extreme case of multiple personality, voices are acted out; they literally become characters. But none of us is immune to their persuasion, finding ourselves as we do repeatedly and unconsciously enacting the same scenes despite our best intentions.

But if we regard these 'states' or 'personas' not as fully articulated, fully functioning people, but as metaphorically equivalent, then their expression is as a mask. And masks can be taken off as well as put on. Indeed in shamanistic societies actors did, in ritual theatre, put masks on, become 'possessed' by the characters they were playing, and then at the conclusion of the ritual, take them off again and return to their 'normal' personality. It shows an ability and talent still demonstrable in modern actors to differentiate, regard and respond to our many selves as masks. Understanding the nature and function of these masks suggests an understanding of ourselves as figures in a story, whereby we might see the significances of events and experiences in terms of plots. Or with reference to the deeper, more universally shared story-lines of our lives, in terms of mythical enactments.

More precisely, the nature of masks leads us to a consideration of how we might reconcile the paradox and ambiguities encountered in our attempts to make distinctions between social and personal identity, or the actor and his mask, and more essentially between appearance and reality. The central paradox encountered when wearing a mask is experienced through its capacity to be simultaneously both concealing and revealing. The covering of the face frees our behaviour because we no longer have to conform to the image we usually project of ourselves. The metaphorical masks of everyday life too can have this transforming effect. Changing our clothes and the wearing of make up are perhaps the most common examples. We not only look different but can experience a change in what we feel and the way we behave. Appearances can, it seems, create realities. Of course our attempts to change what we feel through this physical transformation can fail and may even intensify the very experience we seek to change.

Because a mask can fail to transform our way of experiencing, it has sometimes been considered useful to think of this difference in terms of two different kinds of masks. Peter Brooke for example speaks of these two kinds in the following way. The first he sees in terms of a concealment, of a hiding, even a lie, in that we can discern a difference between the outward appearance and inner reality. What we see is not "in tune with what is going on inside" (Brooke, 1981). These are the kind of masks we meet most often in our everyday life, worn as they are in order to maintain our social face. The second, he sees as one in which the outer appearance is *in* tune with an inner reality. Distinguishing between kinds of masks in this way can, however, be misleading, for it might also be the case that the first kind of mask is in fact also revealing - revealing of a person split two ways.

As such we might regard the difference between these kinds of masks less in terms of some being revealing and some being concealing and rather direct our attention to another underlying dimension. For the tendency to see ourselves in terms of singularity, and various 'either/or' dichotomies, is perhaps our most limiting and most powerful characteristic.

Mask as metaphor implies that every appearance is a reality and likewise every reality is an appearance. The mask is essentially ambiguous, and always of dual nature. Jenkins, (1981) in his article on the use of masks in Bali, describes the mask as "a potent metaphor for the coalescence of the universal and the particular, immobility and change, disguise and revelation". As "living archetypes" masks in Bali are "the interface between the timeless world of myth and the immediate world of fact". Masks thus serve a mediatory role between myth and reality. As personifications of archetypes, masks can be seen to re-present, show us, what Jung called the universal patternings of our psychological experiences. The mask as an archetypal image can thus also be seen as a personification of the psyche's most paradigmatic mode of speech. Like dreams, masks speak to us metaphorically, in images. To recognize that the power of mask resides in its paradoxical quality, and is lost if we believe that it is merely a mask, is also to implicate a different approach to our dreams, an approach whereby every interpretation and explanation must be seen as a kind of fiction.

Turning our attention to the actor now, in relation to his masks, we are able to see more fully the psychological implications and possibilities of using the mask as metaphor. We consider that the actor's capacity to differentiate psychological experience by means of characters or masks, may be seen as a method for recovering and making present the archetypes at play within our everyday experiences.

The actor, by assuming the role of a character, stands as an intermediary figure, situated as he is between identities. Experiencing the multiplicity and paradox of being and not being the character or mask played, the actor-in-performance, as Schechner has pointed out, can be seen as a "paradigm of liminality....All effective performances", he says, "share this 'not- not not' quality: Olivier is not Hamlet, but also he is not not Hamlet: his performance is between a denial of being another (= I am me) and a denial of not being another (= I am Hamlet)" (Schechner, 1981). In psychological terms the actor's mask can be seen to mediate between ego and archetype, between what is personal and what is collective.

One could even say that the actor's ability to distinguish himself from the mask or character possessing him is possible, in other words, because of his state of capacity for entering a schizophrenic-like state. Unlike the schizophrenic though there is not, as is sometimes assumed, a loss of ego functioning, so much as a relativisation of our normal ego, considered in terms of a "letting go" or an unlearning of the ego's habitual ways. In performance consciousness, or double consciousness as it is also described, the actor develops the capacity to stand back and observe his "possession" and must not get taken over by it. The actor thus stands as a metaphor, or a way of seeing, our own potential to distinguish, as David Holt describes, "a continuing and enduring ego from the changing and various personae of the moment" (Holt, 1965).

Psychologically we can understand the development of a performance-like consciousness in terms of the "as if" perspective of play. The experienced reality is given keen description in Winnicot's (1971) concept of "transitional space". Defined as an "intermediate area of experiencing", this reality is not literally true but it is nevertheless experientially real. Thus the reality of the actor as character is that of a figure in a story. Given that this play has long been considered the basis of myth and theatre, as well as psychotherapy, it is perhaps surprising that the actor has not been more directly implicated in our psychological life.

For by seeing ourselves as actors we may see ourselves in the role of many masks. This enables us to re-imagine ourselves and events and experiences against a backdrop of myth and its *many* archetypal figures. If we return to the experience of multiplicity we can see that when we respond to these other figures, or other voices, from our normal ego perspective, which wants always to be centre stage, interpreting all viewpoints in terms of its needs, we respond to conflict oppositionally. This oppositional thinking, based as it is on rational logic, attempts to resolve conflicts accordingly. It is a response which is bent upon seeking a single truth. It must deny other perspectives their truths, must repress them in fact in order to maintain *its* mask. And further, our tendency to identify ourselves only with its mask, what we might call the ego mask, keeps us unconscious of our multiple possibilities. In such an identification we cannot help but continue with our literal enactments.

In summary, we suggest that the development of a performance-like consciousness might be seen as a way of allowing our many selves a more metaphorical expression. Placing this idea in the wider context of story and plot, the development of performance-like consciousness represents an ability to see ourselves as many figures in a story, whereby the significance of events and experiences can be related to a variety of plots. This is unlike Freud, who saw the significance of all stories in terms of only one plot and one character, thus perpetuating the myth of a single author, and more like the newly-emerging Post-Jungian tradition of Archetypal Psychology. James Hillman, the main proponent of this tradition suggests that we re-imagine ourselves in terms of many plots (Hillman 1983). In doing this we might find the kind of dramatic background against which our multiplicity may be validated. The way of the actor's mask suggests to us that to see our conflicts more precisely as "dramatic tensions", of psychological origin and above all necessary to the plot enacted, is an additional perspective worth exploring.

Finally, we might recall Jung's claim that "the gods have become diseases" and perhaps suggest that it is within our contemporary dis-ease, approached as metaphorical mask, that a more authentic identity may be found, one of multiple archetypes. Jung has spoken of our obligation to reverse our rationalistic causal sequence, "and instead of deriving these figures from our psychic conditions, must derive our psychic conditions from these figures.... It is not we who personify them; they have a personal nature from the very beginning" (Jung, 1953). Taking Jung's idea of the collective unconscious to its most radical conclusion we might come to recognize that we can become conscious of not just our personal history, nor just the history of mankind, but of deeper origins. Our identity, expressed in such universal masks, may have to be imagined in other than human terms.

References

Bates, B. *The Way of the Actor*. London: Century, 1986

Breakwell, G. 'Formulations and Searches'. In G. Breakwell (Ed.) *Threatened Identities*. New York, 1983

Brooke, P. 'Lie and Glorious Adjective' (Interview). *Parabola* (Vol. VI, No. 3) 1981

Goffman, E. *The Presentation of Self in Everyday Life*. New York: Doubleday, 1959

Hillman, J. *Healing Fiction*. New York: Station Hill Press, 1983

Holt, D. *Persona and Actor.* Unpublished Doctoral Thesis submitted to the Jung Institute, 1965.

Jenkins, R .'Two-Way Mirrors'. *Parabola* (Vol. VI, No. 3) 1981

Jung, C. *Collected Works.*(Bollingen Series XX, Vol. 13) London: Routledge and Kegan Paul, 1953

Pope, K. 'Fantasy'. In: G. Stricker and R. Keisner *From Research to Clinical Practice.* London: Plenum Press, 1985

Schechner, R. 'Performers and Spectators Transported and Transformed'. *The Kenyon Review* (N.S.3 Part 4), Fall 1981

Winnicot, D. *Playing and Reality.* London: Tavistock, 1971

Double identity: The effect of the acting process on the self-perception of professional actors - *Two case illustrations*

Jacqueline Hammond and Robert J. Edelmann

Department of Psychology, University of Surrey

Aristotle said that a person shown on the stage is of no significance in himself. He merely carries his share of an action whose interest does not lie in his personality. There is something that needs to be acted through. Actors carry that need and the mask they wear underscores the fact that precisely because they are merely acting, they can represent an action which cannot be included within their personality. This sentiment is reiterated by Styan (1975):

> '....either in tragedy, or in farce, the actor immersed in its spirit, stands outside his role, while seeming to believe utterly in its reality.'

But can professional actors really divorce themselves completely from a dramatic role so that it has no effect upon the way they perceive themselves?

Henry and Sims (1970) suggest that professional actors suffer from 'self-image' problems, and that playing a dramatic role gives actors a sense of identity which they would otherwise lack. They found that although the actors initially appeared to show considerable confusion or 'diffuseness' in their identity, when they were retested some weeks into the rehearsal period of a new play, their identity confusion appeared to have decreased.

Fisher and Fisher (1981) argue that 'trying on the identities of others' can be extremely disturbing for professional actors. More recently, DeCosta, Buse and Amdursky (1986) found that professional actors had problems which related to the boundary between themselves and the dramatic roles they played; in other words, where the 'characterisation left off and the individual himself began.'

Despite such studies, there has been a marked absence of in-depth research on the psychological effects of professional acting. This is surprising for a number of reasons:

Firstly, Erving Goffman (1959) whose 'Dramaturgical Model' has so revolutionized social psychological thought since the late 1950s, while drawing parallels between real life and the theatre, hinted that there may be psychological consequences of acting for professional actors when the acting mask is removed.

> An action staged in a theatre is a relatively contrived illusion and an admitted one; unlike ordinary life, nothing real or actual can happen to the performed characters - although at another level of course, something real and actual can happen to the reputation of performers qua professionals whose everyday job is to put on theatrical performances (Goffman, 1955, p. 246).

Secondly, professional actors themselves frequently comment that while playing a dramatic role they often 'become' the part and continue to behave 'in character' offstage. Recently, *The Guardian* (16/9/1989) reported the case of an established British actor who was allegedly 'driven' from his role as 'Hamlet', having talked of the 'demons' in the role and seeing his father in the ghost.

Thirdly, and most importantly of all, the rationale which underlies role theory, role-playing in therapy and psychodrama is that people may come to change their attitudes simply by playing a certain role (e.g., Moreno, 1959, 1964, 1969).

Professional actors are individuals who are continually taking on roles. After all, that is what acting is about - assuming the guise of another character and taking on board others' expectations of how the character should behave. According to Janice Rule:

> To be applauded every night for certain character traits, values and attitudes makes it nigh on irresistible not to carry them over to some

> extent in private life. However, it is not only the applause but the 'living oneself into the part' for weeks on end that makes the separation of stage and home life extremely difficult. (Rule, 1973, p. 54)

But why might such a separation between actors and the dramatic roles they play prove difficult?

From a symbolic interactionist perspective, self-knowledge is acquired through active involvement with others (e.g., Mead, 1934). We learn about ourselves and who we are through the process of socialization. When actors are on stage they are in character. All of their verbal (and much of their non-verbal) communication with the other actors is controlled by the limits of their script. Thus, the information each actor receives about him or herself from the other actors is not about him or her personally, but about the character he or she is portraying. Yet, at least for the duration of the performance the actor has become the character.

The situation is complicated further if one considers Bem's (1967; 1972) self-perception theory. The argument is that self-knowledge is acquired from an individual's observations of his or her overt behaviour and the external stimulus conditions under which it occurs. Actors while they are acting behave as their character should behave and not necessarily as they would behave were they not acting.

The actor's plight is frequently made worse by the media. Actors are often viewed in terms of the characters they portray. This is particularly true of the 'soap' star whose off-screen behaviour is likened to that of his or her on-screen character. And, more often than not, their popularity may be dependent upon them behaving in real life as if they are their on-screen character; or, at least, maintaining that image.

Not only might actors identify with the role they are playing, but the people around actors who do not know them well tend to treat them as the characters they portray. Thus, the hazards that actors may struggle with internally are reinforced by the external world (Rule, 1973).

What might be the consequences if there is a conflict between the actor's self-perception and a dramatic role? According to Wicklund and Brehm (1976) if the self is well-articulated and stable, any discrepant self-presentations may arouse cognitive dissonance. The result should be a feeling of discomfort that leads the individual to any one of several strategies for rectifying the situation. Strategies which have been suggested by Gross et al. (1958) and which might be applied to the actor include:

a conformity to one or other of the polarized expectations (the actor either remains 'himself' or 'herself', or 'becomes' his or her character or public image); or

b a compromise between them (the actor takes on certain of his or her

character's qualities or those belonging to his or her public image); or
c an avoidance of the issue (the actor does not acknowledge that a conflict exists).

The present study specifically addresses the question of identity and role conflict by assessing aspects of self-perception over a 12-18 month period.

This paper details the results from two professional actors who represent part of a larger sample in an ongoing study. When not in work each actor is seen every six weeks. When in work each actor is seen more regularly (usually every two weeks, depending upon the length of the run, the length of filming, etc.).

Subjects

Details of the two actors are as follows: Actor A is 45 years old and female. She has been an actress for 27 years and is well-established within the profession, having considerable experience in deeply dramatic roles both on television, film, in the West End and on Broadway.

Actor B is also 45 years old, and is male. He has been an actor for 23 years and again is well-established, having taken the lead, or supporting role, in a number of television drama series, as well as in the theatre, including the West End.

Procedure

At each session the actor completes a variation of Kelly's (1955) Repertory Grid. At the first session 13 constructs were elicited using a triad format from a total of 14 familial and context-specific elements which will remain constant throughout the duration of the study. The elements are 'someone I like'; 'someone I do not like'; 'how I would like to be'; 'someone 'close' to me'; 'how I see myself'; 'family member (male)'; 'family member (female)'; 'the most successful person I know'; 'my best friend'; 'how I see the character'; 'the director'; 'the last role I played'; 'how I believe the public see me'; and 'my agent'. In addition to the repertory grid, Kuhn and McPartland's (1954) Twenty Statements Test (the 'Who am I?' and a variation of the test, 'Who am I not?') is also completed.

Also at every session, each actor answers a number of questions relating to time spent in rehearsal, length of run and acting technique employed.

Results

From the 14 elements rated by each actor, five elements (considered to be the most important) have been selected for discussion in the present paper.

The first element is 'How I would like to be'. On Actor A's grids (Table 1), her constructs are listed down the left-hand side. She then rated how much she would like to possess each of these qualities on a scale from 1 to 5 (e.g. generous of self would be rated 1, egotistical would be rated 5 and so on).

Table 1.

Element 3: How I would like to be. Actor A:

Constructs:	*Grid number* 1	2	3	4	5
(1) Generous of self v					
(5) Egotistical	1	1	1	1	1
(1) Sensitive v					
(5) Insensitive	1	1	1	1	1
(1) Isolated v					
(5) Not isolated	5	5	5	5	5
(1) Possesses sense of humour v					
(5) Lacks sense of humour	1	1	1	1	1
(1) Not controlled by jealousy v					
(5) Controlled by jealousy	1	1	1	1	1
(1) Fulfilled v					
(5) Unfulfilled	1	1	1	1	1
(1) Centred v					
(5) Uncentred	1	1	1	1	1
(1) Positive v					
(5) Negative	1	1	1	1	1
(1) Careful with money v					
(5) Extravagant	3	3	4	3	3
(1) Patient v					
(5) Impatient	1	1	1	1	1
(1) Warm v					
(5) Cold	1	1	1	1	1
(1) Attractive (as a person) v					
(5) Unattractive (as a person)	1	1	1	1	1
	UE	E		UE	E

UE = out of work, E = in a dramatic role

The numbers along the top of the Table represent the grid number. So far Actor A has completed five grids over a period of approximately three months. On this particular element, there appears to be considerable stability in how Actor A would like to be. The grids completed by Actor B on this element (Table 2) also show stability. He has completed eight grids so far, over a period of approximately seven months, and his constructs are very different from those of Actor A.

Table 2.

Element 3: How I would like to be. Actor B:

Constructs:	*Grid number* 1	2	3	4	5	6	7	8
(1) Happy v (5) Unhappy	1	1	1	2	1	1	1	1
(1) Selfish v (5) Unselfish	3	3	3	3	3	3	3	3
(1) Immature v (5) Mature	3	5	3	4	3	3	3	3
(1) Motherly/fatherly v (5) Not motherly/not fatherly	2	2	2	2	3	2	2	2
(1) Malicious v (5) Not malicious	5	5	5	5	5	5	5	5
(1) Calm v (5) Excitable	2	2	2	3	3	3	3	3
(1) Assertive v (5) Non-assertive	3	3	3	3	3	3	3	3
(1) Musical v (5) Non-musical	1	1	1	1	1	1	1	1
(1) Generous v (5) Mean	1	1	1	2	1	1	1	1
(1) Comical v (5) Not comical	1	1	1	1	1	1	1	1
(1) Stable v (5) Volatile	2	2	2	3	3	3	3	3
(1) Loving v (5) Unloving	1	1	1	2	1	1	1	1
(1) Intelligent v (5) Unintelligent	1	2	2	2	2	1	1	1
		UE				E		

UE = unemployed, E = in a dramatic role
= broken line denotes that actor is in a dramatic role while also in rehearsal for another dramatic role.

The second element is 'How I see myself'. On this element Actor A's ratings (Table 3) are not as stable as are those on the previous element. In particular, her self-perceptions appear to vary as she moves from role to role, although they are more stable within a role (e.g., grid 2 and 3).

Table 3.

Element 5: How I see myself. Actor A:

Constructs:	*Grid number:* 1	2	3	4	5
(1) Generous of self v (5) Egotistical	3	3	2	2	1
(1) Sensitive v (5) Insensitive	2	1	1	2	1
(1) Isolated v (5) Not isolated	5	4	4	4	1
(1) Possesses sense of humour v (5) Lacks sense of humour	1	2	1	2	2
(1) Not controlled by jealousy v (5) Controlled by jealousy	3	3	3	4	1
(1) Tolerant v (5) Intolerant	3	3	3	3	1
(1) Fulfilled v (5) Unfulfilled	2	2	2	3	2
(1) Centred v (5) Uncentred	2	2	2	3	2
(1) Positive v (5) Negative	2	3	4	3	1
(1) Careful with money v (5) Extravagant	5	5	5	5	3
(1) Patient v (5) Impatient	4	4	3	2	1
(1) Warm v (5) Cold	2	2	2	2	1
(1) Attractive (as a person) v (5) Unattractive as a person)	2	2	2	2	1
	UE	E	UE	E	

UE = out of work, E = in a dramatic role

Actor B's ratings (Table 4), on the other hand, are relatively constant, not only within particular dramatic roles, but also across them. This would appear to indicate that, in contrast to Actor A, his self-perception is not affected by the roles he plays.

Table 4.

Element 5: How I see myself. Actor B:

Constructs:	*Grid number:* 1	2	3	4	5	6	7	8
(1) Happy v (5) Unhappy	3	3	3	2	2	2	2	2
(1) Selfish v (5) Unselfish	3	2	2	2	3	3	3	3
(1) Immature v (5) Mature	3	3	2	3	3	3	3	3
(1) Motherly/fatherly v (5) Not motherly/not fatherly	3	2	3	3	3	3	3	3
(1) Malicious v (5) Not malicious	4	3	4	4	4	4	4	4
(1) Calm v (5) Excitable	3	2	4	2	2	3	3	3
(1) Assertive v (5) Non-assertive	4	4	3	3	3	3	3	3
(1) Musical v (5) Non-musical	1	1	1	1	2	1	1	1
(1) Generous v (5) Mean	3	2	3	3	3	2	2	2
(1) Comical v (5) Not comical	3	3	3	3	3	3	3	3
(1) Stable v (5) Volatile	2	3	3	3	2	3	3	3
(1) Loving v (5) Unloving	2	2	2	2	2	2	2	2
(1) Intelligent v (5) Unintelligent	3	3	3	3	3	3	3	3
		UE				E		

UE = unemployed, E = in a dramatic role
= broken line denotes that actor is in a dramatic role while also in rehearsal for another dramatic role.

In terms of how the character being played is seen (element 10), the roles played by Actor A appear to be very different (Table 5). Differences can be seen in her ratings between grids 2, 3 and 4 and 5.

Table 5.

Element 10: How I see the character. Actor A:

	Grid number:				
Constructs:	1	2	3	4	5
(1) Generous of self v (5) Egotistical	-	5	5	5	3
(1) Sensitive v (5) Insensitive	-	3	5	4	3
(1) Isolated v (5) Not isolated	-	1	1	1	2
(1) Possesses sense of humour v (5) Lacks sense of humour	-	5	4	3	2
(1) Not controlled by jealousy v (5) Controlled by jealousy	-	5	5	5	2
(1) Tolerant v (5) Intolerant	-	5	5	5	2
(1) Fulfilled v (5) Unfulfilled	-	5	5	5	2
(1) Centred v (5) Uncentred	-	5	5	5	2
(1) Positive v (5) Negative	-	3	5	5	1
(1) Careful with money v (5) Extravagant	-	2	2	3	2
(1) Patient v (5) Impatient	-	5	5	5	1
(1) Warm v (5) Cold	-	5	5	5	2
(1) Attractive (as a person) v (5) Unattractive (as a person)	-	5	5	5	4
	UE	E		UE	E

UE = out of work, E = in a dramatic role

There is some change across the ratings of Actor B (Table 6), but compared with Actor A, the ratings are more stable. So perhaps Actor B sees the characters he has played, at least during the last 7 months, as being very similar.

Table 6.

Element 10: How I see the character. Actor B:

	Grid number:								
Constructs:	1	2	3	4	5	6	6a	7	8
(1) Happy v									
(5) Unhappy	-	-	-	5	5	5	2	3	3
(1) Selfish v									
(5) Unselfish	-	-	-	2	1	1	1	1	1
(1) Immature v									
(5) Mature	-	-	-	2	3	3	2	2	3
(1) Motherly/fatherly v									
(5) Not motherly/not fatherly	-	-	-	4	5	5	5	5	5
(1) Malicious v									
(5) Not malicious	-	-	-	2	2	2	1	1	1
(1) Calm v									
(5) Excitable	-	-	-	3	4	2	2	4	4
(1) Assertive v									
(5) Non-assertive	-	-	-	1	1	1	1	1	1
(1) Musical v									
(5) Non-musical	-	-	-	5	5	5	5	5	5
(1) Generous v									
(5) Mean	-	-	-	4	5	5	5	5	5
(1) Comical v									
(5) Not comical	-	-	-	5	5	5	4	5	5
(1) Stable v									
(5) Volatile	-	-	-	4	5	4	2	4	3
(1) Loving v									
(5) Unloving	-	-	-	5	5	5	5	5	5
(1) Intelligent v									
(5) Unintelligent	-	-	-	3	2	2	1	3	1
		UE					E		

UE = unemployed [6 = dramatic role in performance], E = in a dramatic role [6a = dramatic role in rehearsal]

= broken line denotes that actor is in a dramatic role while also in rehearsal for another dramatic role.

Element 12 - 'The last role I played': In Actor A's grids (Table 7), the ratings vary not only across roles (as one would expect if this actress is playing very different roles), but also from time to time within them.

Table 7.

Element 12: The last role I played. Actor A:

	Grid number:				
Constructs:	1	2	3	4	5
(1) Generous of self v					
(5) Egotistical	4	3	3	3	2
(1) Sensitive v					
(5) Insensitive	3	1	2	2	3
(1) Isolated v					
(5) Not isolated	1	1	5	4	4
(1) Possesses sense of humour v					
(5) Lacks sense of humour	3	2	2	2	1
(1) Not controlled by jealousy v					
(5) Controlled by jealousy	5	5	5	5	3
(1) Tolerant v					
(5) Intolerant	5	3	2	3	3
(1) Fulfilled v					
(5) Unfulfilled	5	5	5	5	2
(1) Centred v					
(5) Uncentred	5	5	4	3	2
(1) Positive v					
(5) Negative	3	5	4	4	2
(1) Careful with money v					
(5) Extravagant	5	5	5	5	3
(1) Patient v					
(5) Impatient	4	4	3	3	2
(1) Warm v					
(5) Cold	2	3	2	2	2
(1) Attractive (as a person) v					
(5) Unattractive (as a person)	3	3	2	2	2
	UE	E		UE	E

UE = out of work, E = in a dramatic role

So, it would seem that even while she is in a role, the way she sees that role is continually being modified; or, perhaps, she (i.e., her self-perception) is changing with the role and therefore, she sees the role as also changing over time. In Actor B (Table 8) there is stability within a role - yet the roles are seen as being different - contrary to the consistency in his ratings for the character currently being played.

Table 8.

Element 12: The role I played. Actor B:

Constructs:	*Grid number:* 1	2	3	4	5	6	7	8
(1) Happy v (5) Unhappy	3	3	3	3	3	2	5	5
(1) Selfish v (5) Unselfish	2	2	2	2	2	2	1	1
(1) Immature v (5) Mature	2	2	2	2	2	2	3	2
(1) Motherly/fatherly v (5) Not motherly/not fatherly	4	4	4	4	4	4	5	5
(1) Malicious v (5) Not malicious	4	4	4	4	4	4	1	1
(1) Calm v (5) Excitable	3	3	3	3	3	3	4	4
(1) Assertive v (5) Non-assertive	2	3	3	2	3	3	1	1
(1) Musical v (5) Non-musical	4	4	3	4	4	4	5	5
(1) Generous v (5) Mean	3	3	3	3	3	2	5	5
(1) Comical v (5) Not comical	3	2	3	2	2	3	5	5
(1) Stable v (5) Volatile	3	3	3	3	3	3	5	5
(1) Loving v (5) Unloving	3	2	2	2	2	3	5	5
(1) Intelligent v (5) Unintelligent	3	3	3	2	3	2	3	2
		UE				E		

UE = unemployed, E = in a dramatic role

= broken line denotes that actor is in a dramatic role while also in rehearsal for another dramatic role.

Finally, element 13 - 'How I believe the public see me': From her ratings (Table 9), the way Actor A believes the public sees her appears to be affected by the roles she plays. It appears that she expects the public to see her in terms of the dramatic role she is playing at the time.

Table 9.

Element 13: How I believe the public see me. Actor A:

	Grid number:				
Constructs:	1	2	3	4	5
(1) Generous of self v (5) Egotistical	2	3	2	2	1
(1) Sensitive v (5) Insensitive	3	3	3	2	2
(1) Isolated v (5) Not isolated	3	3	2	2	4
(1) Possesses sense of humour v (5) Lacks sense of humour	1	3	2	2	1
(1) Not controlled by jealousy v (5) Controlled by jealousy	3	2	4	3	2
(1) Tolerant v (5) Intolerant	2	3	3	3	2
(1) Fulfilled v (5) Unfulfilled	2	1	3	2	2
(1) Centred v (5) Uncentred	1	1	3	2	2
(1) Positive v (5) Negative	1	2	3	3	2
(1) Careful with money v (5) Extravagant	5	4	4	5	2
(1) Patient v (5) Impatient	4	2	3	3	2
(1) Warm v (5) Cold	2	2	2	3	1
(1) Attractive (as a person) v (5) Unattractive (as a person)	2	2	2	2	1
	UE	E		UE	E

UE = out of work, E = in a dramatic role

However, the way Actor B believes the public sees him (Table 10) does not appear to be affected by the roles he plays. He seems to expect the public to see him for who he is and not in terms of his current and past dramatic roles.

Table 10.

Element 13: How I believe te public see me. Actor B:

Constructs:	*Grid number*: 1	2	3	4	5	6	7	8
(1) Happy v (5) Unhappy	2	2	2	2	2	2	2	2
(1) Selfish v (5) Unselfish	2	2	2	2	3	3	3	3
(1) Immature v (5) Mature	3	4	3	3	3	3	3	3
(1) Motherly/fatherly v (5) Not motherly/not fatherly	4	3	4	3	2	3	3	3
(1) Malicious v (5) Not malicious	4	3	4	4	4	4	4	4
(1) Calm v (5) Excitable	2	2	2	2	3	3	3	3
(1) Assertive v (5) Non-assertive	2	2	2	3	2	3	3	2
(1) Musical v (5) Non-musical	1	2	2	1	2	2	2	2
(1) Generous v (5) Mean	2	3	3	3	3	2	2	2
(1) Comical v (5) Not comical	3	4	4	3	3	3	3	3
(1) Stable v (5) Volatile	2	2	3	2	2	3	2	2
(1) Loving v (5) Unloving	2	2	2	2	2	3	3	3
(1) Intelligent v (5) Unintelligent	3	2	3	3	3	3	3	3
		UE			E			

UE = unemployed, E = in a dramatic role
= broken line denotes that actor is in a dramatic role while also in rehearsal for another dramatic role.

The repertory grid data is supported by the 'Who am I?' statements.

'Who am I?' statements

Actor A's 'Who am I?' statements (Table 11) suggest that her self-perception appears to change according to the roles she plays. For example, in Grid 3 she is confident, positive and on top of her role. In Grid 4 she is out of work again and becoming more negative.

There are also references to the qualities she attributed to the role being played at the time (e.g., reference to torture and pain in Grid 2 - the dramatic character being played was subjected to torture).

Table 11.

Actor A: 'Who am I?'

(Grid 1) (UE)
I am a frightened little girl;
I am someone who is easily hurt;
I am someone who has been judged by a misleading appearance;
I am insecure about my appearance and sexual appeal.

(Grid 2) (E)
I am paranoid, occasionally over-sensitive;
I am acutely aware of what time has done to my body;
I am afraid of being the 'new girl' on the set;
I am anxious about the way the director wants me to play (the character);
I am afraid of torture and pain.

(Grid 3) (E)
I feel confident in my role;
I will make a scene if necessary;
I am on top of my lines.

(Grid 4) (UE)
I am out of work again;
My confidence is steady but up for knocks.

(Grid 5) (E)
I am afraid (co-star) will take against me;
I am afraid of being a disappointment;
I am anxious about my weight.

UE = out of work, E = in a dramatic role

Actor B (Table 12), on the other hand, tends to see himself in terms of his role as an actor and his other everyday roles as a father, and musician. There is also more stability in his self-perception - he describes himself in the same way over several grids (although his self-perception as an actor varies depending upon whether he is in or out of work).

Table 12.

Actor B: 'Who am I?'

(Grid 1) (UE)
I am an actor;
I am a musician;
I am a father;
I am a hedonist.

(Grid 2) (UE)
I am an out-of-work actor;
I am a moody person;
I am a lazy hedonist;
I am a child.

(Grid 3) (UE)
I am a frustrated actor;
I am a loving father;
I am a lazy man.

(Grid 4) (E)
I am a successful actor;
I am a happy parent;
I am a family man.

(Grid 6) (E)*
I am a very busy actor;
I am a word-learning machine.

(Grid 7)
I am a working actor;
I am a vulnerable actor.

UE = out of work, E = in a dramatic role, * = denotes that actor is in a dramatic role while also in rehearsal for another dramatic role.

Discussion

The data presented here is descriptive and part of an ongoing study. However, a tentative interpretation is possible.

It would appear that the two actors presented in this paper are affected very differently by the dramatic roles they play. While Actor A seems to be greatly influenced by her dramatic roles, Actor B does not seem to be. Furthermore, Actor B appears to be far more stable (in the way he sees himself) than Actor A.

To possess such a stable self-perception and sense of identity might be an asset for a professional actor. Certainly Actor B seems to know who he is, and one would expect little or no identity confusion or diffuseness as he moves between dramatic roles. However, according to Wicklund and Brehm (1976), if the self-perception is well-articulated playing a role that is different from oneself can lead to cognitive dissonance. Therefore, Actor B might be liable to suffer from role conflict if he has to play a character who is very different from himself.

Alternatively, such stability could be regarded as inflexibility and rigidity. Thus, perhaps Actor B is not affected by the dramatic roles he plays because he always plays characters who are like himself.

Actor A, on the other hand, appears to possess a less stable self-perception and sense of identity. Thus, perhaps she is more influenced by the dramatic roles she plays because her sense of self is not well-developed. Hence, while she might be expected to suffer less from role conflict, she may be prone to experience identity confusion and diffuseness.

Alternatively, her sense of identity could be regarded as flexible and malleable. She is able, as if she were an empty vessel, to assume the guise and identity of any dramatic role she plays. Such an ability would surely be an enviable asset for any actor.

Of course, it should be remembered that the repertory grid and 'Who am I?' data is based upon each actor's self-report, and may not reflect the perception other people have of them.

It should also be acknowledged that other variables may influence the extent to which actors are affected (or not affected) by the dramatic roles they play. For example, the dramatic role itself. Thus, one might expect an actor to be more affected by playing a deeply dramatic role than by playing a light comedy role.

Similarly, there might be a difference in the extent of influence between a static role (e.g., a role in the theatre in which the actor is repeating the same lines night after night), or a role in repertory theatre (where an actor plays a number of roles for relatively short periods) and a developing role (e.g., in a television 'soap', where an actor is continually developing the character he or she plays, and where that role is usually played for a longer period of time).

Thirdly, with regard to acting technique employed, the actor who favours a Stanislavskian, or 'Method' approach (and who, therefore, attempts to 'become' the part) may be more affected by a dramatic role than an actor who adopts a more distanced, Brechtian approach.

Lastly, it has been suggested that dispositional factors perhaps determine what sort of individual becomes an actor (Hammond & Edelmann, 1990). They might also determine how affected actors will be by the dramatic roles they play.

Interestingly, the scores on a number of personality dimensions of the two actors discussed in this paper vary markedly, particularly on the dimensions of neuroticism, social desirability and shyness (Table 13). Actor A (who appears to be affected by the dramatic roles she plays) is considerably more neurotic, shows greater concern for appearing to be socially desirable and is more shy than Actor B (who appears to be less, if at all, affected by his dramatic roles).

Table 13.

Scores of actor A & actor B on various personality measures.

	Actor A	Actor B
E.P.Q.: Extraversion	13	7
Neuroticism	20	7
Psychoticism	2	3
Lie	3	0
Social Desirability	10	2
Self-esteem	22	15
Self-monitoring		
(a) ability to modify self-presentation	22	22
(b) sensitivity to the expressive behaviour of others	23	19
Concern for appropriateness		
(a) cross-situational variability	27	21
(b) attention to social comparison information	45	36
Private self-consciousness	30	23
Public self-consciousness	20	16
Social Anxiety	14	10
Shyness	17	9
Sociability	15	14

Perhaps a clue to enable us to answer the question whether the self-perception of actors is affected by the dramatic roles they play lies in the findings of an earlier study (Hammond and Edelmann, 1989). On the basis of a series of interviews with professional actors, they concluded that when an actor plays a dramatic role there is not a sudden metamorphosis. That is, the role does not completely take over the actor. Rather, there is a Piagetian (1975) 'assimilation' and 'accommodation' of a dramatic role; with the role bringing to the fore aspects of the actor's self which already existed before the role was played, but of which the actor had not been consciously aware.

In view of this finding, can the argument be taken a stage further to suggest that actors can only play dramatic roles which reflect themselves and portray emotions which already exist within them? Certainly, this would explain the findings of the present study - Actor A has a less stable, flexible and malleable identity and therefore, is able to play wide-ranging dramatic roles; in contrast, Actor B has a rather more fixed and inflexible identity reflected in the relatively similar dramatic roles he plays.

Recently the British actress, Judi Dench, quoting her husband, actor, Michael Williams, said, 'On the stage, you cannot be anything more than you are as a person' (Parsons, 1990, p. 313). Interestingly, such a controversial notion was put forward nearly half a century ago by Fenichel (1946, p. 150) who proposed that an actor cannot play an emotion that he or she has not experienced. Thus, one might conclude that while the good actor believes that he plays his parts, actually he plays himself.

Acknowledgements

The authors are grateful to the Economic and Social Research Council for financial support, and to the anonymous actors for participating in this study.

References

Bem, D.J. (1967) 'Self-perception: An alternative interpretation of cognitive dissonance phenomena'. In *Psychological Review*, **74**, p 183-200

Bem, D.J. (1972) 'Self-perception theory'. In L. Berkowitz (ed.) *Advances in Experimental Social Psychology, Vol. 6*. New York: Academic Press

DeCosta, L., W. Buse & A. Amdursky. (1986) 'Personal myths: living them and pretending them'. In *Dynamic Psychotherapy, Vol 4, No. 2*. Fall/Winter, p 131-139

Fenichel, O. (1946) 'On acting'. In *Psychoanalytic Quarterly, Vol. 15*. p 144-160

Fisher, S. & R.L. Fisher (1981) *Pretend the World is Funny and Forever: A Psychological Analysis of Comedians, Clowns and Actors*. Hillsdale, New Jersey: Erlbaum

Goffman, E. (1959) *The Presentation of Self in Everyday Life.* Harmondsworth: Penguin

Gross, N., W.S. Mason & A.W. McEachern (1958) *Explorations in Role Analysis: Studies of the school superintendancy role.* New York: Wiley

Hammond, J. & R.J. Edelmann (1989) 'Behind the mask: An exploratory psychological study of the professional actor'. Paper given at the London Conference of the British Psychological Society, 20.12.1989

Hammond, J. & R.J. Edelmann (1990) 'The act of being: Personality characteristics of professional actors, amateur actors and non-actors'. Paper given at the First International Conference on Psychology and Performing Arts, 5-7.7.1990

Henry, W.E. & J.H. Sims (1970) 'Actors' search for self'. In *Transaction,* **7**, p 57-62

Kelly, G.A. (1955) *The Psychology of Personal Constructs.* London: Norton

Kuhn, M.H. & T.S. McPartland (1954) 'An empirical investigation of self-attitudes'. In *American Sociological Review,* **19**, p 68-76

Mead, G. (1934) *Mind, Self and Society.* Chicago: University of Chicago Press

Moreno, J.L. (1959) *Psychodrama: Second Volume*; Foundations of Psychotherapy. New York: Beacon House

Moreno, J.L. (1964) *Psychodrama: First Volume* 3rd edition, New York: Beacon House

Moreno, J.L. (1969) *Psychodrama: Third Volume; Action Therapy and Principles of Practice.* New York: Beacon House

Parsons, M. (1990) 'Reflecting nature: A conversation with Judi Dench'. In *The Psychologist, Vol. 3, No. 7.* July 1990 p 312-314

Piaget, J. (1975) *The Development of Thought: Equilibration of Cognitive Structures.* New York: Viking

Rule, J. (1973) 'The actor's identity crisis (postanalytic reflections of an actress)'. In: *International Journal of Psychoanalytic Psychotherapy, Vol. 2,* Part 1 p 51-76

Styan, J.L. (1975) *The Dramatic Experience.* Cambridge: Cambridge University Press

Vidal, J. (1989) 'Demons in the wings'. In *The Guardian,* 16/9/1989 p 23

Wicklund, R.A. & J.W. Brehm (1976) *Perspectives on Cognitive Dissonance.* Hillsdale, New Jersey: Erlbaum

An ecological view of social perception: Implications for theatrical performance

Fairfid M. Caudle

The College of Staten Island, City University of New York

> Suit the action to the word, the word to the action; with this special observance, that you o'erstep not the modesty of nature: for any thing so overdone is from the purpose of playing, whose end, both at the first and now, was and is, to hold, as 'twere, the mirror up to nature; to show virtue her own feature, scorn her own image, and the very age and body of the time his form and pressure.
>
> *Hamlet*, Act III, Scene 2

In this speech preceding the "play within a play" in Hamlet, Shakespeare has touched upon several of the key requirements of acting: that it mirror nature in its gestures, emotional expressions, and the bodily form and gait that communicate a particular age.

How is it that an actor is able to know what these things are? How does the actor mirror them? What determines their impact on the viewing audience? To be sure, resources have been compiled which summarize 'vocabularies' of facial expressions (e.g. Peck, 1987), gestures (e.g. Critchley 1939; Kipnis, 1974; Lawson, 1957 and Mawer, 1932) and make-up (e.g. Baird, 1957/1941; Buchman, 1973; Kehoe, 1969). And, too, there are manuals of instruction on the craft of acting itself (e.g. Chekhov, 1953; and Stanislavski, 1936, 1949 and 1963). And a visit to virtually any library on the performing arts will find an abundance of publications from various disciplines of interest to the performing arts such as anthropology (e.g. Morris, Collett, Marsh & O'Shaughnessy, 1979) and social psychology (e.g. Collier, 1985; Knapp, 1978; Ruesch & Kees, 1972 and Weitz, 1979). However, one would search in vain for a unified theory of acting that both integrates information from the many disciplines that have something to say about communication and, at the same time, provides a framework for the concepts, processes and vocabularies of expression, gesture and movement that the actor brings together in a performance.

Although there exists as yet no comprehensive theory of dramatic communication, there does exist a theoretical perspective that suggests directions that such a theory might take. This perspective originated in the psychology of visual perception and has recently been expanded to include aspects of social perception. I am referring to the point of view that has come to be known as ecological psychology, and the goal of this paper is to suggest how an ecological view of social perception provides insights and unifying concepts of potential value in defining and clarifying the processes through which impact is achieved in theatrical performance.

The ecological view of perception

This point of view has received its main impetus from the work of J. J. Gibson, who has challenged the traditional view of the senses as passive channels of specific types of *sensations* and has instead proposed that the senses function as interrelated *perceptual systems* that orient the perceptual apparatus of the body to detect information from the environment (Gibson, 1966; See Lombardo, 1987, for an analysis of the historical development of Gibson's point of view). Gibson himself proposed that "there is a bewildering variety of ways in which men can *communicate* with other men" (1966, p. 27), noting, for example, that "besides gestures, there are facial expressions, dancing, mimicry, theatrical acting, and making signs or signals" (p. 27). He suggested that a starting point in classifying the many forms of communication is to note that "some communication *conveys information about the world* and some does not". (p. 28). It is the emphasis upon the active role of the perceiver in detecting information within its physical and cultural environment that is the cornerstone of Gibson's point of view.

In his volume entitled *The Ecological Approach to Visual Perception*

Gibson (1979) developed his approach still further. Central to his argument is the adaptive function of perception and the idea that the information in the external world that is of value in guiding behaviour is detected by the organism's sensory systems, which are viewed as having evolved to detect the sorts of information found within the environment in which the organism lives. Gibson has discussed at length the rich information afforded by the environment in its places, objects and substances, and in the events occurring within it. Gibson's perspective differs radically from traditional views of perception in that such information is readily detected without the need for further cognitive processing.

A key concept in Gibson's approach is that of an environmental *affordance*. As Gibson defined them, "The affordances of the environment are what it *offers* the animal, what it *provides* or *furnishes*, either for good or ill" (1979, p 127). Affordances might be thought of as opportunities for behaving or being acted upon that the environment provides. To give an example from the physical environment, our sensory systems readily detect that the ground is firm and thus *affords* support, or that the surface of a lake is not firm and does not afford support but may afford the act of swimming. These characteristics of the environment are readily detected without the need for further thought; a moment's reflection will indicate that it is indeed of value to an organism to be able to detect these things without the need for thinking before acting. With regard to the perception of other people, Gibson noted:

> Animals are ... by far the most complex objects of perception that the environment presents to an observer. Another animal may be prey or predator, potential mate or rival, adult or young, one's own or another's young. Moreover, it may be temporarily asleep or awake, receptive or unreceptive, hungry or satiated. What the other animal affords is specified by its permanent features and its temporary state, and it can afford eating or being eaten, copulation or fighting, nurturing or nurturance ... What the other animal affords the observer is not only behavior but also social interaction. (1979, p. 41-42).

With this observation, Gibson laid the groundwork for the notion that the *behavioural* (and thus *social*) affordances, which indicate a potential for action or being acted upon, constitute one form of information that can readily be detected from the environment.

McArthur & Baron (1983) have argued that the concepts that Gibson specified concerning the relationship between the perceiving organism and its *physical* environment apply with equal precision to the perception of the *social* environment. These authors have pointed out that:

> To fully understand impression formation or causal attribution or other aspects of social perception, we must ultimately identify the nature of the stimulus information that reveals industry, hostility, and the other attributes that we perceive in people. (McArthur & Baron, 1983, p. 215)

Relevance of this view to theatrical performance

The link to theatrical performance can now be stated: We need also to specify the nature of the stimulus information that the actor provides. It is the minute gradations, textures, rhythms and patterns of the voice, eye movements and facial expression, posture and movement, and breathing, that are most readily detected by the audience as emotion, belief, conviction or doubt, attitude, mood, age, or any of hundreds of subtle variations in demeanour. These are in fact the author's "bodyscape." It is the information from these subtle cues that the audience detects and it is these that together can mean the difference between a performance of great impact and a lack-lustre one.

Consider, for example, a photograph of a moment in a scene from *Another Time*, with Albert Finney and Janet Suzman, reproduced in the program of this 1990 production and showing these two actors confronting one another. Despite the fact that this picture is a static display rather than the entire on-going performance event, one can readily detect that the situation is one of great tension and discord. Belligerent facial expressions, confrontational postures, and an actor's clenched fist can be noted. Clearly his actions do not afford approach or affection. Instead they afford threat. The proxemics are also noteworthy: a table has become a barrier, possibly representing an obstacle preventing actual physical confrontation.

It is my view that an ecological view of social perception might provide a framework in which to identify and to organize, in a way relevant to the perspectives of both biology and theatre communication, such characteristics of the social stimuli provided by an actor during a performance. Let me now reiterate some of the most important ecological concepts that McArthur & Baron (1983) have developed within the context of their theory of social perception.

Central concepts of an ecological theory of social perception

Central to arguments concerning an ecological theory of social perception is a focus on the information contained within a stimulus rather than the cognitive processing of such information. MacArthur and Baron have noted that

> Whereas current research in social perception has concentrated on the

> cognitive processing of social information - how schemata, memory and various cognitive heuristics influence the meaning we extract from the social environment - research within the ecological approach will reveal what it is in a person's movements, gestures, voice, and facial appearance that communicates to us that person's momentary intentions, emotional state, or more stable qualities. (p. 216-217)

Clearly, these are the same sorts of information through which an actor creates a character. Elaborating upon Gibson's proposal that an active, exploring organism readily detects and utilizes the rich information found in its environment, McArthur and Baron define an *event* as characterized by "dynamic changes over space and time" (p. 216), and they note that such information is far richer and more substantial than information contained within static stimuli (e.g. drawings or photographs). McArthur & Baron have noted that events

> may be fast or slow (e.g. smiling vs aging), they may be rigid or elastic (e.g. rotating vs stretching), they may be reversible or non-reversible (e.g. rolling vs growing). And, as the foregoing examples illustrate, events occur in the social as well as the physical environment. (p. 216)

Clearly, a theatrical performance can be viewed as an ongoing event that communicates information about interpersonal interactions. Despite the fact that the ability of the audience as perceivers to explore the environment is limited because of fixed seat locations, nevertheless there is a much richer opportunity to detect information than would exist, for example, in a two-dimensional movie. However, it should be noted that even this limitation of fixed seat locations was eliminated in the play *Tamara*, which has played in New York for the past three years. In this play, the action occurs simultaneously throughout a number of rooms, and the audience chooses a character to follow around. Invited to "wear comfortable shoes," members of the audience can treat the unfolding drama as if they were exploring ongoing social events within a rich physical environment. It has not been uncommon for members of the audience to return several times to follow different characters and thus piece together more complete knowledge of the event as a whole.

An important concept for the arguments suggested in the present paper is the notion that, as we perceive events, we are able to perceive those aspects that remain the same for the duration of the event. Things that are perceived as remaining the same have been called *invariants* and comprise two broad categories. One category consists of *structural* invariants, which are aspects of an object's structure, such as shape or colour, that remain the same while it moves (or behaves, in the case of other organisms such as actors).

The second category of invariant is referred to as a *transformational* invariant, which consists of some constant pattern of movement or some other event over time. Both walking and aging constitute transformational invariants in that they consist of patterns of movement or bodily changes that are recognized over a wide variety of shapes and species (McArthur & Baron, 1983). Emotional facial expressions and gestures might be viewed as transformational invariants that are readily detected because of their adaptive relevance in guiding ongoing behaviour.

The communication of emotion throught facial expressions

One topic of great interest to both the actor and the social scientist is the communication of emotion. There is a vast theoretical and experimental literature on the role of facial expression in the communication of emotion. Among the issues that have been explored in the many studies by Paul Ekman and his colleagues is the universality of emotions, and a major finding has been that "observers label certain facial expressions of emotion in the same way regardless of culture" (Ekman & Oster, 1982, p. 147). Consider, for example, two representations of fear (Ekman & Friesen, 1975) and note particularly the raised brows, forehead wrinkles, raised eyelids and open mouth.

Compare these photographs of fear with a sketch, taken from a 1927 book on the art of pantomime (Aubert, 1985/1927), which began by stating that

> the language of action .... is universal; the ways of expressing emotion are identical among different races of mankind. (p. 3)

It is evident that this insight has existed in the world of theatre long before it was confirmed by empirical studies by social scientists, who, sad to say, have paid little attention to the insights and experience recorded by performers and writers on the theatre.

Another topic of great interest to both the social scientist and the actor is whether or not it is possible to distinguish between genuine emotions and those that are intentionally communicated. Research has indicated that, while true feelings can be masked to some extent, there is nevertheless some leakage that can indicate that expressed emotions are not genuine (Ekman, 1985; Ekman & Friesen, 1982; Friesen & O'Sullivan, 1988).

Buck (1984) has argued that facial expressions from genuine and spontaneous emotions are read and understood directly by a receiver, without the need for intervening cognitive judgments, a position that is consistent with an ecological view of social perception. In contrast, intentional emotional expressions, as symbolic representations, do require further cognitive processing to be understood, and they may not elicit the same response as genuinely expressed emotions.

This suggests a dilemma for the actor: Acting is by definition an act of symbolic communication, and so, how is the actor to be perceived as expressing genuine emotions? It is of interest to note that psychologists seeking genuine portrayals of emotion to use in their research have also had this dilemma. In this instance at least, some guidance has been gained from the acting profession:

> When asked to pose an emotion, a person can either deliberately move particular facial muscles, or like a Stanislavski actor, attempt to relive or imagine a situation to create the emotional experience from which the expression will flow. (Ekman, Hager & Friesen, 1981 p. 102)

Compare this with the words of Stanislavski himself, who wrote the following in 1936:

> That type of memory, which makes you relive the sensations you once felt .... is what we call *emotion memory.* Just as your visual memory can reconstruct an inner image of some forgotten thing, place or person, your emotion memory can bring back feelings you have already experienced. (Stanislavski, 1936, p. 158)

In this instance we see some convergence between theoretical and experimental work suggesting a biological basis for the differentiation of genuine and non-genuine emotions, and the suggestion by Stanislavski that emotions should be communicated through reliving events in which such emotions were originally experienced, because, with the memory, one is able to reactivate the same bodily processes that accompanied the emotion when originally experienced. In this connection, consider a cartoon (reproduced in Knapp, 1978, .271) showing former President Richard M Nixon trying out different facial expressions until he gives up in disgust, noting "I just can't get that CANDOR expression." In view of the preceding discussion, we might surmise that he would have been able to reproduce this expression had it been stored in his own "emotion memory" in the first place.

Structural and transformational invariants in theatrical performance

Earlier, it was noted that the detection of invariants is an essential process in perception. We have seen how emotional facial expressions can be viewed as a form of perceptual invariant. Now let us see how this concept is relevant to understanding what is communicated in an on-going theatrical performance.

In developing his ecological position, one of the issues that Gibson struggled with was how to define a picture. He noted that:

> The science of language is well established, but nothing even approximating a science of depiction exists. What artists, critics, and philosophers of art have to say about pictures has little in common with what photographers, opticists, and geometers have to say about them. (Gibson, 1979, p. 270)

What Gibson finally hit on was to define a picture as "an array of persisting invariants of structure" (1979, p 271). He went on to note that "any picture, then, *preserves what its creator has noticed and considers worth noticing*" (1979, p 274, emphasis by Gibson).

Consider, for example, a caricature of a person used as an advertisement for a show. Notice how the invariants of structure that define the individual's face are exaggerated for emphasis. These are the characteristics that the artist noticed and preserved as defining that particular face.

These statements concerning pictures can usefully suggest comparisons with theatrical performances. Whereas a picture is a static display, a theatrical performance is an on-going and unfolding event, with much richer information available to the viewer than that in the static array provided by a picture.

Let us consider one particular type of theatrical performance. The impersonation or recreation of a character already known to an audience. We might define the similarities in *physical* appearance between the actor and the person being impersonated as "an array of three-dimensional structural invariants," as in a photograph of Raymond Massey in a 1938 performance of the play *Abe Lincoln from Illinois*. He wears a beard, stovepipe hat and austere clothing, that even without the performance itself, suggest the character being represented. Numerous additional examples could be given of impersonation, such as the performance currently on Broadway of Robert Morse as Truman Capote in the play *Tru*.

However, keep in mind that looking at a two-dimensional photograph of an actor impersonating someone provides a relatively meagre amount of information compared with what is provided in an ongoing performance. To watch an impersonation in action is a much richer perceptual experience - an event, in ecological terms. We might almost define it as "a multi-dimensional moving array of both structural and transformational, visual and vocal, invariants." Just as a picture consists of those invariants that its creator considered worth noticing and preserving, the invariants selected by the actor for recreation include not only physical appearance but also vocal pitch, accent and inflections, as well as facial expressions, mannerisms and gestures.

Impersonations can suggest their representations with widely varying amounts of information. It is frequently the case that only a superficial resemblance between the impersonator and the character personified is needed to suggest a character, since much can be accomplished with clothing and wigs. Consider recent advertisements depicting Mozart and Shakespeare. The structural invariants selected for reproduction are primarily those of clothing and wigs which suggest the character but fall short of a completely convincing impression.

Consider the many instances in which males have impersonated females. Some are openly outrageous and comic portrayals in which the incongruity of the masculine form in the feminine clothing elicits a humourous response (e.g. Cinderella's ugly sisters (see Lawson, 1957), and the portrayals of the Widow Simone in *La Fille mal Gardee*. Other impersonations of females by males have had as their objective to provide much more convincing portrayals, and in such performances the male assumes not only the clothing but also the voice, mannerisms and gestures of the female. Examples can be seen in the impersonation of a female by a Kabuki performer (see Hanna, 1988), in the oriental mistress in Mme. Butterfly, and in the female impersonators in *La Cage aux Folles*. In each of these examples of impersonation, it is both the structural and behavioural invariants that have been selected by performers to be recreated.

Attention to resemblances which might also be viewed as structural invariants, or the potential for creating them through make-up, may have considerable influence in casting decisions. This is illustrated, for example, in photographs of actors in two performances, in 1941 and 1986, of Noel Coward's *Blithe Spirit*. There is a striking resemblance, both in physical appearance and in gestures, between Cecil Parker in a 1941 picture and Simon Cadell in a 1986 picture.

The same applies to the actors cast in Herb Gardner's 1986 play, *I'm Not Rappopor*t. Hal Linden in 1986 and Jack Klugman in 1987, had hair and facial features with readily discernible similarities.

Perceptual attunements and perceptual learning in the dramatic arts

One concept of ecological psychology that has not yet been mentioned is the idea of *attunement*. As McArthur and Baron (1983) have noted, the ecological view hypothesizes that perceptual systems have evolved to be sensitive to particular types of information that have meaning and relevance to adaptation, a consequence that might be termed "biological preprogramming in response to evolutionary pressures" (McArthur & Baron, 1983, p 218).

One category of information in which humans and other species seem particularly attuned is that associated in some way with aging. As McArthur and Baron (1983) have noted, the morphological changes associated with aging can be viewed as a transformational variant occurring over time. These changes are 'invariant' in the sense that the changes in skin texture and bodily shape that connote aging are relatively invariant from one individual to another.

However, the size and shape of facial features also provide structural invariants that communicate the quality of babyishness. The ethologist Konrad Lorenz proposed that juvenile features such as large heads and eyes trigger nurturing behaviour and affection through innate releasing mechanisms (Lorenz, 1971).

It is of interest to the present discussion to note that the presence of juvenile facial characteristics in adults has also been found to influence the social perception of adults. Adult faces characterized as babyish were perceived as more honest, warm and kind, whereas angularity in facial features resulted in lower ratings of warmth and honesty (Berry & McArthur, 1985; 1986. See Caudle, in press, for further discussion of such facial characteristics). One might hypothesize that such facial features also have some influence in casting decisions. It is unlikely that the angular-jawed James Cagney, noted for his gangster and tough-guy roles, would ever have been cast in the role of the mild and retiring 'Mr Peepers', played by the baby-faced actor, Wally Cox.

Dramatic roles often call for a character to age; this might occur over the course of filming a movie, or it might occur during the course of a single on-stage performance. In either case, both the actor and the make-up artist must recreate the transformational invariants in facial features and other characteristics that will be perceived as aging by the viewer.

Compare the 'before' and 'after' pictures, in a make-up manual (Kehoe, 1969) of an actor aged for a television production. This transformation from a young man into an aged one makes extensive use of such devices as latex protheses that simulate the aging skin around the neck. This particular make-up is finely detailed since it was designed for use in a television production with close-up shots. However, even the exaggerations needed in order for stage make-up to withstand the lights and distance from the audience are based on the selection of prominent invariants to emphasize.

Within the context of the make-up artist's skill, consider another concept important to an ecological position, the influence of perceptual learning on attunements.

McArthur and Baron (1983) have characterized perceptual learning as being:

> revealed when one compares the forest that is seen through the eyes of

> a naturalist to the forest seen through the eyes of a city dweller. Whereas the naturalist will differentiate - that is *see* many levels of structure, the city person may never see anything more than an uniform and boring mass of green. (1983, p 218)

One need only look at the many precise instructions for shading, texturing, colouring and contouring, and the many products available to achieve these goals, to realize that those trained in make-up have learned to make much finer discriminations than those who have not been so trained. It would appear that the same sort of process applies to many others involved in the theatre, such as lighting designers and set designers, among others. In fact, this process of perceptual learning is very likely central to becoming an actor. The actor becomes sensitized, as it were, to the fine nuances of facial expression, voice, gesture and movement; the make-up artist, to facial and bodily textures and contours; the set designer, to the objects, furnishings and patterns that evoke a particular time or place. All of these things might be viewed, collectively, as the ecology of theatrical performance: that is, all of the stimulus information about emotions, characterization, time and place that is presented for the audience to detect.

Conclusion

This paper has sketched only the barest outlines of an ecological view of social perception as it relates to theatrical performance. It has, I believe, demonstrated the potential value of this framework for the development of a comprehensive theory of dramatic communication. In preparing this paper from the perspective of a psychologist, I find that I have undergone the process of perceptual learning myself in the sense that I have become attuned to the wealth of knowledge and expertise concerning communication and social perception that has been recorded concerning acting, dance, mime, make-up and other aspects of theatrical performance. Clearly, social scientists have as much to learn from those associated with the theatre as the latter stand to gain from the application of psychological concepts.

References

Aubert, C. (1985) *The Art of Pantomime* (E Sears, Trans.). Salem, New Hampshire: Ayer Company (Original work published 1927)

Baird, J.F. (1957) *Make-up: A manual for the use of actors, amateur and professional* (revised ed.) New York: Samuel French (Originally published 1941)

Berry, D.S. & L.Z. McArthur (1986) 'Perceiving character in faces: The impact of age-related craniofacial changes on social perception.' *Psychological Bulletin*, **100**, p 3-18

Buchman, H. (1973) *Film and Television Makeup*. New York: Watson-Guptill Publications

Buck, R. (1984) *The Communication of Emotion*. New York: Guilford Press

Caudle, F.M. (In press) 'Communication and arousal of emotion: Some implications of facial expression research for magazine advertisements.' In S. Agres, J. Edell & T. Dubitsky (Eds.) *Emotion in advertising: Theoretical and practical explorations*. Westport, Connecticut: Greenwood Press

Chekhov, M. (1953) *To the Actor, on the technique of acting*. New York: Harper & Row

Collier, G. (1985) *Emotional Expression*. Hillsdale, New Jersey: Erlbaum

Critchley, M. (1939) *The Language of Gesture*. London: Edward Arnold

Ekman, P. (1985). *Telling Lies: Clues to deceit in the marketplace, politics and marriage*. New York: W.W. Norton

Ekman, P. & W.V. Friesen (1975) *Unmasking the Face: A guide to recognizing emotions from facial clues*. Englewood Cliffs, New Jersey: Prentice-Hall

Ekman, P. & W.V. Friesen (1982) 'Felt, false and miserable smiles.' *Journal of Nonverbal Behavior*, **6**, 238-252

Ekman, P., W.V. Friesen & O'Sullivan, M. (1988) 'Smiles when lying.' *Journal of Personality and Social Psychology*, **54**, 414-420

Ekman, P., J.C. Hager & W.V. Friesen (1981) 'The symmetry of emotional and deliberate facial actions.' *Psychophysiology*, **18**, 101-106

Ekman, P. & H. Oster (1982) Review of research, 1970-1980. In P. Ekman (Ed.) *Emotion in the Human Face* (2nd ed.) New York: Cambridge University Press

Gibson, J.J. (1966) *The Senses Considered as Perceptual Systems*. Boston: Houghton Mifflin

Gibson, J.J. (1979) *The Ecological Approach to Visual Perception*. Boston: Houghton Mifflin

Hanna, J.L. (1988) *Dance, Sex and Gender: Signs of identity, dominance, defiance and desire*. Chicago: University of Chicago

Kehoe, V. J-R. (1969) *The Technique of Film and Television Make-Up* (rev. ed.) London: Focal Press

Kipnis, C. (1974) *The Mime Book*. New York: Harper & Row/Colophon Books

Knapp, M.L. (1978) *Nonverbal Communication in Human Interaction* (2nd ed.). New York: Holt, Rinehart and Winston

Lawson, J. (1957) *Mime: The theory and practice of expressive gesture with a description of its historical development*. London: Sir Isaac Pitman and Sons. Republished by Dance Horizons, Brooklyn, New York

Lombardo, T.J. (1987) *The Reciprocity of Perceiver and Environment: The evolution of James J Gibson's ecological psychology.* Hillsdale, New Jersey: Erlbaum

Lorenz, K. (1971) *Studies in animal and human behavior,* (Vol. 2) (R. Martin, Trans.). Cambridge, MA: Harvard University Press

Mawer, I. (1932) *The Art of Mime: Its history and technique in education and the theatre* (2nd ed.). London: Methuen

McArthur, L.Z. & R.M. Baron (1983) 'Toward an ecological theory of social perception.' *Psychological Review,* 90(3), 215-238

Morris, D., P. Collet, P. Marsh. & M. O'Shaugnessy (1979) *Gestures, their origins and distribution.* New York: Stein and Day

Peck, S.R. (1987) *Atlas of Facial Expression: An account of facial expression for artists, actors and writers.* New York: Oxford

Ruesch, J. & W. Kees (1972) *Nonverbal Communication: Notes on the visual perception of human relations.* Berkeley: University of California Press. (Original work published 1956)

Stanislavski, C. (1936) *An Actor Prepares* (E.R. Hapgood, Trans.). New York: Theatre Arts Books

Stanislavski, C. (1949) *Building a Character* (E.R. Hapgood, Trans.). New York: Theatre Arts Books

Stanislavski, C. (1963) *An Actor's Handbook: An alphabetical arrangement of concise statements on aspects of acting* (E.R. Hapgood, Ed. and Trans.). New York: Theatre Arts Books

Weitz, S. (Ed.) (1979) *Nonverbal Communication: Readings with commentary.* New York: Oxford

What's on between the actor and his audience? Empirical analysis of emotion processes in the theatre

Elly A. Konijn

Department of Theatre Studies, University of Utrecht

Diderot states in his *Paradoxe sur le comédien* (1959; 1773) that in order to have the greatest emotional effect on the spectator, the actor has to be in complete control of his acting behaviour and should not be emotional on stage. This concerns the classical question as to whether it is a necessary requirement for the actor to be emotionally involved with his character at the moment of rendering the role in front of an audience. Nowadays we can recognize the actor's dilemma in Stanislavskian and Brechtian theories, which are opposed on this point (Emmet, 1975; Roach 1981). Stanislavsky (1936) proposes that the actor "lives his role", that he gets into the skin of his character, whereas Brecht (1967-8) says that the actor has to play his character with distance. The paradox of acting is still a central thesis in theatre research. This study is directed at empirically investigating the processes of emotion management in actors playing a character.

In the 18th century there was a big gap between theatrical practice and theatrical theories. The theories mainly consisted of stringent rhetorical rules

(Barnett 1987; Rougemont 1988). The lifelong conflict between two leading French actresses, Mlle Clairon (1798) and Mlle Dumesnil (1800), concerning the naturalness of their staged characters' emotions is often mentioned by Diderot (1959). The context of the 18th century is important to an understanding of Diderot's paradox (Proust, 1984; Hobson, 1977; Szondi, 1984). At that time psychology was not yet a scientific discipline, but psychological ideas were imbedded in philosophical ideas. In the 18th century the deistic view was prevailing. An emotion was something coming from heaven, from the Lord (Wartofsky, 1952; Vartanian 1949; Barzun 1986).

Social psychology of emotion

In current theories of emotion two main streams can be distinguished. On the one hand there are the *peripheral feedback* theories, first stated by William James in 1884. It says, stated briefly; when you give expression to a smile you will get the feeling of being happy. For peripheral emotion theory the experience of physiological changes *is* the experience of having an emotion. Schachter and Singer (1962) added that physiological changes incite an individual to seek a cognitive interpretation of their aroused state. Physiological changes together with finding an environmental explanation leads to the experience of having an emotion. Crucial to peripheral emotion theories is the notion that physiological feedback is prior to emotions and possible accompanying cognitions (Zajonc, 1984; Ekman, Levenson & Friesen, 1983). On the other hand there are *cognitive* emotion theories (Sartre, 1939; Lazarus, 1984; Frijda, 1986; 1988) which state that without mental processes you cannot have any emotions; emotions are related to the situational meaning structure. Cognitions come first and the physiological changes follow. Depending on regulation processes the subject will have the experience of an emotion and give expression to it.

In order to explore the processes of emotion management in actors playing a character in front of an audience, theories from the psychology of emotion will be applied to the theatre. Related problems can be found in the area of 'public speaking behaviour' studies and 'stress and human performance' studies (e.g. Baldwin & Clevenger, 1980; Houtman, 1990; Pruyn, 1986; Sanders, 1983; Dimsdale, 1984). The theoretical frames in those studies are social facilitation and inhibition (SFI) theories and stress models (Zajonc, 1965; Bond & Titus, 1983; Sanders, 1983). These theories assume a relationship between stress, personality characteristics and the quality of performance. In general these theories predict stress on performers confronting an audience, hence influencing the quality of performance (Zajonc, 1965; Zajonc & Sales, 1966). A meta-analysis of the SFI-phenomenon (Bond & Titus, 1983) and Dimsdale (1984) show that the relationship between performer and public is dependent on task-characteristics, in particular, the degree of difficulty or complexity. Some studies use simple tasks requiring only quantitative efforts (e.g. speed), while other studies use complex tasks demanding cognitive information processing and the quality of performance is what counts (e.g. accuracy). An audience will heighten the stress level only if the performance concerns a complex task, hence impairing the accuracy of performance (Bond & Titus, 1983). Furthermore, an audience will have facilitating effects on dominant (i.e. well-learned) responses (Zajonc, 1965). Individual differences or appraisal processes further influence the experienced stress level and its consequences on performance (Sanders, 1983; Steptoe, 1983; Lefcourt, 1976). In particular, feelings of control of the task performance are important. Likewise, expert and novice performers differ in the way they appraise the situation (Fenz & Jones, 1972). Depending on the kind of task (complex vs simple and dominant vs subordinate) and personality characteristics (individual differences) the heightened stress level will have either a positive (Zajonc & Sales, 1966; Bond & Titus, 1983) or a negative effect on the quality of performance (Piperek, 1981; Bond & Titus, 1983). A social psychology of emotion and performance can therefore be helpful to explicate theatrical processes.

Diderot's paradox empirically approached

First, we have to find out who are the really great actors, because Diderot clearly distinguishes between good, middling and worse actors. The paradox of acting applies to the really great actors, according to Diderot (1959; 1773). Is a great actor nowadays the same as a great actor was in the times of Diderot? Are the really great actors the ones who gain most prizes? Are they the ones most applauded by critics? Or do we have to ask the audience? In articles, interviews, etc., references are made to 'the greatest actors of the time', but no criteria are given.

The second research problem is how to ask spectators about the emotions they feel while watching a performance and compare them with the emotions the characters are portraying? As Diderot states it, a theatre performance aims at an emotional effect, but perhaps nowadays directors want a different effect on the spectators. Recent research in theatre studies use a broad range of psychologically based instrumentation. An overview on audience research is given by Schoenmakers (1990). From these studies we may conclude that it is possible to ask spectators about their emotional experiences while watching a theatre performance.

The third problem concerns the actor's emotions on stage. How can we or the actor distinguish whether he is portraying a real emotion or a put-on emotion. Can the actor distinguish between emotions resulting from his profession as an actor, for instance, being upset by the audience or certain critics, and the emotions his character must have? Can the spectator distinguish between put-on emotions and real emotions on the other side of the proscenium? According to Diderot, spectators will say the actors are portraying real emotions when they are really good actors. For then, the actor will portray the emotions of the character in such a way as to make the spectator believe they are real emotions.

Diderot's statement was empirically investigated in 1888 by the psychologist W. Archer. He circulated a questionnaire concerning the crucial question whether the actors really experience real emotions when acting. Independently of Archer the French psychologist Binet performed a similar study in 1896 and came to the same conclusions as Archer. In general the actors and actresses did answer that their tears, blushing, pallor, perspiration and so on were real on stage.

Emmet (1975) criticized Archer's study, pointing out that being able to put on the outward manifestations of emotion proves nothing more than the possession of a well-developed expressive instrument. Kepke (1963) used Q-methodology and Wayne-Smith (1971) used the semantic differential to investigate identification of actors with their characters. No actor-character identification could be determined. Alekseev (1985) and Collum Dovard (1977) investigated the emotional capabilities of actors in their personality structures. Observation and interviewing techniques are used in a study on actor-director interactions (New, 1964). Perky (1976), Jackson & Latané (1981) and Weisweiler (1983) studied the effects of audience presence on actors. Perky (1976) found some effects of audience variation (positive, neutral and negative audiences) on the quality of acting and non-verbal behaviours of actors. Jackson & Latané (1981) found decreasing effects on actors' subjective stress reports as the number of co-actors increases and increasing stress levels proportional to size and status of audience. Weisweiler (1983) found differences in physiological measurements of professional actors between rehearsals and performances. Furthermore, actors have been used in recent years in psychological experimentation for general psychological purposes (e.g. Ekman, Levenson & Friesen, 1983).

These studies provide various theatrical theories with empirical evidence. However, the actor's dilemma whether to feel or not to feel on stage still causes heated debates among theatre practitioners and researchers (Emmet, 1975; Roach, 1981). As an illustration of how modern methods may be used to unravel the paradox of acting in the near future, I will now describe a study of actors' stage fright and performance.

An empirical study of stage fright and performance

The starting point of this study was a remark often made by actors during rehearsals: "Wait until the audience arrives...". With this remark actors suggest that their presentation will be much better during public performances compared to rehearsals. On the other hand, stage fright may worsen an actor's performance in front of a live audience. Following the theoretical considerations above three assumptions guide this explorative study.

1 The presence of evaluative spectators induces stress on actors performing a complex task (Bode & Brutten, 1963; Bond & Titus, 1983). Rehearsals and public performances offer natural opportunities to manipulate stress-levels, which have been measured by means of continuous heart rate recordings (Van der Molen, Somsen & Orlebeke, 1985; Weisweiler, 1983; Piperek, 1981;) and questionnaires (Jackson & Latané, 1981).
2 Stage fright is modulated by the cognitive appraisal of the actor (Sanders, 1983; Dimsdale, 1984). In particular the effects of control or lack of control over the environment are apparent in the cardiovascular system (Steptoe 1983). Therefore individual differences are measured by means of the Locus of Control variable (Rotter 1966; Lefcourt, 1976).
3 The quality of the performance will be influenced by the presence of an audience (Zajonc, 1965; Bond & Titus, 1983). Quality of performance is assessed by self-ratings as well as the ratings of four expert observers (Perky, 1976).

Procedure

Subjects
Subjects were four Dutch amateur actors (two male and two female) of about the same age (around 20) who participated voluntarily. They had no arousal-inducing habits (like coffee-drinking or smoking). The procedure was repeated with the same subjects during two dress-rehearsals (no audience) and three public performances so that circumstances were comparable.

Instruments
The LOC-variable was measured with an adapted version of Rotter's I-E scale (1966; Lefcourt 1976). All 26 participants in the theatre project were used as a comparison group. The 40-item questionnaire was filled in about one week before the first night performance. Consistency reliability (Cronbach's α) is low (α = .59) but split half reliability is .75 (Spearman Brown corrected for test length).

Quality of an individual actor's performance was measured with a 28-item questionnaire. A modified Dutch version was developed after a questionnaire in Perky (1976) (see Appendix). To avoid certain demand characteristics items are both positively and negatively formulated.

Immediately after each performance this Quality-list was filled in by the actors for their own performance (self-reports) and by four expert observers. The expert observers were members of the theatre company hierarchy. During rehearsals and an experimental try-out they were trained in judging acting qualities. Nevertheless, they did not agree with each other because the interrater reliability was low; neither the p.m.c.-coefficient nor Cohen's Kappa (computed for performances separately) exceeded .20. The internal consistency of the Acting-Quality list was high: Cronbach's = .96 and split-half reliability .97 (Spearman Brown, corrected for test length).

Stress has both a psychological and a physiological component (Cox, 1978; Steptoe, 1983). Questionnaires served as a measure of psychological stress (Jackson & Latane, 1981), for which Items 9 and 14 and the first question below item 28 from the AQL were used.

Heart rate frequency and variability were used to measure the physiological component (Van der Molen et. al., 1985; Payne & Rick, 1986; Mulder, 1986; Kamphuis & Frowein, 1986). Heart rate was recorded by portable Heart Rate Monitors (HRM) developed at the Free University of Amsterdam and could afterwards be connected to an Apple IIe computer for graphical and statistical examination. The HRM measures interbeat intervals (IBI; distance between beats in msec.). A greater interval indicates a lower level of heart rate frequency (formula is 60.000/msec. IBI = beats per minute (BPM)). Thus the Figures have to be interpreted upside down.

Heart rate variability may also be used as a stress indicator (Mulder, 1986; Kamphuis & Frowein, 1986; Grossman & Wientjes, 1986). Because interbeat intervals are recorded the variability of heart rate can be computed precisely. Reduction of energy (power) for blood pressure regulation occurs with an accumulation of mental load and is reflected in the .10 Hz heart rate variability spectrum, which is computed by means of Fourier spectral analyses. This gives an indication of the mental load imposed by acting.

Theatre Play

The stage production "Bende" from a Dutch theatre company "De Opmaat" (Groningen) took about one hour playing time and served as the research environment. In all 26 young people participated in different performances. The parts of the four actors under investigation were sufficiently comparable and each had some sort of little monologue. During a dress rehearsal (reh-1) and a take-up rehearsal in the midst of the playing period (reh-2) measurements took place without an audience. During the first night performance (perf-1), the second (perf-2) and the fourth performance, about a month later (perf-3), public performances were recorded. A training session was held during a dress rehearsal one week before the first-night performance. Except for the expert observers, audiences were not aware that any research was going on.

Analysis

The results of the LOC-, Quality- and Stress measurements were analysed on an individual and a group level. For subsequent analyses of heart rate measurements we selected five periods of 5 minutes each. These were two periods backstage (non-acting); about a quarter of an hour 'before' and 'after' the performance, and three periods on stage (acting); the first 5 minutes ('beginning') the last 5 minutes of performance ('end') and 5 minutes during the 'applause'. These moments were chosen because of the comparability of activity and stage presence of the four subjects.

Results

Individual differences in locus of control were too small to perform further analyses, so it was not possible to relate individual differences to Quality and Stress results. Compared to the group mean, the four actors tended (non-significantly) toward the internal end of the LOC-scale (group mean = 2.19, individual scores; 2.10, 2.00, 2.20 and 1.78).

Figure 1 is a graphical comparison of the means of self-reports and experts' judgements of Quality of Acting. This shows that in general actors ascribe to their own performances a higher quality than do expert observers. Furthermore, the quality of acting was generally better during performances than during rehearsals. Statistical testing of differences in the Quality of Acting between the separate rehearsals and performances was done (only for the expert ratings) by means of analysis of variance for repeated measurements (ANOVA-BMDP2V) with one factor (performance) and five levels (reh-1, reh-2, perf-1, perf-2, perf-3). Significant differences were found at the 5% level: F(performance) = 4.24, df = 4, p = .0228. Thus, quality of acting was judged significantly better during performances than during rehearsals. There was, however, no significant difference between the first dress rehearsal (reh-1) and the opening night performance (perf-1).

Results of the psychological stress measurements are shown in Figure 2. Before and during rehearsals little psychological stress was reported, compared with during performances. Figures 1 and 2 show a similar pattern so there may be a comparable subjective element concerned in reporting the Quality of Acting and psychological stress.

The limitations of personal report are shown nicely in that subjects' reported that the audience presence hardly made them nervous (Item 14), whereas their heart rate rose quickly as soon as they came on stage during

Figure 1.

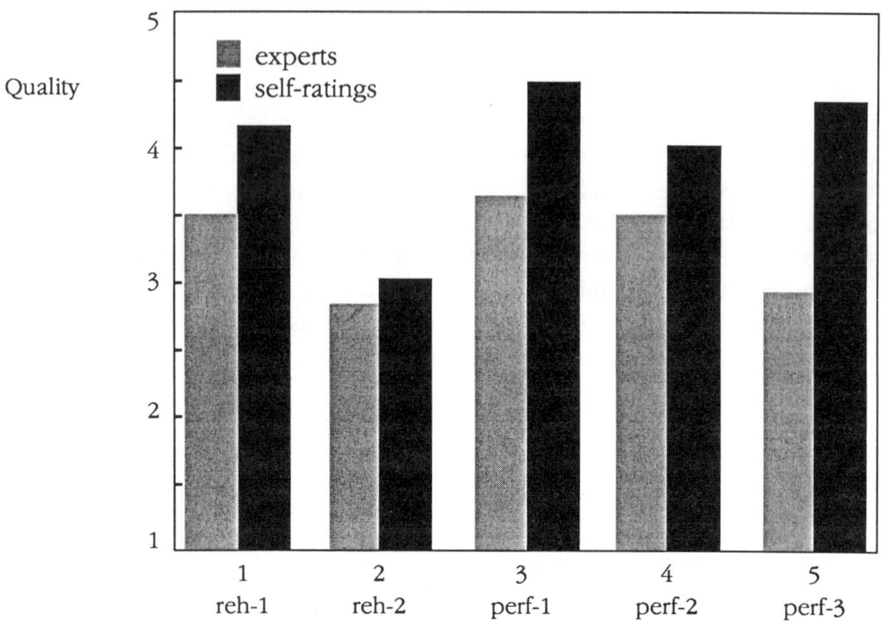

Figure 2.

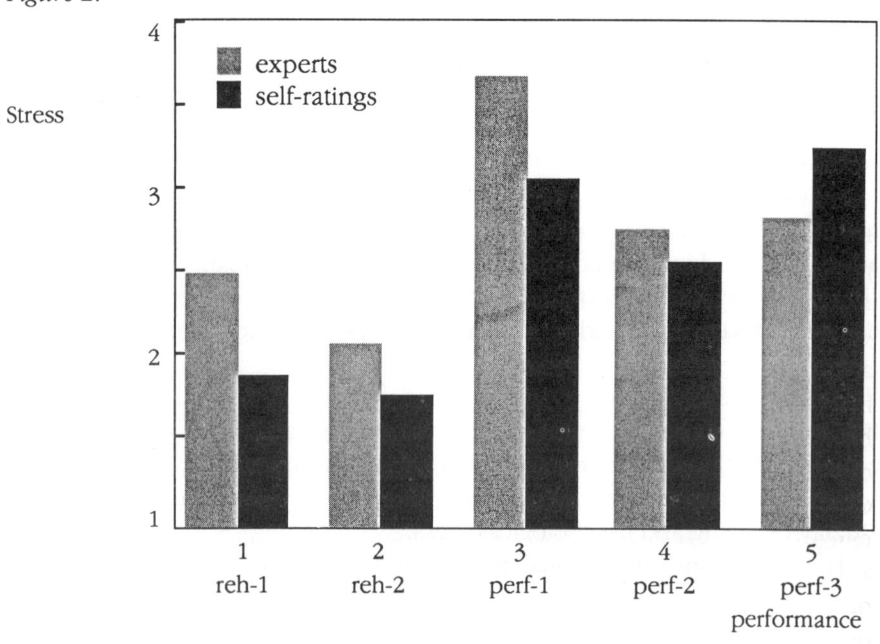

performances (Figures 3 and 4). The raw data of the continuous heart rate recordings are graphically shown for one actress in Figure 3. This shows recordings of the first measured rehearsal (reh-1) and the opening night (perf-1).

Figure 3.

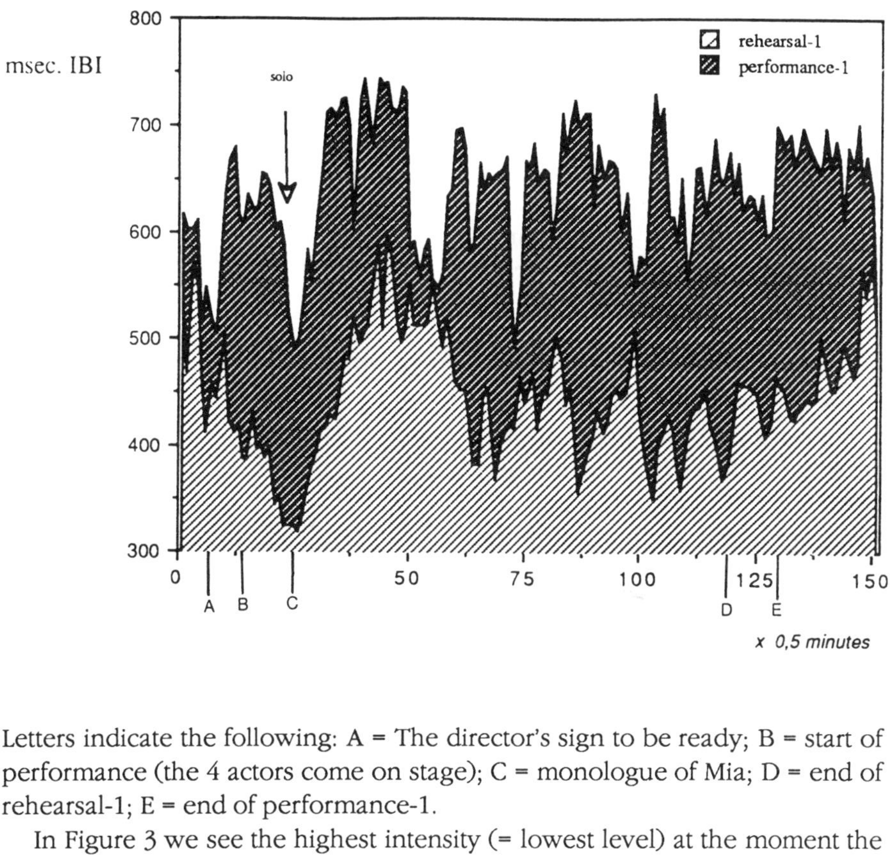

Letters indicate the following: A = The director's sign to be ready; B = start of performance (the 4 actors come on stage); C = monologue of Mia; D = end of rehearsal-1; E = end of performance-1.

In Figure 3 we see the highest intensity (= lowest level) at the moment the actress is performing a monologue. For several minutes heart rate rises to 180 beats per minute (BPM). Averaged for the first 5 minutes of performance her heart rate is 151 BPM against 94 BPM during the same period of the dress rehearsal. Averaged over the four actors the same periods show 141 BPM during the first performance (perf-1) and 96 BPM during the first measured rehearsal (reh-1). Prior to the confrontation with the audience, heart rate is already increasing. When the actress is coming on stage heart rate rises quickly and it slows almost as quickly when she is going backstage. Overall patterns are the same for rehearsals and performances, i.e. the same

Figure 4.

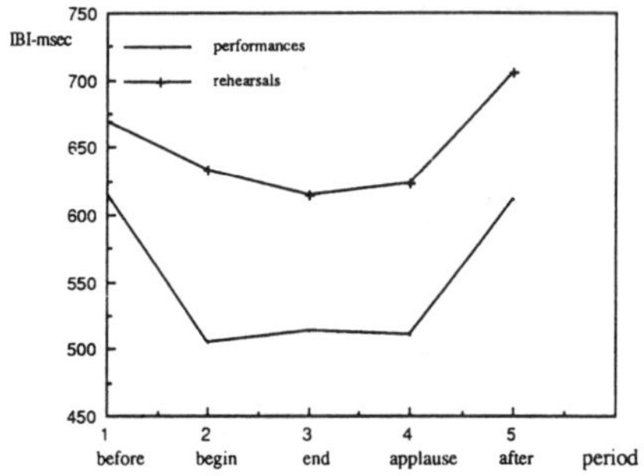

Figure 5.

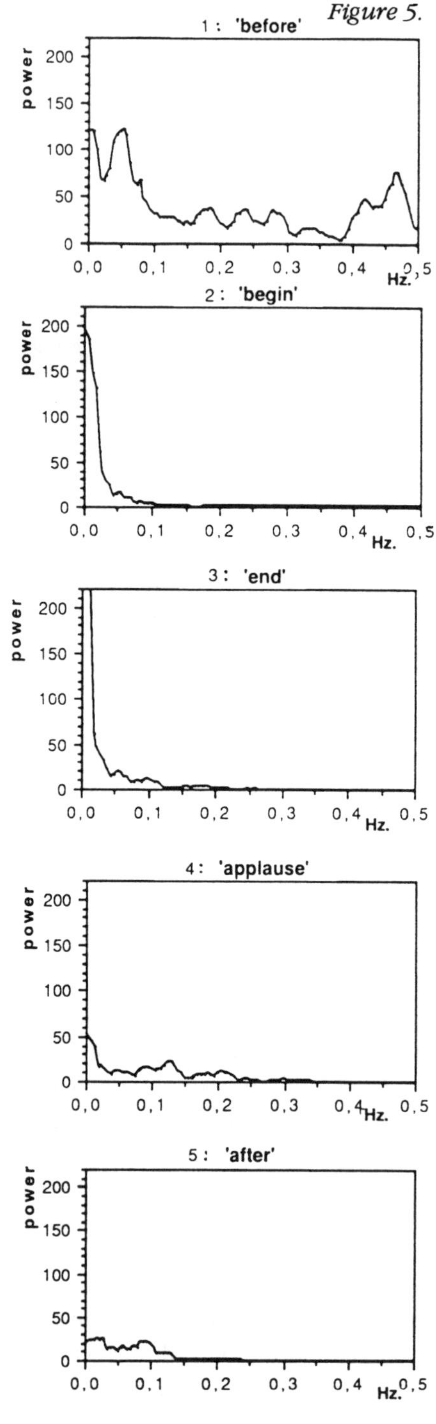

moments show heightened or lowered stress-levels. Because the length of the rehearsal is less than the length of the performance (resp. 52 and 58 minutes) the peaks and troughs of heart rate level are not exactly parallel.

Figure 4 shows mean heart rate frequencies of the five selected periods for the two rehearsals and three performances. Heart rate levels are higher for performances. Statistical testing was done by averaging across subjects and periods. The resulting mean HR-levels were subjected to an ANOVA-analysis for repeated measurements. The two factors performance and period, with five levels each, both had significant effects at the 5% level ($F_{performance}$ = 11.75, df = 4, p = .0109; F_{period} = 11.70, df = 4, p = .0183; after correction on degrees of freedom with Greenhouse Geiser Probability). No significant interaction effect was found.

Figure 5 shows the results of the Fourier analyses of heart rate variability. In the first picture (before performance) there is a reasonable amount of power at the .10 Hz spectrum (ranging from .05 to .15) indicating a low level of mental load. In the second (beginning) and subsequent phases there is a considerable reduction of the the power in the .10 Hz spectrum, indicating a considerable increase of mental load. No significant differences between rehearsals and performances or between the five selected periods was revealed by Analyses of Variance over the power levels. However, acting in general appears to demand a considerable mental load.

Conclusion

In conclusion, amateur actors do experience extremely high stress levels during public performances and this seems to improve their performance.

Results support the conclusion of Bond & Titus (1983) that audiences induce stress on actors performing a complex task; however, it didn't impair but rather improved the quality of performance. This also supports the thesis of Zajonc (1965) that, after a long-lasting rehearsal period, acting in a public performance belongs to the dominant set of responses, which are thus facilitated by the presence of an audience. Furthermore, the results support the idea of positive stress in challenging situations as offered by Lazarus and Folkman (1984).

Interestingly, comparable high heart rate levels were found with professional actors in Munich (Weisweiler, 1983). Unfortunately, quality of performance or personality characteristics were not taken into account. A study with professional musicians in Vienna also showed high heart rate levels during public performances and similar differences from rehearsals (Haider & Groll-Knapp, 1981). Contrary to our findings, the Vienna musicians performed worse during public performances than during rehearsals according to themselves (no observers were used) (Piperek, 1981).

Perhaps the only emotion that really matters to the actor is the tension of work-related stress (e.g. stage fright). Maybe the magic of a good actor is that he is one who can manage this work-related stress in such a way as to make the audience believe it belongs to the emotions of the character and get them involved with these supposed emotions. Theatrical communication is a two-way reciprocal process but until now empirical theatre research has consisted mainly of audience and reception research (Schoenmakers, 1990). The focus has been on the emotional impact of theatrical performances and films. In the present research project emphasis is not only on the spectator but on the production side as well; in particular, the actor is the subject of study.

The paradox of acting (Diderot, 1773) is still a central thesis not only in hermeneutic theatre studies but also in the empirical study of theatrical processes. A social psychological orientation may be helpful to explicate theatrical processes as illustrated in the above reported study of actors' stage fright and performance. Also, recent theoretical and technical developments permit more precise measurement and data processing. The time has arrived to confront Diderot's paradox with empirical analysis.

Acknowledgements

The actors' stage fright and performance study is carried out under the supervision of Prof Dr M.W. Van der Molen (Dept. of Psych., Univ. of Amsterdam). I am grateful to him and also to Drs H.C.M. Vorst, Drs W. Wijker (both of Dept. of Psych., Univ. of Amsterdam) Dr I.L.D. Houtman (Dept. of Human Movement Sciences, Free Univ. Amsterdam) and Drs E.S.H. Tan (Dept. of Theatre Studies, Univ. of Amsterdam). The Diderot study will be the subject of a dissertation with Prof Dr H. Schoenmakers (Dept. of Theatre Studies, State Univ. Utrecht) as supervising promotor.

Preliminary results of the empirical study are published in Konijn, E A (in press) 'Waiting for the audience: empirical study of actors' stage fright and performance'. In: Prof H. Schoenmakers (ed.) (in press) *Performance Theory, Audience and Reception Studies* Utrecht/Munich; Tijdschrift voor Theaterwetenschap, Dept. of Theatre Studies, Utrecht, The Netherlands.

References

Alekseev, N.P. (1985) 'An experimental study of the emotionality of theatre-college students.' *Soviet Psychology, Vol.23.* 59-72

Archer, William (1888) *Masks or Faces? A study in the psychology of acting.* London: Longmans, Green & Co

Baldwin, S. & T. Clevenger (1980) 'Effects of speaker's sex and size of audience on heart rate changes during short impromptu speeches.' *Psychological Reports,* **46**, 123-130

Barzun, Jacques (1986) 'Diderot as philosopher.' In: *Diderot Studies, Vol. XXII,* 17-27. Geneva

Barnett, Dene (1987) *The Art of Gesture: the practices and principles of 18th century acting.* Heidelberg: Winter

Binet, A. (1896) 'Reflexions sur le paradoxe de Diderot', *L'Annee Psychologique 1896,* **3**, 279-295

Bode, D.L. & E. Brutten (1963) 'A palmar sweat investigation of the effect of audience variation upon stage fright.' *Speech Monographs,* **30**, 92-96

Bond, C. & L.J. Titus (1983) 'Social Facilitation: a meta-analysis of 241 studies.' *Psychological Bulletin,* **94(2)**, 265-292

Brecht, Bertolt (1967-8) *Gesammelte Werke 15: Schriften zum Theater I* (W. Hecht, Ed.). Frankfurt am Main: Suhrkamp Verlag

Clairon, Hyppolyte (1969; 1798) *Memoirs of Hyppolite Clairon, the celebrated French actress: With reflections upon the dramatic art* 2 vols. New York: Benjamin Blom

Collum Dovard, K. (1977) 'The empathic ability of actors: a behavioral study' In: *Diss. abstr. international literature and art, Oct. 1977, Vol. 38 (4A)*, 174

Cox, T. (1978) *Stress.* London: Macmillan Education Ltd

Diderot, Denis (1959; 1773) 'Paradoxe sur le comédien.' In: Paul Verniere (Ed.). *Diderot: Oeuvres Esthetique* Paris: Editions Garnier Frères 291-380

Dimsdale, J.E. (1984) 'Generalizing from laboratory studies to field studies of human stress physiology.' *Psychosomatic Medicine*, **46 (5)**

Dumesnil, Marie-Francoise (1800) *Mémoires de Marie-Francoise Dumesnil, en response aux mémoires d'Hyppolite Clairon; suivis d'une lettre de célèbre Lekain* Paris: Dentu

Ekman, P., R.W. Levenson. & W.V. Friesen (1983) 'Autonomic nervous system activity distinguishes among emotions.' *Science* Sept 1983, Vol. 221, No. 4616, 1208-1210

Emmet, Alfred (1975) 'Head or heart: the actor's dilemma.' *Theatre Quarterly, Vol. 18*, 1975 15-21

Fenz, W.D. & G.B. Jones (1972) 'Individual differences in physiologic arousal and performance in sport parachutists.' *Psychosomatic Medicine* **34**, **1**, 1-8

Frijda, N.H. (1986) *The Emotions*. New York: Cambridge University Press

Frijda, N.H. (1988) 'The Laws of Emotion.' *American Psychologist, May 1988, Vol. 43, No. 5*, 349-358

Grossman, P. & Wientjes (1986) 'Respiratory sinus arrhytmia and parasympathetic cardiac control: some basic issues concerning quantification, applications and implications.' In: P. Grossman, K.H.L. Jansen & D. Vaitl (Eds.) *Cardiorespiratory and cardiosomatic psychophysiology.* New York/London: Plenum Press

Haider, M. & Groll-Knapp, E. (1981) 'Psychophysiological investigation into the stress experienced by musicians in a symphony orchestra.' In *Stress and Music.* M. Piperek (Ed.). Vienna: Wilhelm Braumuller

Hobson, M. (1977) 'Sensibilité et spectacle: le contexte medical du "paradoxe sur le comedién" de Diderot.' *Revue de metaphysique et de morale*, **82**, 145-164

Houtman, I.L.D. (1990) 'Stress and Coping in Lecturing: a study on stability of stress responses, individual differences and stress moderators.' Amsterdam: Free University (Diss.) Dept. of Human Movement Sciences

James, W. (1884) 'What is an emotion?' *Mind, Vol. 9*, 188-205

Jackson, J.M. & B. Latané (1981) 'All alone in front of all those people: Stage fright as a function of number and type of co-performers and audience.' *Journal of Personality and Social Psychology*, **40**, **1**, 73-85

Kamphuis, A. & H.W. Frowein (1986) 'Assessment of mental effort by means of heart rate spectral analysis.' In: J.F. Orlebeke, G. Mulder & L.J.P. Van Doornen (Eds). *Psychophysiology of cardiovascular control: Models, methods and data.* New York: Plenum Press

Kepke, A.N. (1963) 'A study of communication of perception of character among actors, director and audience, using Q-methodology.' (Diss .)

Lazarus, R.S. (1984) 'On the primacy of cognition.' *American Psychologist, Vol. 39, No. 2,* 124-129

Lazarus, R.S. & S. Folkman (1984) *Stress, Appraisal and Coping*. New York: Springer

Lefcourt, H.M. (1976) *Locus of Control: current trends in theory and research.* Hillsdale, New Jersey: Lawrence Erlbaum Associates

Mulder, G. (1986) 'Attention, effort and sinusarrhythmia: how far are we?' In: J.F. Orlebeke, G. Mulder & L.J.P. Van Doornen (Eds.) *Psychophysiology of cardiovascular control: Models, methods and data.* New York: Plenum Press

New, G.R. Jr. (1964) 'Play production as a democratic group process.' *Speech Monographs,* **32**, 312

Perky, S.D. (1976) 'Effects of positive and negative audience response on actors' nonverbal performance behavior and on their attitudes.' Dissertation: Bowling Green State University

Piperek, M. (1981) *Stress and music: Medical psychological, sociological and legal strain factors in a symphony orchestra musician' profession.* Vienna: Wilhelm Braumuller

Proust, J. (1984) 'Interpréter Diderot aujourd'hui.' In: E. de Fontenay & J. Proust (Eds.) *Interpréter Diderot aujourd'hui.* Paris: Centre Culturel International de Cerisy-la-Salle, Le Sycomore, Colloque de Cerisy S.F.I.E.D., 9-17

Pruyn, A.T.H. (1986) *Performance and activation under social evaluation.* Delft: Eburon (Dissertation, Univ. of Groningen, Dept. of Social Sciences)

Roach, J.R. Jr. (1981) 'Diderot and the actor's machine.' *Theatre Survey, Vol. 22,* 51-68

Rotter, J.B. (1966) 'Generalized expectancies for internal vs external control of reinforcement.' *Psychological Monographs,* **80**, 1-28

Rougemont, M. de (1988) *La vie théatrale en France au XVIIIème siècle.* Paris: Librarie Honore Champion

Sanders, A.F. (1983) 'Towards a model of stress and human performance' *Acta Psychologica,* **53**, 61-99

Sartre, J.P. (1939) *Esquisse d'une théorie d'émotion* Paris: Hermann (Dutch translation, L.M. Tas (1963) *Magie en emotie* Meppel: Boom)

Schachter. S. & J.E. Singer (1962) 'Cognitive, social and physiological determinants of emotional state.' *Psychological Review,* **69**, 379-399

Schoenmakers, H. (1990) 'The spectator in the leading role. Developments in reception and audience research within Theatre Studies: Theory and Research.' In: W. Sauter (Ed.). *Nordic Theatre Studies: New Directions in Theatre Research.* Special International Issue: proceedings of the XIth FIRT/IFTR Congress, 93-106. Stockholm/Copenhagen: Munksgaard Ltd

Stanislavski, K. (1936) *An Actor Prepares* (trans. E. R. Hapgood). New York: Theatre Arts Books

Steptoe, A. (1983) 'Stress, Helplessness and Control: the implications of laboratory studies.' *Journal of psychosomatic research*, **27**, **5**, 361-367

Szondi, P. (1984) 'Denis Diderot: théorie et pratique dramatique.' In: J. Starobinski, J. Chouillet, G.E. Lessing et al (Eds.) *Diderot (Diderot et le theatre).* Paris: Comedie Francaise, Grands Dramaturges, 33-62

Van der Molen, M.W., R.J.M. Somsen & J.F. Orlebeke (1985) 'The rhythm of the heart beat in information processing.' In: P.K. Ackles, J.R. Jennings & M.G.H. Coles (Eds.). *Advances in psychophysiology, Vol. 1,* 1-88 Greenwich: JAI press

Vartanian, Aram (1949) 'From Deist to Atheist: Diderot's philosophical orientation 1746-1749.' *Diderot Studies, Vol. 1* 47-64

Wartofsky Marx, W. (1952) 'Diderot and the development of materialist monism' *Diderot Studies, Vol. II.* 279-330 (O. Fellows et al. Eds.) Geneva: Librairie Droz S.A.

Wayne-Smith, R. (1971) 'Actor-Character personality identification in a theatre production.' *Empirical Research in Theatre*, **1**, **1**, 29-38

Weisweiler, H. (1983) *Die Belastung des Schauspielers an seinem Arbeitsplatz.* Munich: Münchener Universität, Theaterwissenschaft (Dissertation)

Zajonc, R.B. (1965) 'Social Facilitation' *Science*, **149**, 269-275

Zajonc, R.B. (1984) 'On the primacy of effect.' *American Psychologist, Vol. 39, No. 2* 117-123

Zajonc, R.B. & S.M. Sales (1966) 'Social Facilitation of dominant and subordinate responses.' *Journal of Experimental Social Psychology*, **2**. 160-168

Appendix

ACTING-QUALITY-LIST
(translation of the Dutch version in Konijn 1988)

What do you think of tonight's performance as a whole ?

a. Performance flowed smoothly	agree	|--|--|--|--|--|	disagree
b. This was a good performance	agree	|--|--|--|--|--|	disagree
c. Timing was precise	agree	|--|--|--|--|--|	disagree
d. It was problematic tonight	agree	|--|--|--|--|--|	disagree
e. There were technical difficulties tonight	agree	|--|--|--|--|--|	disagree

What do you think of tonight's individual performance of Gi ?

1. Gi's performance flowed smoothly	agree	|--|--|--|--|--|	disagree
2. Gi maintained concentration throughout performance	agree	|--|--|--|--|--|	disagree
3. Gi sang well tonight (or: used his voice in the right manner)	agree	|--|--|--|--|--|	disagree
4. Gi felt in control of his performance	agree	|--|--|--|--|--|	disagree
5. Gi's timing was precise	agree	|--|--|--|--|--|	disagree
6. Gi did not pay attention to ensemble interaction	agree	|--|--|--|--|--|	disagree
7. Gi's cue pick-up was precise	agree	|--|--|--|--|--|	disagree
8. Gi played badly	agree	|--|--|--|--|--|	disagree
9. Gi was nervous	agree	|--|--|--|--|--|	disagree
10. Gi's interaction with the audience was bad	agree	|--|--|--|--|--|	disagree
11. Gi's performance was broad	agree	|--|--|--|--|--|	disagree
12. Gi was at his best tonight	agree	|--|--|--|--|--|	disagree
13. Gi's stage-fighting went well	agree	|--|--|--|--|--|	disagree
14. Gi became nervous through the audience	agree	|--|--|--|--|--|	disagree
15. Gi danced badly	agree	|--|--|--|--|--|	disagree
16. Gi had line problems	agree	|--|--|--|--|--|	disagree
17. Gi played with guts	agree	|--|--|--|--|--|	disagree
18. Gi's acting had no believability	agree	|--|--|--|--|--|	disagree
19. Gi enjoyed his performance	agree	|--|--|--|--|--|	disagree
20. Gi was really in character tonight	agree	|--|--|--|--|--|	disagree
21. Gi could be heard well	agree	|--|--|--|--|--|	disagree
22. Gi reacted well to the audience	agree	|--|--|--|--|--|	disagree
23. Gi played insecure	agree	|--|--|--|--|--|	disagree
24. Gi dared to time well	agree	|--|--|--|--|--|	disagree
25. Gi had continuity in his performance	agree	|--|--|--|--|--|	disagree
26. Gi had his weak moments tonight	agree	|--|--|--|--|--|	disagree
27. Gi's character came across clearly	agree	|--|--|--|--|--|	disagree
28. Gi had mastered his role	agree	|--|--|--|--|--|	disagree

- Do you think Gi was nervous before performance went on ?
  very much |--|--|--|--|--| not at all
- Did there happen something special or disturbing during performance ?
  (if 'yes', then 'what was it ?)
- Did there happen something special or disturbing during the day or evening ?
  (if 'yes', then 'what was it ?)
- Did you like the audience tonight ?

The manipulation of the audience by director and actor

Nicholas Arnold

Department of Performing Arts, Leicester Polytechnic

To begin with some caveats. When discussing the arts, we should not operate the pseudo-Romantic notion which marginalizes the artist as a flawed being with a damaged psyche. It is equally important not to read the terms acting and actors as synonymous with performance and performers. Moreover, I am using, as a model, conventional narrative-text-character based theatre. The next stage to this would be to test some of the notions put up against New Theatre: anti-authorial, anti-textual, image-based, deconstructive, with its emphasis on the creative autonomy of the performer. Finally, it is important to distinguish director/actor manipulation from authorial. In Shakespeare's 'King Lear', when Gloucester is blinded on the stage, the event is textually prescribed. The director and performers can only control how it is shown, not what is shown.

Under normal circumstances, an audience's view of a live performance is pan-optic. The eye is free to rove over the whole performance space, and even to leave it and examine the environment in which the performance takes place. And yet, an account of a performance by an audience member - and often, a consensus by the whole audience (which is to say, in reality, an account of the reception of a performance), will be optically and auditorily focused, and highly selective of incident and narrative significance. This strongly suggests that there are forms of manipulation of the watchers, to create, and shift, a focus of attention.

But, despite the popularity of such notions as the performer's 'control' or 'domination' of an audience, an audience does not watch against its will. Any performer knows that the conventional active/passive relationship between actor and audience is, in fact, a constantly shifting relationship between equals, signalled and sustained by a continuous interchange of messages between the two parties, which re-adjusts the relationship as the performance is developed in time and space. Paradoxically, an audience actively seeks a 'passive' role in the relationship, in order that the theatrical event may take place. And, equally, the performer needs to be as receptive as the audience. The audience is not dominated: it is involved in a complex reciprocity with the performers. Any manipulation thus takes place within contractual parameters which the audience has tacitly agreed, and which it ultimately controls. If the rules are broken, the audience ceases to 'play the game'. It becomes restless and dissatisfied. Its physical rhythms begin to cut across, and interfere with, those of the performance (Wilson, 1985, p. 64) and, in extreme cases, it leaves the auditorium, and asks for its money back.

In a very real sense, the audience manipulates the director and actors, since it holds this Damoclean sword above their heads. Many of the signals which the performers are so eager to pick up from the audience are those which tell them that they are still 'on track'. We thus begin from a position of manipulated performers, since the first rule of audience manipulation in the performing arts is to ensure that the performers do not break the rules. Most have failed: Handke (1971); the Living Theatre (e.g. the audience contact experiments in *Paradise Now*). Some have succeeded: (e.g. Ariane Mnouckine, with *1789*).

The audience is therefore active *ab initio* in the theatrical contract - but what kind of a deal does it set up?

Buying a ticket is willingly giving up a portion of your liquid assets, and making a self-limiting commitment to a certain place and time in the future. (Re-introducing an element of choice means losing your money.) On arrival, the theatre foyer provides for only a very limited range of activities. You can deposit your coat, have a drink, have a pee, and look at the front-of-house displays. In the auditorium, it is necessary to accept further limitations. You have to sit - frequently in a designated position, which orients you in a certain direction (being fixed to the floor, unlike domestic furniture). Finally, all the lights are extinguished, except in a specific zone, where all future activity is located. But it is the audience's decision to accept these limitations on freedom. It is an active process of self-denial, in return for which a performance is supplied. This is an important point, and one which suggests that the audience not only acquiesces in such manipulative subordination, but enters a social and psychological mode where acquiescence and passivity is experienced as a norm, and autonomous activity is deviant. There is a positive psychological pleasure in entering into, and being in, this state of delightful bondage. Manipulation of the audience may be aided by this subliminal emotional orientation.

Within this web of obligation and mutual anticipation sits the production itself. The director monitors the reception of the production which is being made. This role is justified by the fact that he or she will ultimately not be a participating performer. However intimately directors may be involved with their actors in rehearsal, the object of this relationship is to elicit elements which the director then retires from the performing area to judge. Directors thus exercise external influence over a wide variety of devices to focus the audience's attention. There is a nominal hierarchy, at the top of which the director sits - thus notionally controlling the creation of the whole visual, aural, temporal, spacial, rhythmic, dynamic and emotional experience; through approval, application and alteration of scenic design, costume, lighting design, sound effects, speed of scenes and scene-changes, position, delivery and physical relationship of the actors and so on. But to see this as the trappings of dictatorship is to overlook the fact of the construction of the reality of the performance by the audience. If a shared, and agreed, construction of reality is desirable, then someone must ensure that the signals are clear, the codes are recognized, and that attention is directed towards them.

The notion of the director as tyrant, in opposition to the aims and best interests of the performers, is understandable, if distracting.

At every level, the director's materials are created by people, who have their own autonomous creative perceptions and recipes, which, nevertheless, have to be incorporated into a specific whole. A brick does not care how it is mortared into a wall. The same cannot be said for a composer, who finds that the theme she has written for Falstaff in Love has been assigned to introduce the Anne Page scenes (*The Merry Wives of Windsor*). But the composer is not in possession of the other elements of the picture. It is most difficult for actors. Performing is a complete, coherent, and systematic experience: yet somebody else keeps insisting that this coherence be destroyed, by incorporating other elements, or eliminating something of what has already been created.

The director is torn between the desirable aesthetic picture, and the accurate human one - even at the purely visual level. Usually these two concerns combine. The placement of figures in a performance space is said to be 'right' when they are in spatial relationships and positions which signal their role, status, relationship and expected behaviour. The emotional satisfaction at this visual picturing of human intangibles is construed as, and may be, aesthetic pleasure.

The actor has a difficult task, because the physical statements which are selected as encoding a social reality for the audience's reception and construction may not, in physical actuality, be either real or accurate. They may be stylized, stereotyped, inflated, invented. It does not matter, as long as they function accurately. But the actor has the task of physically incorporating them, and making them cohesive and coherent, of bridging the gap not only between the inchoate elements and the coherent whole, but between the unfettered realm of ideas and the insistent reality of the performance area.

By contrast, one of the director's most important tasks, in the sphere of audience manipulation, takes place prior even to the beginning of rehearsal. This is the analysis of the primary structures of the text, and the conception of primary images, attitudes or dynamics, to support and project these structures in performance. For example, many people, if asked to describe Shakespeare's *Julius Caesar*, can usually provide a coherent and pointed account until Caesar's assassination. After this, the narrative not infrequently contracts to a mention of Mark Anthony's speech to the Roman people, and of many concluding battles. A similar account is frequently given by actors and directors. The text tells us different. The assassination of Caesar takes place less than half way through the play, and it is not even an isolated event, since it is closely followed by the murder of Cinna the poet. Such juxtapositions are an insistent and all-pervading feature of the piece, which does not rise to a single climax, but is a chain of twinned scenes, linked by dyads of similarity and difference to the preceding and succeeding ones. An audience watching a production prepared according to these structural perceptions receives quite different signals of priority and meaning.

Notwithstanding the control of preparation and reception by the director, the actor controls production. Any good director works from what the actor gives, because it is not possible (except perhaps for Tadeusz Kantor) for directors to materialize on stage and polymorphically embody their internal, Platonic interpretations. (The semioticians of the Prague School were well aware of the annoying power of the actor to modify, or even completely discard, the signals prepared in rehearsal, and were correspondingly more at ease with, for instance, traditional Chinese theatre, with its indices of lexically specific performance codes. (Brusak, 1976)).

The actor needs this structurally implicit, and procedurally explicit, independence and power. A production is prepared under one set of circumstances. It is performed under another set, which varies night to night, moment to moment. The messages must, therefore, be continuously re-encoded, so that they are received in the desired way, under differing conditions. It is, of course, at this point, that the performance 'realizes' itself, via the actor. Up to now, it has merely been a complex of well-founded conjectures, lacking the audience as the vital articulatory component. Once the structure is completed, via this articulation, it is not unusual for the actor to discover, with the director, that they have made a Frankenstein's monster, simultaneously having to assess the potential of the beast and learning how to ride it.

It is also up to the actor to use manipulative devices to achieve the focus demanded by the director, and implied in the text of the writer. An actor may be dressed in red, while all others are in black, be at the top of a flight of stairs in a spotlight, the recipient of the gaze and gesture of the entire company: but if the actor does not, firstly, engage techniques to acknowledge this focus, and then further techniques to maintain it, the focus loses significance, and will disappear. It can be superficially supposed that such techniques are in play when we recognize the employment of unusual and significant intonation, gesture and timing. But such things are merely stereotypical and highly stylized representations of a notion of theatricality. Every actor is aware of the subtle, but absolute, 'gear change' which the organism undergoes when moving into 'performance mode', before articulating the performance proper. Eugenio Barba uses the term 'pre-expressivity' to identify the condition, and has produced a useful taxonomy of its features (Fowler, 1986). He describes them at the macro-level of physical embodiment into the cultural form, but distinguishes them by their universality, and their lack of separate lexical significance, in any specific performance aesthetic. But the basis of pre-expressivity is clearly at the level of subliminal micro-shifts and micro-signs, which Konrad Lorenz (1952) hinted at when writing of the perceptive clarity of animals. The transformation is actuated by mental decision and volition, not via a physical technique, and the result is not self-perceived kinaesthetically (because the physical changes have been subliminal) but as a change of condition, which is experienced emotionally. This is perfectly reasonable, since the change at the physical level is such that the whole deportment has departed, subtly but absolutely, from that which is employed in normal life. Barba describes it as the transition from 'daily' to 'extra-daily' behaviour. The audience, similarly, reacts at the level of feeling to these subliminal signs which, although small, are none of them assignable to any domestic lexicon, and which therefore resonate with the potency of that-which-has-yet-to-be-assigned-meaning (Wilson, 1985, p. 18).

It is frequently said that performers manipulate their audience's emotions, and that they 'use' their own emotions as if they were finite, accessible tools in a technical repertoire. As well as being a fairly red herring, this is inaccurate, since we are not in contact with the emotional condition of the performer and its use, but only with what can be perceived externally.

We have a personal commitment to maintaining our centrality in the performance exchange, and, clearly, a component of this will be an emotional commitment. As we construct our version of the performance, we may experience sensations which we interpret as emotional response. All except the most banal and least satisfactory scenarios are situationally complex. One of the aspects of Macbeth's hopelessness towards the end, is that it is pitiable, as well as satisfactory. If this aspect is 'foregrounded' in performance, the audience is likely to recognize this perspective, and respond emotionally. But the response will usually be sympathetic, not empathic. When Gloucester's eyes are put out, the emotions presented on stage are rage, pleasure, terror. We usually feel anger, disgust, pity. Empathic responses are more usually evoked through language, with its poetic capacity to convey inner states. Emotional response is thus a product of the audience's awareness of the performance event. (As Berthold Brecht understood perfectly. What he attacked were emotional responses which replaced, or suborned, the audience's awareness. This is manipulative, and can be seen in film of Hitler's speeches, or an American presidential election campaign.)

So, as well as considering our emotional response as a factor determining the direction and duration of our attention, we need to look at two fundamentals of the acting process itself, at the responses which they elicit, and at their role in maintaining and extending the performance collaboration: mimesis and active interpretation.

The mimetic representation of reality sensorily activates our capacity to respond, physiologically and psychologically, both sympathetically and empathically. This does not require all the elements of the actual event represented to be reproduced. To see a sharp knife pulled through clutching hands does not need the welling of stage blood. Kinaesthetic transference ensures that we experience an empathic wince of phantom pain in our palms, and we are feelingly sympathetic to the victim's picture of agony, hands doubled under armpits, teeth bared in a rictus. This disposes of any notion of 'the willed suspension of disbelief' at this stage of the performance experience. It is clearly extremely difficult to disbelieve. The more so, since the mimetic process is simultaneously self-reinforcing for the actor. The potency and continuity of the performance activity is enhanced by the same, but, in this case, self-referential, messages of the physical and emotional results of such actions, coming to the actor as to the audience.

Mimesis is also attention-grabbing in its own right. It combines the wonder of transformation, of skin-turning, with the awesome paradox of two beings simultaneously inhabiting the same organic dimension - with the attendant psychic and psychological queries of identity and determinacy. It is *magique concrete*, and its practitioners draw the eye and the brain, as they embody the protean discourse of theatricality, and roll up notions of reality and illusion.

This entrainment of the audience into the liminal regions of fascinated uncertainty is zin the actual process of carrying a performance forward through time. Performing involves a continuous series of decisions about the portrayal of circumstance. It is thus a process of active, or creative interpretation 'on the hoof'. These decisions and potential changes are, anyway, immanent within the form, as it is a live art, and dependent on assumptions and presumptions about the fixity of the future environment, which are negated by our instinctive apprehension of entropy. The heart-attack may strike, the trousers may fall down. And the audience is subconsciously aware that it is deeply implicated, as it cannot predict its own reaction to what has not yet occurred. Thus the audience, quite literally, does not know what will happen next. (No more do the actors. The two groups have to work together on this one.) And as well as variety within conventional codes, the performers cannot be trusted (no more than can the audience) not to move outside, and present new proposals for performance. Not for the sake of difference, but because new ends need new means.

The necessary manipulations of live performance thus stretch the 'ground rules' of the production of art, so that the audience cannot rely on previous assumptions about how the material they are about to receive will be presented. They need to pay attention! Thus, as it is as many levels, and in many contexts, the performance becomes an exercise in risk, constantly testing its own basis, sawing away at the branch it sits on. The audience are involved in this risk. It is nerve-racking! And the longer they stay around, the more they are involved in a collaboration towards success.

References

Brusak, K. (1938) 'Sign in the Chinese Theatre' in L. Matejka & I.R. Titunik (Eds.) *The Semiotics of Arts* (1976) Cambridge, Ma: MIT Press

Fowler, R. (1986) (Ed.) Papers of the 4th Session of the International School of Theatre Anthropology. Holstebro: Norsk Teaterlaboratorium

Handke, P. (1971) *Offending the Audience* (M. Roloff, Trans.) London: Methuen

Lorenz, K. (1952) *King Solomon's Ring* (M.K. Wilson, Trans.) London: Methuen

Wilson, G. (1985) *The Psychology of Performing Arts*. New York: St Martin's Press

The influence of the medium on creativity in dance and fine art

E.C. Haworth & J.T. Haworth

Department of Psychology, University of Manchester

Traditional theories of artistic creativity emphasize the importance of conscious artistic intentions to portray perceived ideas, truths or essences (Ingarden, 1972). The working methods of many artists, however, are often at variance with the view that the idea is the main driving force in the production of the artwork, and that the artist is producing an analogue for an important idea. While the initial perceived idea can be important in artistic creativity, the matrices of ideas that an artwork contains can come about through a process of interaction of the artist with the artistic medium (e.g. dance or paint and canvas). This view of the creative process in art is articulated by Merleau-Ponty (1962), who emphasizes the importance of pre-reflexive thought and a more primordial contact with the world to produce art as 'enriched being' (Haworth, 1989).

On this latter view, the medium of the artwork is an integral part of the work, and the medium and its handling is as much a part of the artistic process and product as the initial idea which an artwork may portray. The choice of medium and the way in which it is handled can have a significant influence on the artwork and the ideas it contains. The lived experience of the artist can feed into this process of interaction with the medium; and artistic expression can involve a release of 'feelings' through interaction with the particular medium, whether this is the movement of the dancer or the manipulation of the paint and brush by a painter.

Themes

One of the great themes of artworks is the interplay between the world and the spirit: the search for images of those states of mind embodied in nature that exist beyond consciousness. These may be concerned with the grandeur of the world. There can also be a desire to explore and express spiritual yearnings and dissatisfaction of the self. Observations of the self reflected against aspects of grandeur with which one's spiritual existence may resonate, can result in unsatisfactory comparisons. The search for fruitful images of man and nature may stimulate expressions of disenchantment including a concern with violence and revolt.

Violence as a theme within an artwork is not necessarily a single matter, but rather an integration with other aspects. Violence may be present as a social comment, but may also concern itself with an integral part of life and the emotions concerned. For instance, Picasso's violent images, such as 'Guernica', become a protest against war, whilst Bacon provides images of psychological torment, and the choreographer Pina Bausch's *Bluebeard* appears to be concerned with an 'intimate' element of violence, namely sexual violence.

With the paintings of Bacon and Picasso, one is able to 'ponder' on the extent of the theme, as the viewer is able to return again and again to the artworks, perhaps revealing further integration with other aspects of violence. In contrast, Bausch's treatment of the subject matter through dance provides an immediate sexual image with the viewer drawn into the battle between a man and a woman. Here one enters a personal world of emotional and sexual turmoil, and a world that is happening at that moment.

Painters

Picasso's 'Weeping Woman' provides a semi-permanent crystalisation of thought, emotions and lived experience, expressing both realistic and emotional sensations. It was produced in relation to the atrocities of war, in particular the bombing of Guernica. Indeed it has been considered a postscript to 'Guernica', Picasso's famous monochrome large scale painting, embodying all the tragic mood of war. The strident colours in 'Weeping

Woman' are typical of the Expressionists. Kirchner and other German expressionists wanted direct communication by jolts of colour and shape, preferring the German Gothic to the classical backgrounds, amplifying the distortion of shape. The work of many of these artists drew directly on the violence of their time where their work has been viewed as gestures of revolt.

The colour range in Picasso's 'Weeping Woman', from warm golden yellows to acid green and blacks and vivid reds, presents an emotional and symbolic representation of both the exquisite and the terrible, similar to many of Van Gogh's paintings. For Van Gogh, "nature was to him both the exquisite and terrible. It consoled him, but it was his judge" (Hughes, 1980). His method of painting with strong swirling brushstrokes, as in 'Landscape near Montlejour' (1988) signified the vibrant energy of the world, the thumb print of a powerful and violent God. Similarly, his juxtapositions and use of colour could be used to express the terrible passions of humanity. Van Gogh, in fact, opened up the modernist syntax of colour to admit pity and terror as well as pleasure.

In Picasso's 'Weeping Woman', the distorted head with its acid colour modelling is juxtaposed against a warm background perhaps signifying terrible and uncalled for violence disrupting the normal ambient course of life. The deliberate reduction in depth between the background and the foreground emphasizes a sense of immediacy, yet the powerful image as a symbol for violence is one which echoes across time. It has been noted that the dissonant colours "help to elevate the dramatic conflict to the timelessness of myth." (Jaffe, 1988). Through colour, Picasso has produced a violent image, not a pure replica of war, but an emotional symbol which will continue to provoke through time. The painting shows controlled, structured expression. The paint has a raw, powerful effect, being thickly and strongly applied in places with boldly drawn lines. The emotional expression by the artist appears to have been a considered development, as many variations of the 'Weeping Woman' were produced and doubtless many were discarded or reworked.

Francis Bacon, "whose main ambition was to be a painter of the tragic figure, telling a truth about human events the camera could not" (Hughes, 1980), is much concerned with violence. He, however, renounced expressionism, preferring instead a detached clinical gaze, viewing the human body as available to inspection, sex and political concern. The environments in his paintings, according to Hughes, suggest a loss of will; the dingy walls of rooms that might be detention chambers, the rack-like beds that turn into grills, the assembly of vaguely medical looking tubes, the closed rooms and unidentifiable furniture, nasty in texture and colour: these are an arena for violence. And in the best of Bacon's art, as Hughes points out "the paint has a dreadful materiality as though the grainy cellular structure of the pigment were a smear of tissue". All this lends itself to an image of psychological torment; a far more introverted and private violence than Picasso's almost outward condemnation of society.

Bacon uses the back of primed canvas, which has a rougher, more absorbent surface. He has said he wants a technique as "raw as possible", and such a surface is sympathetic to his aims and the effect it has on his image. Bacon's use of his medium to produce this rawness provides an image of 'raw' emotions. One can almost picture the torment inside the human head through his use of materials. Bacon (1985) has said that his image is realized through "the transforming effect of cultivated accidents of paint". Andrew Durham, commenting on this, says that these words "provide a key insight into his painting technique: that series of physical acts by which the images in his mind in a kind of pool of consciousness become manifest in a plastic image". It appears as though Bacon is trying to work through his own personal conflicts by his actions on his medium. The image crystallizes or emerges as the work proceeds, perhaps relieving his own personal torment.

The background in 'Figure Writing in a Reflected Mirror', is typical of many of Bacon's works in that it consists of large areas of colour which provide a setting for the figure. The background is applied quickly using acrylics or household emulsion. The actual image is more subtly treated using oil colours which can be applied directly or used as thin washes. The properties of the paint are sometimes altered by adding sand or dust, and it may be worked into with the fingers, sanded down, or impressions of cloth made into it, to which pastel can then be applied. All this adds to the rawness and intricacy expressing this psychological violence in contrast to Picasso's bold, structured work, enhancing the way in which he treats the theme.

Dance

Pina Bausch's dance *Bluebeard* is controversial, violent and sexually explosive, heralding it as a landmark of twentieth century dance. It is based on Bartok's one-act opera *Duke Bluebeard's Castle.* Like Bacon, Bausch concentrates her choreography around psychological aspects of violence; the fierce sexual struggle between man and woman full of pain and guilt and loneliness from which there is no escape. As with the image of suppression in Bacon's figures in a room, with the one closed space representing no escape from psychological torment, Bausch provokes this same element of suppression. The stage area represents one setting; a garden, grey and dismal in colour with one window which appears to lead nowhere. The image created is one which is claustrophobic in nature with no escape from the emotional and physical violence. In dance one is able to portray a true or realistic setting which enhances the feeling of the violent event happening at that moment in time rather than a replica.

With dance as a medium, realism can be portrayed because movement, an everyday action, is the major element. In a sense, the physical violence can be portrayed realistically, such as the action of ripping a dress, or dragging the body, or slapping the face. Movement does not always need to be abstract, but can concentrate on everyday physical actions to portray the subject matter. This real action can conjure the desired sympathetic effect from a viewer, but may not be the only method that a choreographer will use. In some instances, as with the work of the dance company DV8, a simple stroke of the face can create a more intense or menacing sensation of violence than an explicitly violent action. In each case, an emotional content is set up by the movement on the stage, whereby the movements can be a release of emotions whether these movements are abstract in nature or realistic. As Best (1974) has stated, "Movement of the human body has alway been a medium for expressing the emotions" for "the existence of an emotion is the external physical behaviour of the person who is feeling the emotion".

Bausch uses the notions or realism and emotionalism to create a desired effect. With Bausch's continuous use of real, physically violent actions, the viewer has a sense of being a bystander to the immediate action; the action is being carried out in front of an audience. Because of the strong element of truth in movement, the emotions protrayed by the dancers appear as true. Hence as the movements are violent in nature and the emotions are true to the movement, emotions revealed are true to the subject matter. In this way, a choreographer can expect a specific response from an audience to the elements of realism and emotionalism provided by the artwork. The response may be different in each person, *but* each person will be affected in some way.

In *Bluebeard*, there is a strong use of everyday gestures such as hand movements to the face, and stroking the hair. These gestures are taken to their extremes becoming slapping and ripping hair movements. The image created is one which is grotesque in nature as the spectator has seen the violent movement originate from a simple everyday action. The dancers constantly break into throwing themselves against the wall and floor. This physical violation is juxtaposed with the main female figure standing in the centre moaning and clutching her head. The juxtaposition of real physical violence with the mental torture creates a powerful image as the two extremes are brought together.

Another of Bausch's choreographic elements appears to be the notion of shocking the audience into an emotional response. Throughout the piece, Judith is constantly physically violated by Bluebeard. The movements appear sexually violent, ripping at her body, throwing her to the ground and attacking her, all in a realistic fashion. With Bacon and Picasso, the reality of the violence appears more subtle and abstract. However, through facial expression and vocal noise, the mental torment of Judith is also portrayed. Bausch repeats movements throughout, each time making them bigger and more violent, enhancing their emotional content. This use of repetition perhaps plays on the notion that "art rests on the fact that deep feelings pattern themselves in a coherent way all over life and behaviour" (Best, 1974). Thereby, the repetition of movement could echo the pattern of emotions in life.

Bausch integrates music into her piece which dance as a medium allows. Throughout, Bluebeard returns to the tape-recorder on stage and switches the opera on and off. The music echoes the movement, rising to a peak with the dynamics of the dance. This particular choice of music seems to add little to the theme of the piece; perhaps a more violent auditory and visual image could have been created, as in *Clockwork Orange*, where external physical violence was juxtaposed with the melodic tones of Beethoven's Fifth Symphony.

Improvisation

In Bausch's *Bluebeard* the handling of the medium in connection with the theme of violence appears to rely on a specific element of truth. However, this element of truth is not only determined by the subject matter, but is also an integral part of the creative process of the medium of dance. As indicated earlier, the creative process can be influenced by the way in which an artwork is handled. Indeed, the creative process can determine what direction an artwork takes and the final product itself.

To produce a final 'dancework' one method used during the creative process is *improvisation*. If, as with the theme of violence, real emotion is being dealt with, emerging from the performance in the form of movement, a significant influence on the artwork can be that at no point during the rehearsal is any movement restriction placed upon the performer in terms of being 'choreographed upon'. Rather, in this approach, the creativity in terms of movement should allow for complete freedom of expression. Improvisation can become a useful tool for the performer, not only for the material content it produces but also as a method to enhance the emotional truth in performance. "Improvisation is not just a matter of splashing about in self-indulgent euphoria as outsiders often suspect, for it aims at bringing the actor again and again to his own barriers, to the point where in place of newfound truth he normally substitutes a lie" (Brook, 1988). It is not enough to just have a subject matter, as this only inspires ideas. Instead, through an understanding of one's medium, a development of the ideas inspired by the subject matter can be produced. In some instances, through the creative process, whole new avenues can be opened leading to a final product which is far removed from the initial ideas concerned, one which is true to the subject matter and not pre-conceived. Through the use of improvisation, the final product is not only that of the director or choreographer, but each dancer plays an important role in contributing his/her creative skills. In this way, the artwork must begin with a loose framework as each dancer may interpret the theme differently, thereby producing material or an emotional content that leads the artwork in a whole new direction.

In order for artistic expression to be released truthfully through the creative process of improvisation, emotions realized through the artist's particular medium must be allowed to be portrayed freely. Rather than being produced by an outside influence the whole process can be based upon 'inner focus', to enable the movements to come from within. Recalling set gestures or movements can cause restriction seeming to reproduce actions rather than drawing on any deep creativity. Bausch moved away from any recognizable dance moves during the creative process, relying on emotional mental images such as hidden fears and mental scars to provoke movement from her dancers. As Brook (1988) considers, the actor "is reaching inside himself for an alphabet that is also fossilized, for the language not of invention but of his condition therefore revealing a performance that he thinks to be spontaneous but is filtered and monitored many times". Creative improvisation has a sense of 'breaking free' from 'conditioning', producing the concept whereby the movement improvisation is based around a 'feeling' or 'quality'.

However, with the theme of violence, recalling past experiences in connection with this subject matter can become disturbing for the performer. During the creative process, physical and mental breakdown can occur when the performer allows himself to delve into past emotions with no detachment. Although an emotional, expressive performance requires a great deal of physical and mental exploration, the performer must not allow the emotions to fully 'take over' and believe that emotional commitment and unhesitating self-exposure are all that really count. Rather the artist "is called upon to be completely involved while distanced - detached without detachment" (Brook, 1988). Indeed, during this process, there is a need for an outside eye to direct and control the emotional involvement. For a director to be involved in manipulating the creative process to a final product, emotional content does not need to be forced on the dancers to produce material, but rather guided and monitored. Bausch invites her company to produce the material around a given emotion involving complex explorations. But as director, she is able to stand aside and control the emotional involvement. Brook also considers this issue, concluding that "the director must sense where the actor wants to go and what it is he avoids, what blocks he raises and to his own intentions. No director injects a performance. At best a director enables an actor to reveal his own performance".

To produce a final product, continuous creative exploration produces a stream of on-going ideas. These 'matrices' of ideas can lead in several different directions and in most cases the director plays an imperative role in the manipulation of the ideas by the constant input which gently directs the pathway during the creative process.

For a group of dancers working together the director's role is important in feeding in initial ideas which provide for a realm of creative exploration, but, also important, is the ensemble quality in which these dancers work. Improvisation sessions do not need to rely fully on the individual creativity but can allow for a "group of people to come together and begin to find a way of responding directly to one another" (Brook, 1988).

Working as an ensemble allows for the creative process to become richer as one idea feeds off another and each individual interprets a certain concept in his own individual way. If one performer produces a movement unexpected, but true, the others may take this up and respond on the same level. With the use of the ensemble quality a specific bond is created between performers which allows not only for a creative open-minded attitude "developing a collective sense of responsibility for the quality of an improvisation" (Brook, 1988), but also an awareness of the group as a whole during performance.

Conclusions

Bacon, Picasso and Bausch have produced through their different mediums, the theme of violence as a symbol of emotional and psychological torment rather than a replica. Bausch has used realistic movement, but it has always been side by side with a psychological concept. Although her work has produced a picture of sexual violence, it is not one which is a complete physical replica. The emotions behind the violent actions have clearly been created by the juxtaposition of 'real' and 'expressive' movement. With Picasso's juxtapositions of colour, the image of violence is expressed immediately. This initial shock element created by clashing colours in a structure produces the effect of a calculated controlled image of violence. Picasso appears to echo the effect of a calculated controlled war upon society by his method of use of his medium. Bacon, although working with the same medium as Picasso, allows the theme of violence to be treated in a different manner. The personal and psychological appears stronger, and his emotions appear to be expressed rather more than those of society.

From both mediums, dance and painting, it is apparent that the artist has had to juggle with his own emotions and feelings as well as creative perceptions. Each artist has developed personal truth with elements of expression, through interacting with the different media to produce artworks which are both responsive to the times and of enduring significance.

It is clear from the work of these artists that the creative process in dance and fine art involves a complex interaction between thought, emotion and activity, and that as indicated by Merleau-Ponty (1962), the medium has a significant influence on the artwork. The medium is not just a substrate to carry or portray a pre-conceived idea, as traditional theorists, such as Ingarden, maintain.

References

Bacon, F. (1985) Exhibition Catalogue, Tate Gallery, London. London: Thames and Hudson

Best, D. (1974) *Expression in Movement and the Arts.* London: Lepus Books

Brook, P. (1988) *The Empty Space.* Middlesex: Pelican Books

Haworth, J.T. (1980) 'The embodyment theory of prereflexive thought and creativity'. In: K.J. Gilhooly, M.T.G. Kearne, R.H. Logie and G. Erdos (Eds.) *Lines of Thinking, Vol. 2,* 203-215 London: Wiley

Hughes, R. (1980) *The Shock of the New.* London: BBC Publications

Ingarden, H. (1972) 'Artistic and Aesthetic Values'. In: H. Osborne (Ed.) *Aesthetics* London: Oxford University Press

Jaffe, L.C.H. (1988) *Picasso.* London: Thames and Hudson

Merleau-Ponty, M. (1962) *Phenomenology of Perception.* London: Routledge and Kegan Paul

PART II
Performers – Personality and Problems

Toward an understanding of the performing artist

Shelley Reciniello

SRA Associates, New York

Psychological study of creativity has, in the past four decades, explored a vast amount of phenomena and has, consequently, contributed greatly to the understanding of creativity as a cognitive function with certain specifiable personality characteristics. Research in the area, for the most part, has been thorough, conscientious, adventurous and, in fact, quite creative. However, there appears to have been an exception regarding research conducted in the area of the performing arts. Within this area, the creativity of the actor and the dancer, in particular, have yet to be adequately explored.

There are many reasons for this apparent neglect. The first concerns the obvious difficulty involved in such a pursuit. In both acting and dancing, there is no tangible creative product. The playwright does produce the play, and the choreographer does create the dance, but in performance, the actor and the dancer are the living instruments of their art. Whereas creativity research in other fields could explore the person, the process, or the product, here, more or less, the person is the process and the process is the product.

Another reason that is often cited as justification for the lack of psychological study of the actor is the unsubstantiated claim that dramatic art is not a creative art, but rather an interpretive art (Wallach & Wing, 1969; Rubin, 1974). Supporters of this claim argue that creativity is not a factor in dramatic art since actors rely on the script's words and ideas and not on their own. Likewise, psychological theories and studies of dancers that can contribute to an understanding of the creative ability of these performers are rare, and this is also partially due to the interpretive versus creative art controversy. In the case of the dancer, it is often resolved by referring to the choreographer as "creative" and the dancer-performer as "interpretive" (Nadel & Miller, 1978).

That a dramatic creation involves more than the words and ideas of the script and that it is dependent on the creativity of the individual actor, is made obvious by the many diverse performances of one role by different actors. In the words of Lee Strasberg (1964):

> Each time we see an actor in a part we are really seeing an actor creating a new character. He may get his ideas obviously from the author, in the same way that a painter who paints a certain object in nature is receiving his ideas and impressions from that object, but what he does is dependent intrinsically on his own creative capacity, on his own imagination, on his own understanding, on his own skill. (p. 83)

Perhaps the most interesting as well as the most destructive reason that the creativity of the actor and the dancer has not been more adequately explored, involves an approach emanating primarily from the psychoanalytic tradition that seeks merely to identify the similarities between performer and madman and to expound upon theories of exhibitionism, narcissism and weak self-identification. The act of making comparisons between the madman and the genius has an ancient history in all realms of creativity, but nowhere is it more fruitful than in considering the idiosyncrasies of the actor and the dancer.

This stance has resulted in several analytically influenced accounts and studies of actors and dancers (Aaron, 1986; Bergler, 1960; Blum, 1976; Chyatte, 1949; Fenichel, 1946, 1960; Freud, 1963; Gabbard, 1979a, b; Golden, 1940; Drake, 1950; Kaplan, 1965; 1969; Miller, 1938; Taft, 1961; Weissman, 1961) that include a simplistic, reductionist, treatment of the creativity of these performers, a lack of enquiry into the abilities necessary for creative dramatic and dance performance, and a marked tendency to stress the similarities between performers and deviants rather than to search for distinguishing differences. Many of these studies, in fact, used instruments designed to assess psychopathology and hence, resulted in descriptions of artists in psychopathological terms.

The antitheatrical prejudice

It is appropriate to review a theory that may provide some understanding of the origins of these unfortunate trends. The theory has been espoused by Barish in a book entitled *The Antitheatrical Prejudice* (1981), wherein he traces the roots of ambivalence toward the theatre and a distrust of actors and plays, beginning with the time of Plato up through the present day.

According to Barish, Plato feared the potential political influence of the theatre and the great power of the theatre to create change. Because of all this, all drama and theatre were banned from the Republic in order to prevent a threat to the body politic. Whereas later thinkers would see the so-called transmutation of unacceptable impulses into art as therapeutic, Plato was in favour of total supression of any artistic desires. Furthermore, Plato was distrustful of actors whom he felt mimicked the traits of others in order to ward off their own failures and limitations. Despite Plato's opinions, the stage did thrive in ancient Athens and it played a noble role in the religion of the state. Plato's views, however, served to create an ambivalence toward the players and their plays. They were tolerated and even appreciated, but it was understood that they were to have no place in the ideal state of the future.

In early Rome, Barish continues, disapproval of the theatre was more clearly defined and it peaked during the days of the Empire. Although the theatre was extremely popular, it was simultaneously considered disreputable and disgraceful. Actors were denied all civil rights, could not engage in military service, could be beaten at will by the police, were forbidden to leave their profession for another, were forced to have their children become actors, and were banned from attending plays as audience members. Barish comments:

> The law thus created and maintained a hereditary disgraced caste, whose members were cruelly persecuted and yet at the same time forbidden to take up any honourable calling. Like prostitution, the stage had come to be thought of as a necessary evil. As it was evil, its practitioners had to be humiliated and punished for their part in it. But as it was necessary, they had also to be prevented from making their escape from it, since its continuance needed to be guaranteed. (p. 42)

Furthermore, it was regarded as scornful for an actor to accept money for performances. Actors were treated as criminals and low-lifes and it is possible, Barish believes, that a vicious circle was created wherein only those types had nothing to lose by becoming actors.

The Christian Church added a new twist to the actors' dilemma by excommunicating them. In order to receive the sacraments, such as marriage, for example, an actor would have to renounce his profession, which was an act forbidden by the state. An actor, therefore, was often put in the humiliating and dangerous position of denying his profession one day in order to be married, and resuming it the next in order to remain alive. According to Barish, Christianity was also quite suspicious of the actor's motives in impersonating others. From the early Christian writings of Tatian and Tertullian, he notes that they have attributed "to the actor a kind of didactic identification with his roles, or at least with his scurrilous roles. When he portrays madness or sodomy, he is giving his audience lessons in how to do it." Furthermore, Barish states: "In the world of Tertullian's polemic, the difference between art and life has no status .... To portray a murder is as wicked as to commit one" (p. 45-46). The actor is seen as someone who commits mortal sin by lying about who he is and when he pretends to be someone evil he enhances the offence. On the other hand, if he pretends to be someone good, he's adding insult to injury by daring to be someone he could never be. Barish also points to another argument begun by Tertullian and echoed throughout the centuries which "involves the claim that actors deserve to be hated by all right-thinking people because the law already proscribes them. An existing injustice thus becomes its own justification" .50).

Other examples of the antitheatrical prejudice appear in later years in the writings of St John Chrysostom and St Augustine, but seem to quiet down a bit during the Middle Ages where the theatre was primarily church drama in the form of passion plays and the like. However, the banner was held high again in the 16th and 17th centuries with the rise of Puritanism. Barish describes Prynne's Histriomastix as "a gargantuan encyclopedia of antitheatrical lore which scourges every form of theatre in the most ferocious terms (p. 83). The publishing of this collection in 1633 appears as the climax of a movement which began in the mid-16th century and ended with the closing of the theatres in 1642.

Just as the writings of Marlowe and Shakespeare seemed to call forth the rantings of the Puritans, so too says Barish, did the popularity of Racine and Moliere in France stimulate the rage of the Jansenists. "Plainly the theatre comes to be felt as subversive, and its subversive possibilities felt as a real threat, when it counts for something in the emotional and intellectual life of the community" (p. 191). The Jansenists of the 17th century pointed to French legislation of the 16th century which equated actors with whores and whoremasters, forbidden to receive the sacraments and denied Christian burial. Barish claims that Nicole, a great spokesman of the time, followed the tradition of Plato which espouses the belief that in order to play the more violent feelings of man, the actor must be subject to them in himself. This contradicted the view of Tertullian and others that actors were hypocrites and liars. To 17th century France, actors were even more to be despised because they weren't liars but were sincere in the vile emotion they displayed. This is a striking example of "damned if you do, damned if you don't".

Perhaps one of the strongest attacks launched against the theatre comes surprisingly from Rousseau. Barish interprets Rousseau's primary objection as follows:

> if society is cursed at the root by its theatrical origins, if it is itself only a perpetual charade of illusion, created by self-interest and self-love, the theatre proper quintessentializes the evil. It takes a man already conditioned to be a hypocrite and an exhibitionist and makes him one by profession. .258)

An actor represents to mankind, therefore, all that is base in his nature - selfishness, vanity, deceptiveness.

Diderot, it is interesting to note, takes exception to the view of his time that actors are sincere in the emotions they portray. Rather, he sees them as imitators who lack sensitivity of any kind, the practitioners of a very convincing craft. Although Diderot admires the talent, he does not admire the actor. Barish states:

> In Rousseau's eyes, the actor's trade corrupts him, alienating him from his true self. Diderot reverses the order: for him, the actor lacks a self to begin with, and it is because he has no character of his own that he is able to assume so many imaginary ones .... And Diderot goes on to paint a harsh picture of the indigent rake (or the abandoned courtesan) turning to the stage as a last resort, there heightening the public's scorn for the profession, and, in response to that scorn - however mingled, in some cases, with adulation - sinking deeper than ever into self-hatred, and perpetuating in his own treatment of others the ruinous treatment he has received from the world. (p. 281)

Rousseau concurred with the Romans, the Puritans and the Christians that the role of women in the theatre was particularly contemptuous. Agreeing with his predecessors that actresses be equated with prostitutes, he argues that acting was not a feminine activity, being the polar opposite of the activities of a wife and mother. Barish points out that Rousseau succeeds, therefore, in making an antitheatrical and an antifeminist argument, one and the same.

Rousseau's influence was strong and it was not until the French Revolution that the bans against actors were lifted. However, the conservative wing of the French Church stuck to its persecution until the latter part of the 19th century. Following Plato's example, Auguste Comte (1865) exiled the theatre from his utopia of the Positivist movement though he was one of the most avid theatre-goers of the time. The latter 19th and early 20th centuries continued with such hypocritical demonstrations of the anti-theatrical prejudice. Barish points to statements of writers, especially writers for the stage such as Shaw, Conrad and others, who seemed to be stuck with the dilemma of how to produce plays without actors. Barish concludes his book with a chapter entitled "The Theatre Against Itself" which is where he believes a great part of the prejudice has come to rest. The playwrights and critics of our time, with their emphasis on the natural versus the theatrical, run the risk of stripping the theatre of that which it needs to exist. Barish summarizes the current state of the antitheatrical prejudice as follows:

> The battle of the theatre, in its more superficial sense, has been won long ago. Actors now win knighthoods in England, inhabit the seats of government in America, and are revered as sages in France. But the antitheatrical prejudice, tenacious, elusive and protean in its own right, and springing, as it seems, from the deepest core of our being, seems to have taken refuge in the theatre itself, as well as in certain outposts of psychoanalysis and certain philosophies of existence. (p. 475)

Barish offers many possible explanations for the antitheatrical prejudice. One that is pertinent to the present discussion involves, ironically, a psychoanalytic interpretation of the prejudice as it appears to exist in the minds of several psychoanalysts (Aaron, 1986; Bergler, 1980; Blum, 1976; Fenichel, 1946; Freud, 1942; Gabbard, 1979a, b; Kaplan, 1965, 1969; Weissman, 1961) who have presented disparaging views of the actor. Barish writes:

> Does the theatre derive some of its hypnotic power from a reverse transposition? Does the greediness of our gaze point to a buried memory of the earlier thirst to be gazed at, and our satisfaction when that thirst was slaked? Is our desire to sit as beholders merely the other side of the coin of our wish to be beheld, our unacknowledged exhibitionism? If so, perhaps the antitheatrical prejudice reflects a form of self-disgust brought on by our conflicted longing to occupy the center of the stage once more. (p. 476)

There seems to be something lurking beneath the obsession of those, as Barish puts it "in certain outposts of psychoanalysis" besides a dedication to their field that causes them to judge the actor so harshly, and to painstakingly place his every movement on stage and off within a web of narcissistic and exhibitionist interplay. Barish has perhaps pointed to a possible answer. They so strongly despise the actor's narcissistic displays because they despise their own. They write, after all, with a bravura of style from such an opinionated stance that it could certainly be called narcissistic, and what they write is published (exhibited) and not kept in obscurity. They perhaps will argue that they are engaged in writing, in philosophizing, and not focusing on themselves. The actor, likewise, is engaged in acting, in creating, in focusing on himself/herself when necessary since he is the instrument of his art. Not like the personality researchers who focus on the person in his/her entirety, the analysts have placed the focus on the person in his/her limitations. They see the work as merely an outgrowth of these limitations and they are stuck with the repercussions of their choice. Perhaps because they were afraid to admit, along with Freud, that before this question they would have to lay down their arms, they took to what they knew best, the dark side of human nature.

The theatre's audience, which is made up not only of the spectators but the writers, the critics, the producers, and, alas, the analysts, is all too willing to accept the image of strength and self-assurance the actor possesses in his role as real. As Freud wrote: "The charm of the child lies to a great extent in his narcissism, his sufficiency and inaccessibility; just as does the charm of certain animals which seem not to concern themselves about us, such as cats and other large beasts of prey .... It is as if we envied them their power of retaining a blissful state of mind - an unassailable libido-position which we ourselves have since abandoned" (1963, p. 70). Perhaps it was a moment of self-confrontation for Fenichel when he wrote of the actor, "Like the whore, he is held in contempt but secretly envied" (1946, p. 156). The analytic theories of the actor seem, therefore, to reveal more about those writing them than about the actor and his art. After surveying what has been written, researchers Bahs and Stockwell (1972) conclude: "Our knowledge of the relationship of the personality of the actor to his performance remains limited. We have no information regarding how specific personality characteristics affect an actor's abilities to perform or to achieve excellence on the stage" .16).

The dancer

That the dancer also suffers from bias is quite evident. Robert Joffrey (1978) explained, "Dance is perhaps the least understood of the performing arts" (p. 134), and this consequently applies to the dancer. The dancer's seemingly narcissistic involvement with the body and emphasis on nonverbal expression is extremely suspect in a culture that is both overly verbal and wary of its own narcissistic tendencies. Similar to the antitheatrical prejudice, dancers have suffered through history, frequently being aligned with actors and subject to the same persecution (Barish, 1981). Like the theatre, the dance itself has also enjoyed periods of adulation and elevation over the centuries, while at the same time the dancer was often condemned for being exhibitionistic and narcissistic. In discussing the dancer's supposed narcissism, Nadel (1978) writes:

> The dancer is constantly involved with the imperfections of his human form; through the power of the mind, he attempts to achieve an understanding of himself and his instrument. The thought process can involve picturing the skeleton, working with images or lines of action in the body, lying or standing still picturing the perfect placement, or working out mentally the perfect phrasing for a movement sequence.
>
> Concentration on oneself can be a narcissistic exercise, but this is merely another imperfection to overcome. When the body can be looked at as an object or vehicle for the will of the mind, the narcissistic inclination can be controlled. Meditative thought directed towards the self is vital to the dance (p. 15).

Therefore, the self-focus of the dancer, as with the actor, is merely a concentration on the instrument of the art. It is when others seize on this, and focus merely on the personality of the dancer instead of on the work, that the theories of narcissism and exhibitionism become empowered. The dancer and choreographer Erick Hawkins claims that this is an old phenomenon: "This great distortion which was inherent in the beginnings of ballet was that the person of the dancer was exhibited and not the art, the inner art, as seen through the dancer. It is part of the cult of personality of the West" (1978, p. 344).

Hawkins makes another valuable observation which may also help explain why the study of the dance and the dancer has never been properly undertaken. The majority of dancers are women, and women as artists have never enjoyed much acceptance. Hawkins writes:

> Just as the woman in our culture was looked upon in the words of Simone de Beauvoir as 'object', so her place as an 'object' was transferred to the stage. Since in real life the woman was accepted and approved as 'object', so she was approved by the male audience as 'object' on the stage. When the man entered upon the stage as a dancer with its emphasis on charm and physical display, he too was regarded as 'object'. But in our culture a man with a man's work to do cannot be an 'object'. So here was the impasse (p. 344).

Women in the traditional role of object which was only enhanced by the themes of the ballet, and men in the untraditional role of object with their sexuality in serious question, were not considered artists, and consequently, not worthy of analysis.

The approach

This digression into antitheatrical prejudice was deemed necessary in order to place the lack of informative psychological research on the actor and the dancer within an historical framework, and to present the possibility that such a condition may be indicative of a larger state of affairs. Despite this trend, there have been some studies of actors and dancers from diverse fields of psychological investigation that have contributed to a better understanding of actors and dancers. (Barron, 1972; Fried, 1964; Hatterer, 1965; Neacsu, 1972a, b, 1974; Neascu and Marcus, 1972, 1974; Marcus, 1974; Parsons and Lindauer, 1980; Schreppel and Lindauer, 1976; Stacey and Goldberg, 1953; Natadze, 1958; Metcalf, 1931; Collum, 1976; Motkov, 1983; Alekseev, 1985; Clements, Dwinell, Torrance and Kidd, 1983; Alter, 1984a, b; Alter et al, 1972; Nadel and Miller, 1978; Brennan, 1982, 1983; Manley and Wilson, 1980; Koffka, 1942).

An attempt was made to integrate some of this work. Perhaps the most impressive of these studies was Barron's (1972) interviews and personality assessments of student actors and dancers. Barron has long distinguished himself in other research as an investigator and admirer of artists, searching for the nuances of differences that existed between artists and madmen rather than compounding the similarities. Barron's work is drawn from the tradition he helped establish at the Institute of Personality Assessment and Research (IPAR) in the 1950s. The IPAR interview approach, which has yielded a large body of information about writers, painters, architects, creative mathematicians and musicians, was identified as the most appropriate approach and was modified for this study.

The design of this study was also influenced by the work of Fried (1964) and Hatterer (1965) in the area of clinical intervention with artists; Parsons and Lindauer's (1980) comparisons of the aesthetic characteristics of actors and dancers; and a series of studies on creative dramatic acting by Neacsu and Marcus (Neascu, 1972 a, b; Neacsu and Marcus, 1972, 1974; Neacsu, 1974; Marcus, 1974) at the University of Bucharest in Romania. It is noteworthy that the Neacsu and Marcus research was undertaken because Romania is a socialist country in which only those who demonstrate creative dramatic ability are admitted to drama school. The government presented Neacsu and Marcus with the task of operationalising factors involved in dramatic ability so that an effective screening process could be instituted.

A decision was made for the moment to investigate members of the acting and dance professions. Working professionals, students, and famous actors and dancers were targeted. The creativity of these performers could not be assessed at this time; that step awaits a larger, more empirical study.

It is desirable, however, that research on the performer be expanded from the personality assessment represented in this initial venture into an assessment of the kinds of skills necessary in the performing arts. Studying only the personality of a creative individual and not his/her work and talent or skills causes an improper emphasis to be placed on the person to the neglect of the process and the product. Instead, as Neacsu and Marcus (1972) and also Bahs and Stockwell (1972) have noted, we need to know how the personality variables interact with the creative talents required to become a professional actor or dancer.

In summary, this research is best conceptualized as a preliminary investigation of the actor and the dancer under the mantle of the psychological study of creativity. The pursuit of this kind of research has the following broad goals:

1 to provide psychologists with more information about the creative process as it exists in theatre and dance;
2 to assist performing artists and theatre and dance educators in understanding the intersection of creativity and personality, and in gaining clearer insight into the complex relationship between the performer's goals and needs and societal demands and expectations;
3 to assist clinicians in their work with performers. Many performers seek therapy to help them cope with the difficulties of their lifestyles. The more that is known about performers, the better therapy can be attuned to their needs and concerns.

It should be added at this point that the interest of psychologists in the study of the performing artist has increased greatly over the last decade. The recent work of psychologists, such as Wilson (1989), and the research being presented at this conference is most encouraging.

Method

Subjects

A total of 464 actors and dancers participated in the research:

138 professional actors - working performers from Broadway, off-Broadway, off-off Broadway, repertory, TV and film (drama, comedy, musical comedy).

122 professional dancers - performers from major dance companies, Broadway, TV and film (ballet, modern, jazz/tap).

82 student actors - studying full-time, pursuing a professional career in dance.

106 student dancers - studying full-time, pursuing a professional career in dance.

Procedure

Twenty-page questionnaires were distributed to schools and companies of performers. Participation was voluntary and questionnaires were completed privately and returned in enclosed stamped return envelopes. Questionnaires were anonymous and confidential. They were:

1 Fitzgerald's Experience Inquiry - an instrument measuring Schachtel's concept of openness to experience as it relates to regression in the service of the ego.
2 The Gough Adjective Checklist;
3 Sixty interview questions including an adaptation of Helson's Childhood Activities Checklist.

Interview questions included a series of exploratory questions focusing on the performer's perception of his/her art form and its relationship to society which sought to investigate the effect the interpretive versus creative art controversy and the psychoanalytic focus on the personality of the artist have had on the performer. The following interview questions were analyzed for this submission:

1 Are you proud of being an actor (dancer)?
2 Have you ever been embarrassed to tell people that you were an actor (dancer)?
3 In any of your theatrical business dealings have you ever been treated unfairly as an actor (dancer)?
4 What do you think society as a whole thinks of actors (dancers)?

Results and discussion

Proud

Actors and dancers were asked if they were proud of being actors and dancers. Overall, 97% said yes, 1% said no and 2% said yes and no. This question seems to call forth a response based on one's professional identity, hence yielding a high level of affirmative responses. Clements et al (1983) obtained similar results when administering the Something About Myself Test (SAM) to actors, and claimed confirmation of "widely held notions about individual actors in theatre: one, that they do not think of themselves as artists concerned with providing works of art; two, that they prize their individuality, sensitivity, self-direction and critical capacities; and three, that they possess intellectual curiosity, imagination and the desire to recombine things and ideas in innovative ways".

Embarrassed

Performers were asked to answer the following questions: Have you ever been embarrassed to tell people that you were an actor (dancer)?
____ Yes ____ No. If yes, why? ________. Overall, 47.5% of the actors compared to 28.5% of the dancers said yes, 40.6% of the males compared to 35.6% of the females and 39% of the professionals versus 36.2% of the students.

Actors and dancers, professionals and students, males and females were compared by a three-way ANOVA. Actors scored significantly lower (more embarrassed) than dancers ($F(1, 433) = 16.34$, $p < .0001$) and female dancers scored significantly higher (less embarrassed) than male dancers and male and female actors ($F(1, 433) = 5.58$, $p < .05$). A three-way ANCOVA controlling for both age and education maintained both effects.

In sum, actors are more embarrassed than dancers to admit to their profession. As far as females are concerned, female actors are more embarrassed than female dancers. As far as dancers are concerned, males are more embarrassed than females. Regarding actors, females are more embarrassed than males. An eight group one-way ANOVA further clarified that female professional dancers were the least embarrassed and significantly different from all other groups ($F(7, 433) = 3.71$, $p < .001$).

It is understandable that actors are more embarrassed than dancers to admit to their profession. The training involved in dance leads to a more tangible product - leaps, bounds, leg extensions, etc. - that are easily recognized, accepted and applauded. This creates in the dancer a more immediate sense of identity. He/she can admit to a certain level of physical and movement prowess that he/she is proud of and that can be easily demonstrated. The actor, on the other hand, has no such immediate tangible proof to offer that he/she can act. Neither his/her body's condition or a two-minute display of his/her craft would suffice to convince anyone. In the words of Earle Gister, Director of the Davis Center for the Performing Arts at City College in New York, "I think that by the same token people who perceive and look at theatre are equally ill-equipped to ascertain the skills and the techniques required of the performer" (1978, p. 135).

The professional actor also has to contend with those who claim to be actors though lacking training or skill. Saying "I act" can be as convincing as saying "I talk" to an uninformed audience. Gister summarizes it by saying: "At least in dance, if you can't move and use space properly and have a whole sense of tension, form, shape, you don't even try it. You don't even get up and put your foot on the stage before a public. But in theatre, there are all kinds of people who are willing to put their feet and their emotions and everything else on the stage before they are ready" (p. 135-136).

The time and commitment involved in the training of a dancer is also more widely understood and respected. On the other hand, there is a popular notion that anyone can act, which is enhanced by the examples of ex-football players and models beginning film and TV careers. The training and process involved in creative acting is still much of a mystery to the general public and appears much like play when compared to the physical hard work of the dancer, which, to a degree, is likened to the athlete's training.

Stereotypes of the performer may also be gender-specific and these may in turn be different for dancers and actors. As stated, actors of both sexes have to struggle with admitting to their profession - either they will not be believed or if they are believed, they may be regarded as immature and frivolous. The male actor, in addition, may be regarded as somewhat of a charlatan, con-artist, fast-talker, ladies' man, but still may win a certain amount of respect for his "charm". The actress will pay a higher price. Her morals may be questioned along with her intelligence. The female dancer, on the other hand, especially the ballet dancer, is widely held in high esteem. Her physical dexterity is admired and the image she projects is one of woman on a pedestal, pure and utterly feminine. It is possible that the ballerina versus the actress can provide, for some, another variation of the madonna-whore theme.

Sexual orientation may enter into the differential assertion of embarrassment by male and female dancers. The cultural stereotype is that dance is feminine and that male dancers are most probably homosexual. Male dancers obviously make a commitment to dance despite the stereotype. The commitment is made early and yet some of the ambivalence may remain and surface in response to a question about "embarrassment".

Alter et al (1972) had questioned dance students about why there were not more male dancers. Responses spoke of societal pressures, an "immense social negativism" that the dancer must constantly face, that the dancer would be "considered feminine" and that he would probably experience some sense of "isolation" (p. 104-105). Erick Hawkins (1978) wrote of his own ambivalence and about the state of dance as it exists for a male dancer: "After I had started my first dance training in New York, for two years I did not write to my family what I was doing. When a young man has arrived at his vocation and is put in the terrible position that his vocation in the world's eyes is a questionable one for a man, you can see what trouble he is in" (p. 342).

Hawkins describes taking a summer off from his training to search for a solution to his dilemma. He travelled throughout the southwest, near where he was raised, observing Indian dancing. "I had seen men use dance as part of their worship, part of their way of coming into harmony with their own life .... That through dancing the people were protected, and the young men initiated into manhood" (p. 343).

From this Hawkins reached a new understanding of what dance meant to him and the place of dance for men in our society. He writes:

> Once the dance of men in our theatre is not partial, piecemeal, a triviality, mere virtuousity, mere romantic daydream, mere narcissistic display, mere exhibitionism of private neurosis, mere adjunct to the display of women's charm, it would be honored and would be a worthy vocation .... It is the specialization in our dance in which it is not demanded of men dancers that they be complete men and complete artists, carrying on their art in relation to everything else in the world, that has given dancing for men its bad name and its insignificance .... Dance for men in America has no prototype underlying ritual and myth such as the matador in the Spanish bullfight has to give him his challenge, his commitment, his worth and his honor .... A man dancing will have to go far beyond entertainment .... The man dancing in America no matter how long it takes will have to find this archetypal image; that the man dancing in the theatre is showing man becoming man. (p. 344)

In summary, 47.5% of the actors and 28.5% of the dancers admit to having been embarrassed to tell people that they were performers, whereas 97% of the performers said that they were proud of being actors and dancers. The question of being proud to be a performer calls forth a response based on the artist's professional identity. The question of being embarrassed, on the other hand, calls forth memories of incidents, specific experiences wherein performers would have experienced some sort of private or public humiliation if they acknowledged their profession. The difference in the responses to these questions points not to a contradiction between being proud or being embarrassed but rather suggests a conflict at times between a personal professional identity and perceived societal expectations and acceptance.

Unfair

Performers were asked to indicate if they had ever been treated unfairly in any of their professional business dealings. Overall, 60% said yes, 40% said no ($N = 416$). Actors and dancers, professionals and students, males and females were compared by a three-way ANOVA and a three way ANCOVA controlling for age and education. Both analyses confirm that actors, 72.1% claim to have been treated unfairly significantly more times than dancers, 47.9%, ($F (1, 406) = 23.26$, $p < .0001$) and that professionals, 69%, were significantly different from students, 46.2%, ($F(1, 406) = 21.41$, $p < .0001$). No significant difference was found between males, 62.9%, and females, 57.2%.

That 60% of all performers claim to have been treated unfairly is not surprising given the nature of the business, wherein, contrary to the public's belief, the performers are usually the low group on the totem pole. The stories recounted by performers in response to this question ran the gamut from casting couch propositions, to unclean, vermin-ridden dressing rooms, to being replaced without notice, to being fired from a show the performer opened in, won awards for, and made a hit. That dancers were treated less unfairly than actors may be due to the fact that most dancers have security as members of a company. The theatre, for the most part, also has greater opportunities for making money than most dance companies and unfairness often stems from these opportunities.

That professionals experienced more unfair treatment than students may be a product of more experience and, therefore, more opportunities for unfair treatment, and perhaps a certain optimism and willingness on the part of young performers to accept less than fair treatment in exchange for a role. This is quite obvious in the non-Equity theatre productions in which students usually perform until they become union members.

Society

Performers were asked to respond to the question, "What do you think society as a whole thinks of actors (dancers)? The majority of performers believed society's view of the performer was unrealistic, inaccurate, negative, or at best ambivalent. A qualitative analysis of these responses was very revealing about the apparent conflict between the self-image of many performers and perceived societal opinions and expectations. Responses were grouped into categories which summarize the general themes proposed by the performers. Although there was some overlap and one response could possibly fit into several categories, each response was classified according to a list of criteria and placed in only one category. The following is a representative sample of quotes from performers. Since the categories were somewhat different for actors and dancers, they are presented separately.

Actors

N = 220

No response (blank, unintelligible)	7
No opinion on performer's part	3
"Who cares what society thinks?"	3
	13

Remaining = 207

A. Love/hate

1 These actors believe society as a whole has strong, ambivalent feelings about performers. Society both loves them and hates them. N = 25

"They revere and have contempt for them."

"Society think of actors as commodities, at once heroes and yet dispensable."

"They tend to hold us in awe and think of us as somewhat eccentric. I think we may frighten many people because on a deep spiritual level they sense their own connection to the forces of the psyche and the imagination. When that frightens them they tend to belittle us as a profession."

"A strange mixture of both awe and raised eyebrows. I think they're fascinated - but feel that we're prone to be unstable and a bit lacking in the 'morals department'."

"I think as much as society might adore those actors up there on stage or screen, they think actors as a species are immoral. Someone once said they think of us as gods and live with us as if we are whores."

2 A second group of actors also cited a love/hate relationship by listing various reactions from different members of society. N = 16

"Opinions run the gamut from glamourous to degenerate."

"They're either impressed or distrustful - not much middle ground."

"Glamour, larger than life heroes, bums, spoiled children, overpaid, oversexed gypsies."

"They have a totally romanticized view. Glamourous, sinful, egotistical or some worship them. Basically they don't see us as human beings."

"I think people have lots of different ideas about actors - many are in awe, many envious, many think they are flakes, many think they are totally bizarre, unstable - without any moral fibre. Many people have a lot of respect for actors - many people have little respect for them. I think most people think there is 'something different' about actors."

B. Lack of respect

1 Many actors stressed that it is only the famous, hence successful actor, that society respects. Those who can't find work are viewed quite negatively. Again, a dichotomy of thought is represented. N = 31

"I think they have respect for those who have 'made it' - are in a successful TV show, movie, play - and are making money. I think they think the rest of us who are still building our careers, struggling at times, are starry-eyed kids who should wise up and find a real career."

"It's a business of recognition - people tend to regard and respect you on your visibility."

"I think society sees actors either as egotistic blow-hards or as poor misguided losers, unless, of course, they are of the celebrity status. Then they are just too wonderful for words."

"Lay people seem to see actors in terms of a whole battery of stereotypes, e.g. if they don't recognize you (film, TV etc.) they think you're a phoney or at least 'strange'. If they *have* seen you, particularly on TV, they think you're wonderful but still strange."

"Most people don't respect most actors. Society forces each actor to prove his worth or value either by performance or credits."

"Actors who are truly great, they very rightfully adore and stand in awe of. Actors who are celebrities, they think they possess. Actors whom they've never heard of, but are seeing for the first or second time, they barely notice. They'll wait until they read about them in *People* magazine or see them in a successful movie."

2 Some actors believe that society has no respect for acting as a profession. N = 9

"On the whole acting is looked upon as not a very hard job and actors don't need skills to do what they do. More often now, I'm running into people that think acting could be a nice pastime, but not a real job because you're not with a company for 30 or more odd years and you never know if tomorrow you'll be working."

"Regardless of the fact that most American heroes and heroines are actors, I feel that actors are still considered below other 'professionals' such as doctors, lawyers, even business people. Perhaps it's because it's so risky - financially and in terms of lifestyle. Perhaps because we generally see things in an unconventional way."

"They think they're bums that should get real jobs."

"They look down on them - acting isn't a steady paying job."

"For the most part, unless you are a "Star", I believe society is indifferent towards actors. I don't believe acting as a profession is taken too seriously by society. I do know many (non-actors) who believe acting means playing around or people that are only in acting while they're searching for a worthwhile money-making career."

"Many think it's just a hobby - not too serious."

C. Envy

1 Some actors felt that society envies them. N = 10

"I think most people would like to try it."

"Life in the limelight is something everyone envies to some degree."

"I say most people don't understand what we are all about; but everybody, I feel secretly, wishes they could get up and do what we do."

"They are jealous that they don't have the courage to pursue the field themselves."

2 Others pointed to a society living vicariously through them. N = 5

"Society thinks of actors as being bigger than life. Society lives vicariously through performers."

"Society lives vicariously through the actor, movies, theatre, records, tapes, videos, etc. Yet, they like to see us fall, get bad notices, become drug dependent and so on. The *National Enquirer*, for instance, is a success because society loves to read about what they think the 'real' life of an actor or entertainer is like. We (actors) can't survive without society, nor they without us."

"Society looks up to actors as fantasy figures who don't lead real lives. The actors are the characters they play. The actor can experience the life that the audience cannot."

D. Glamorous view of the profession

1 Many actors believe that most of society has an unrealistic glamorized view of the acting profession and do not see the reality of the actor's life. N = 26

"Society has a glamorous view of actors. Many think it is easy and happy-go-lucky. The majority do not understand the real struggle and challenge of being an actor."

"Highly paid for little work. Public sees only the glamour and the glitz."

"I think there is a general idea that actors lead a fairly glamorous life and this is often appealing to the 9-to-5 office worker. People, I find, are usually fascinated by actors and their life-styles - often disregarding the discipline and sacrifice it requires to become an actor."

2 In addition, some actors believe that people equate being a celebrity with being an actor. N = 10

"The majority of society confuses untalented celebrities with actors."

"Generally people don't know how to distinguish between *actors* and people who act. We see a lot of non-actors and/or 'personalities' in the media, and too much of the time there's a lot of attention and respect paid to people in glamorous positions who aren't actors at all."

"The only actors that people in general know of are the successful ones. So they base their opinion on that. They think acting is glamorous, high-paying and a piece of cake."

"I think the majority of the population think that only people who are 'stars' are actors. The average person has probably never met an average actor. Their only exposure to actors are the ones they see on TV or film and then they are the character they play - not a real person."

"I haven't the faintest idea since society rarely sees actors. It sees celebrities."

3 Because society glamorizes or romanticizes the profession, many actors believe that society has no real understanding of what acting as an art form actually is. N = 10

"They think of movie stars or TV or soap stars. They think the hardest part of being an actor is learning all those lines. 'How do you learn all those lines?' They have, for the most part, no idea what living a part entails."

"As a whole they think it's only hard work as far as finding a job. They don't realize the mind and heart bending it takes to develop a role. 'You were great,' they'll say, 'How do you memorize all those lines?' as though that's all there was to it."

"I don't think society thinks of actors as actors but rather as personalities, larger than life people who entertain. They don't think of the craft that goes into a performance."

E. Disdain

1 A great many actors felt that society feels quite negatively about actors. Some focused on a strong sense of general disdain. N = 20

"They have no identity themselves."

"Bums."

"I believe society thinks of actors in a negative way, i.e. drug addicts, prostitutes. But also as flaky, strange characters and neurotics."

"They think that they are all weird, gay people who are show-offs and obnoxious."

"Rogues and vagabonds."

"Flakey, anti-establishment, wild, crazy."

"Third-rate citizens."

"The consciousness of the majority regarding actors is limited, narrow and conservative, with belief systems about us going back to ancient times."

2 Some focused on an ancient view of actors as egotistical and/or immoral. N = 13

"Freeloaders. Most think actors lead the fast immoral life. Fast women, drugs, booze. They don't understand that you can be a good performer and not do those things."

"They are egotistical, money-hungry, immoral individuals."

3 Others cited a popular view of our society that actors are immature and childish. N = 17

"That we're children, unreliable, crazy, over-emotional, lucky and over-sexed. I think most people resent actors because they think somehow we're having fun they aren't having in their lives. I think it's probably true; but they fail to see us *work* at it."

"Frivolous children - not real people. Many people are jealous."

"Exotic but irresponsible creatures."

F. Different

A few actors saw society's opinion as being more neutral, that actors were just "different." N = 8

"A struggling lot of beings that live a separate reality from the rest."

"I think there's a mystique about them. People see them as 'different' somehow, but don't always know if it's a good or bad difference."

G. Admire/respect

A few actors believe society feels positively about actors.

2 felt society admired them;

3 believed society respected them;

2 believed that respect for actors was increasing in our society.

Dancers

N = 228

No response (blank, unintelligible)	12
No opinion on performer's part	3
"Who cares what society thinks?"	6
	21

Remaining = 207

A. Love/hate

1 These dancers believe society as a whole has strong ambivalent feelings about dancers. Society both loves them and hates them. N = 21

"They love them on stage. They question it any other place."

"Society thinks it's wonderful and exotic and special. However, society also subconsciously says that if someone is going to get away with doing what they like for their whole lives, society will have to extract the price of low pay. Society also resents, consciously, our freedom and happiness."

"I think society is in awe of dancers, but they think we are stupid and we don't have to work hard."

"Society is fascinated and horrified by dancers. Fascinated because they are mysterious creatures in their own little world and horrified because all mysteries or things that are not easily understood give vent to peculiar stories or myths."

"I think society thinks we are weird and crazy for going through all of the work it takes to be a dancer. But people love to go see us in a show."

"They think that they aren't very smart and that they couldn't be anything important. They think the men are homosexual, yet they admire us for our grace, courage to perform and dedication."

"In one sense they worship us. In another sense they don't really think we're working and they don't take us seriously."

"We are the muses. We are a fantasy. Risk-takers. Sluts. Thoroughbreds. We have beautiful bodies. We are a frill in life. Entertainment on Saturday nights."

2 A second group of dancers. N = 12

"I think society separates dancers from the real world or business world, with a portion of society having a great respect for dancers while the other portion of society looks down on us."

"I think there are mixed feelings. Some think a dancer is an exhibitionist, a dreamer, gay. Some realize that a dancer is a hard-working person."

"They think we're beautiful, special, perhaps eccentric and some people think we're probably a little dumb. Too physical and not intellectual enough."

"Some think they are stupid; some see dancers in a romantic way, 'Isn't it exciting to be a ballerina!'; some see us as deprived of normal lives, starving ourselves."

"Certain people think we are goofing about playing or not being realistic about earning a living in the real world. The rest either really admire dancers for doing what they love or the feats they can perform/accomplish, or for the hard work involved."

B. Lack of respect for dance

1 Some dancers stressed that it is very successful or famous dancers that society respects. Those who can't find work are viewed quite negatively. Again, a dichotomy of thought is represented. N = 5

"Being a Broadway dancer, I've noticed people look up to you as a dancer - as long as you have work in a good or popular show."

"Unless a dancer is in a ballet company (or Broadway show) I think most people discount it as a profession or as something valid."

"We are bohemian, homosexual, irresponsible and strange. If you're a rich and famous artist, however, you are admired."

2 Some dancers believe that society has no respect for dance as a profession. N = 40

"Society thinks that dance is not a real career. They think it's all fun and games."

"'What will you do when you stop?' They think this career is very short-lived and, since we don't make *any* money, they are afraid for our future. They think what we do is glamorous and fun. I don't really think they know how difficult this career is."

"Recently they have been given greater respect and acceptance, but still not what they deserve. I teach dance and get paid very little - that's a sign of society's respect."

"Many people have asked me if I was too stupid to do anything else."

"Most people consider dancing (as a career) to be a passing fancy. Something to *play* at. And a dancer will grow out of the childhood fantasies of being a dancer. There is never enough credit given to a dancer as being an artist."

"They think it's a beautiful art; however they have the misconception that all, or mostly all, dancers are dumb, empty people, who aren't really 'working', don't have a 'real' job."

"I think society thinks much like my mother and father. They have a hard time explaining what I do. It produces no product, pays meagrely and wears people out and down at an early age. It is a nice hobby, but nothing to be taken seriously. Why should dancers be paid since they like their work so much?"

"A profession with no future, no stability, a waste of time."

3 Because society glamorizes or romanticizes the profession, many dancers believe that society has no real understanding of dance as an art form or the amount of hard work involved. N = 20

"I'm not sure how seriously we are taken. 'Oh isn't that wonderful', but there isn't much of a sense of what is involved or how totally the work absorbs one."

"I think the general population looks upon dancers as *fluff* - something to watch but not very important. I don't think they are aware of the amount of very difficult work (physical and mental-creative) involved."

"The average person does not understand the dedication, discipline and sweat to produce something that looks so pretty and so easy."

"I suppose it bothers me that so many people are ignorant to the incredible amount of work a dancer puts in a day."

4. Many dancers believe that dance is seen as entertainment only and that dancers are taken solely at face value. N = 23

"Many stereotypes exist - gorgeous bodies but stupid upstairs. Many people don't realize dancers have minds and feelings and are human just as anyone else."

"Nice but not important."

"Generally, many are very impressed with the physical abilities of dancers, but do not realize that there is so much more behind the dancer as a whole."

"We are certainly not a necessity, so people could give or take us."

"I don't think that society thinks of dancers at all. If they did we would have more fundings for the arts. If anything we are not thought of, our feelings are not thought of."

"Most people have no idea what modern dance is in its many forms, and thinks of dancers as those decorative things one sees at a musical comedy or at the ballet. Therefore, most people think of dancers as entertainers rather than artists."

C. Envy

Some dancers felt that society envies them. N = 8

"Many are envious of the physical beauty but take great joy in watching dancers."

"In a way I think they envy us to some degree to have the ability to do things with our bodies that they cannot. In another way I think they find us a bit unusual because of the lifestyle and dedication we possess and they don't understand."

"In the US, I think people often think of dancers as not having 'settled down' yet. At the same time, they *all* wish they 'could' do it. In actuality, they probably could if they wanted to as much as I do. That's ironic."

"I think everyone wishes they could dance and are closet dancers. I've especially noticed this after performances."

D. Disapproval/disdain

These dancers cited the many negative opinions they believe society has of dancers, running the gamut from disapproval to disdain. N = 34

"Weird, freakish and a bunch of lesbians and homosexuals."

"Dumb! Narcissistic."

"Lazy bums who have nothing better to do than twiddle on our toes all day."

"Mindlessness and homosexuality."

"That dancers in show biz are wild. And all male dancers are gay."

"Airheads. They don't view them as intelligent, creative human beings. Are very judgemental of dancers and often stereotype them as sleazy, sexy and weird."

"Silly, selfish, self-absorbed people."

"They think of them as indulgent, consumed, unconscious of others (needs or concerns)."

E. Different

Some dancers saw society's view as being much more neutral - that dancers were just "different". N = 10

"As a breed apart."

"Different."

"Out of touch, a different breed of people - specialized people."

"Society puts dancers in a class by ourselves. They really don't look at us as being a part of their class or group. We are in a world by ourselves."

F. Admire

Several dancers felt that society thinks positively about dancers. N = 13

"I think society loves dancers. They think we're different than just business people."

"Society is impressed by dedication, self-discipline, sacrifice."

"I think they have a tremendous admiration for us. But I don't think they understand what we are doing and why we do it."

"I think society admires the discipline, strength, stamina, dedication."

G. Respect

1 Several also felt society has respect for the ability, dedication and discipline of dancers. N = 12

"I think that society respects dancers because they work the hardest out of everyone in the profession and are not paid what they deserve for the dedication they have to their art."

"I think that society can really respect dancers for their self-discipline and beauty."

"I believe dancers are respected by most of society, but many are not aware of the realities faced by the dancers. Dance is basically misunderstood by society in general."

2 Some dancers felt that society is changing in its opinion toward dancers and respecting them and their abilities." N = 9

"I think we're in a time where dancers are being thought of more as artists - they're being more accepted now, which is great. I also think that people think dancers are special people."

"As times are changing, people are accepting dance as a hard-earned profession that takes more tolerance than most jobs."

"Society is becoming more aware of the hard work dancers go through from the many movies and TV shows playing. They see that dancing is not just getting up on the stage and having fun - that there is a lot of blood, sweat and tears. And yes, they do respect our dedication to this art."

"Better now than ever before - the stigma is being lifted."

Although the majority of both actors and dancers believe that society does not view their professions positively, it is notable that 34 dancers compared to 7 actors felt that society did admire or respect members of their profession. This, of course, was not a quantitative analysis, but this observation echoes the earlier explanation of why dancers may be less embarrassed to admit to their profession than actors. One of the reasons cited was that the product and process of the dance with its athletic component is more easily recognized and appreciated by the public than that involved in acting.

Conclusions

As the history of the antitheatrical prejudice has shown, there is validity to the performers' wariness of societal opinions, demands and expectations. The price they pay for acknowledging this conflict is to feel at odds and not entirely accepted by the society in which they live and to which they wish to make a contribution.

It becomes, then, an issue of the performer feeling marginal or peripheral to society. The identity of an artist is acknowledged and owned with pride by the performers themselves, but the relationship of the performer to society remains unclear. Depending on situation and circumstance, the performer may feel less than a legitimate, contributing member of the community. Hence, embarrassment sometimes ensues. The late director Alan Schneider (1978) once stated:

> I think that we are on the verge of having a national theatre, consisting of a nationwide theatre and a nationwide attitude toward the theatre .... I feel more optimistic and more hopeful of the opportunities and, therefore, of the need for bettering our training and making more possible that first step: Some way of helping young people into a profession which they respect. The only time I've ever seen American actors respect themselves as performers was on a trip to the Soviet Union, which the Arena Stage Company and I embarked on three years ago. Suddenly, they felt that they were not just actors, not just workers, not just rogues and vagabonds. They were artists and they were important to society. (p 180)

If performers are to feel essential to society, their role and place in society must be clarified. Psychological research, which seeks to describe the creative process as it exists in the theatre and dance and to explain the intersection of creativity and personality in the actor and the dancer, can do much towards this goal.

References

Aaron, S. (1986) *Stage fright: its role in acting*. Chicago: University of Chicago Press

Alekseev, N.P. et al. (1985,) 'An experimental study of the emotionality of theatre college students.' *Soviet Psychology, 23 (3)*, 59-72

Alter, J. (1984a) 'A factor analysis of new and standardized instruments to measure the creative potential and high-energy action preference of performing arts students: A preliminary investigation.' *Personality and Individual Differences, 5 (6)*, 693-699

Alter, J. (1984b) 'Creativity profile of university and conservatory dance students.' *Journal of Personality Assessment, 48 (2)*, 153-158

Alter, J., D. Denman & F. Barron (1972) 'Dancers write of themselves and dance education.' In: F. Barron, *Artists in the Making* 86-112. New York: Seminar Press

Bahs, C.W. & J. (1972) 'Relationship of perception of the body to pantomimic ability. I: Body-Cathexis.' *Empirical Research in Theatre, 2,* 16-29

Barish, J.A. (1981) *The Antitheatrical Prejudice.* Berkeley, California: University of California Press

Barron, F. (1972) *Artists in the Making.* New York: Seminar Press

Bergler, E. (1960) 'On acting and stage fright.' *Tulane Drama Review, 4,* 159-164

Blum, R. (1976) 'A psychoanalytic profile of the actor: perspectives on career developments.' *Western Speech Communication, 40,* 178-188

Brennan, M.A. (1982) 'Relationship between creative ability in dance and selected creative attributes.' *Perceptual and Motor Skills, 55,* 47-56

Brennan, M.A. (1983) 'Dance creativity measures: a reliability study.' *Research Quarterly for Exercise and Sport, 54 (3),* 293-295

Chyatte, C. (1949) 'Personality traits of professional actors.' *Occupations, 27,* 245-250

Clements, R.D., P.L. Dwinell, E.P. Torrance & J.T. Kidd (1983) 'Evaluation of some of the effects of a teen drama program on creativity.' *Journal of Creative Behavior, 16 (4),* 272-276

Collum, D.K. (1976) 'The empathic ability of actors: a behavioural study.' Doctoral dissertation: Florida State University

Drake, F. (1950) 'A study of the personality traits of students interested in acting.' *Speech Monographs, 17,* 123-133

Fenichel, O. (1946) 'On acting.' *Psychoanalytic Quarterly, 15,* 144-160. Reprinted in *Tulane Drama Review,* Spring 1960, *4*

Freud, S. (1942) 'Psychopathic characters on the stage.' *Psychoanalytic Quarterly, 11,* 455-476. Reprinted in *Tulane Drama Review,* Spring 1960, *4*

Freud, S. (1963) 'On narcissism: an introduction.' In P. Rieff (Ed.) *General Psychological Theory* (56-82). New York: Collier Books. (Original work published 1914).

Fried, E. (1964) *Artistic Productivity and Mental Health.* Springfield, Illinois: Charles C Thomas

Gabbard, G.O. (1979a). 'The creative process of the actor.' *Bulletin of the Menninger Clinic, 43 (4),* 354-364

Gabbard, G.O. (1979b) 'Stage fright.' *International Journal of Psychoanalysis, 60,* 383-392

Gister, E. (1978) 'A symposium: the individual artist.' In: W. McNeil Lowry (Ed.) *The Performing Arts and American Society* 130-180. Englewood Cliffs, New Jersey: Prentice-Hall.

Golden, A. (1940) 'Personality traits of drama school students.' *Quarterly Journal of Speech, 26,* 564-575

Hatterer, L.J. (1965) *The Artist in Society.* New York: Grove Press Inc

Hawkins, E. (1978) 'Why does a man dance, and what does he dance, and who should watch him?' In M.H. Nadel & C.N. Miller (Eds.) *The Dance Experience* 342-345. New York: Universe Books

Joffrey, Robert (1978) 'A symposium: the individual artist.' In: W. McNeil Lowry (Ed.) *The Performing Arts and American Society* 130-180. Englewood-Cliffs, New Jersey: Prentice-Hall

Kaplan, D. (1965) 'Homosexuality and the American theatre.' *Tulane Drama Review, 9*, 10-55

Kaplan, D. (1969) 'On stage fright.' *Drama Review, 45*, 60-83

Koffka, K. (1942) 'The art of the actor as a psychological problem.' *American Scholar, 11*, 315-326

Manley, M. & V. Wilson (1980) 'Anxiety, creativity and dance.' *Dance Research Journal, 12 (2)*, 11-22

Marcus, S. (1974) 'Substitutive imagination and scenic projectivity.' *Revista de Psychologie, 20 (1D)*

Metcalf, J. (1931) 'Empathy and the actor's emotions.' *Journal of Social Psychology, 2*, 235-238

Miller, C.H. (1938) 'Value of certain standard tests for a study of dramatic talent.' *Journal of Social Psychology, 9*, 437-449

Motkov, O.I. (1983) 'A study of the dependence of creativity appearance on personality characteristics.' *Novye Issledovaniya v Psikhologu, 2 (29)*, 19-24

Nadel, M.H. (1978) 'The spirit of the dance.' In M.H. Nadel & C.N. Miller (Eds.) *The Dance Experience* 15-17. New York: Universe Books

Nadel, M.H. & C.N. Miller (Eds.) (1978) *The Dance Experience.* New York: Universe Books

Natadze, R. (1962) 'On the psychological nature of stage impersonation.' *British Journal of Psychology, 53 (4)*, 421-429

Neacsu, Gh. (1972a) 'Capacity of scenic expression as a relation between expressivity and creative mental elaboration.' *Studia Psychologica*, 1972, *14 (2)*, 142-148

Neacsu, Gh. (1972b) 'The unity of transposition and expression - the fundamental index of dramatic talent.' *Revue Roumaine des Sciences Sociales: Serie de Psychologie, 16 (1)*, 3-15

Neacsu, Gh. (1974) 'Vocal expressiveness as an indicator of dramatic talent.' *Revista de Psichologie, 20 (2)*, 153-165

Neacsu, Gh. & S. Marcus (1972) 'The psychological structure of dramatic talent.' *Revue Roumaine des Sciences Sociales: Serie de Psychologie, 16 (2)*, 133-140

Neacsu, Gh. & S. Marcus (1974) 'Methodological bases for dramatic aptitude testing.' *Revue Roumaine des Sciences Sociales: Serie de Psychologie, 18 (1)*, 15-24

Parsons, C. & M. Lindauer (1980) 'Dance and theatre: their psychological importance and the aesthetic characteristics of their participants.' *Psychological Documents, 10 (4)*, 1-24 (Ms. No. 2143)

Rubin, S.R. (1974) 'Components of aesthetic activities and interests: toward a multifactor theory.' Unpublished doctoral dissertation: Columbia University

Schneider, A. (1978) 'A symposium: the individual artist.' In: W. McNeil Lowry (Ed.) *The Performing Arts and American Society* 130-180. Englewood Cliffs, New Jersey: Prentice-Hall

Schreppel, E. & M.S. Lindauer (1975) 'Introversion-extraversion in actors' self-images and perceptions.' In: M.S. Lindauer (Ed.) *Research in Psychological Aesthetics and the Arts: a personal collection.* Brockport, New York: Brockport State College

Stacey, C. & H. Goldberg (1953) 'A personality study of professional and student actors.' *Journal of Applied Psychology, 37(1)*, 24-25

Taft, R. (1961) 'A psychological assessment of professional actors and related professionals.' *Genetic Monographs, 64*, 309-387

Wallach, M. & C. Wing, Jr. (1969) *The Talented Student.* New York: Holt, Rinehart & Winston Inc

Ward, D.T. (1978) 'A symposium: the individual artist.' In: W McNeil Lowry (Ed.) *The Performing Arts and American Society* 130-180. Englewood Cliffs, New Jersey: Prentice Hall

Weissman, P. (1961) 'Actor/playwright - both share potential for neurotic acting out.' *Psychoanalytic Quarterly, 30*, 549-567

Wilson, M.J. (1989) 'Professional actors and their attributions for their successes and failures.' Unpublished doctoral dissertation: New School for Social Research

The act of being: Personality characteristics of professional actors, amateur actors and non-actors

Jacqueline Hammond & Robert J. Edelmann

Department of Psychology, University of Surrey

> 'Actors - they'll seduce your daughter and possibly your wife. And what's more they don't pay their bills, everybody knows that. And they don't wash very often, and they swear terribly in public. They scratch their balls, and they drink a great deal' (Charlton Heston in Bates, 1986 p. 19).

Such a sardonic self-image, although somewhat exaggerated, reflects the way professional actors are frequently regarded by those who stand outside the profession.

While by some, particularly their fans, actors are idolatrously revered, by others (e.g., the media), they are treated with suspicion. More often than not, actors are seen as being 'different', as deviating from the conventional and perhaps, therefore, the 'normal'.

Unfortunately, psychology has done little to alter, or indeed to investigate seriously, the professional actor stereotype. Of the few psychological studies which have been conducted on the personality of professional actors, most have suggested that actors tend to lack a firm sense of self (Henry & Sims, 1970). Others have concluded that actors have 'poorly integrated, largely hysteric and schizoid personalities. They are exhibitionistic and narcissistic, having much pent-up aggression. They are passive, vulnerable to stress, tend to be overly anxious and have impaired body images. Their major defences are regression, projection, denial, isolation and reaction formation. Last, homosexuality is a major area of pathology.' (Barr et al., 1972).

Fisher & Fisher (1981) claimed that professional actors tended to be more exhibitionistic and more impulsive compared with non-performers. Furthermore, they found that professional actors' scores on the EPQ were consistent with the EPQ norms for various occupational groups which place actors in the 'hysterical' (i.e. extraverted and emotional) quadrant of the major two-dimensional framework.

Thus, the sum total of previous research adds up to a not very flattering interpretation of the professional actor's alleged behaviour. Whether such behaviour is the result of dispositional factors, or a product of the acting profession itself is clearly open to question.

Layder (1981), for example, argues that much of the seemingly neurotic behaviour associated with professional actors is the result of the eccentricities of the acting profession (e.g., the response to 'competitive individualism' and constant close surveillance; and the high unemployment and the temporary nature of work when it is attained).

Bates (1986) also takes this approach and maintains that much of the actor's behaviour is a natural response to the vagaries of the acting profession itself.

Therefore, can we conclude that the actor's behaviour is purely situationally-specific, or are dispositional tendencies important?

Certainly, an unbending commitment to acting appears to have been present in actors at a very early age (approximately 10 years old, Hammond & Edelmann, 1989).

Inevitably, however, before the acting process and its effect upon professional actors can be looked at in greater depth, a question which needs to be addressed is whether professional actors differ from non-actors in terms of personality and the way they perceive themselves.

Goffman's (1959) parallels between real life and the theatre would have us believe that individuals in everyday life 'act' according to their everyday roles just as professional actors act in dramatic roles. But can similarities really be drawn, or is there something unique about the personality and self-perception of the professional actor? Hence, this study set out to look at the way professional actors perceive themselves on a number of personality dimensions and whether their self-perceptions differ in any way from those of two comparison groups of amateur actors and non-actors.

Of all the personality characteristics attributed to the professional actor, perhaps the most frequently applied is that of extraversion. It is a common assumption that to be an actor you have to be an extravert. Certainly that was suggested in the Fishers' (1981) study. Thus, the EPQ was selected for the present study.

Consistent with the notion that all actors are extravert is the belief that actors have big egos, are self-centred and self-involved. In view of this self-esteem was assessed. This refers to the degree to which one values oneself - and, although not necessarily related to strength of identity, it measures the extent to which one might cope with threats to one's identity.

That some people appear to be better able than others to manage the way they present themselves was highlighted in the early 1970s by Snyder (1974). He suggested that their success depends upon their ability to monitor their own performances when signals from others tell them that they are not having the desired effect. This ability Snyder labelled as self-monitoring. A decade later Lennox & Wolfe (1984) revised Snyder's theory and included an additional scale of concern for appropriateness. Both self-monitoring and concern for appropriateness were assessed in the present study.

Professional actors need to feel disinhibited (at least while they are acting). That is, their inhibitions (particularly social ones) have to be lowered in order for them to feel 'free' to express themselves fully. Actors cannot afford to be encumbered with social constraints (Hammond & Edelmann, 1989). In view of this, social desirability was measured in the present study. While similarities have been drawn between social desirability and lying (e.g. Meehl & Hathaway, 1946), the inclusion of a measure of social desirability in the present study was to assess the need of the subjects to obtain approval by responding in a culturally appropriate and acceptable manner (i.e., in a socially desirable way).

It might be assumed that professional actors should be privately self-conscious. That is, they attend to the private and hidden aspects of themselves. But are they publicly self-conscious? One might expect that in order to be able to perform in front of a group they would not be. Thus, private and public self-consciousness and social anxiety were assessed in the present study.

Another common assumption about actors is that they are extremely sociable people and certainly not shy. Of course, shyness is not low sociability. Whereas sociability is the tendency to affiliate with others and to prefer being with others to remaining alone; shyness describes the reaction to being with strangers or casual acquaintances where one feels awkward or uncomfortable. So, shyness and sociability can independently affect how an individual behaves in a situation. An actor who appears not to be shy while he is acting could be the opposite in real life, when the asking mask is removed. Thus, the present study also assessed shyness and sociability.

Subjects

161 subjects took part. Of these, 51 were professional actors (27 males and 24 females) who were currently appearing on either television, radio, film or stage (a number in the West End of London); 58 of the subjects (27 males and 31 females) were amateur actors who belonged to and performed in amateur dramatics companies in the South East of England; 52 of the subjects (7 males and 45 females) were non-actors who said that they had never acted in the dramatic sense. They comprised teachers, bank officials, estate agents and sales staff of several departmental stores.

All the subjects were English-speaking. The mean age of the professional actors was 43.4 (age range: 24 to 69 years) for the males, and 43.9 (age range: 23 to 65 years) for the females; the mean age of the amateur actors was 41.8 (age range: 23 to 64 years) for the males, and 42.2 (age range: 18 to 62 years) for the females; and the mean age of the non-actors was 32.3 (age range: 19 to 58 years) for the males, and 38.3 (age range: 18 to 65 years) for the females.

Questionnaires

Each of the subjects was given a set of 6 standardized questionnaires to complete. The questionnaires were:

1 *The Eysenck Personality Questionnaire* (EPQ; Eysenck & Eysenck, 1975). This is a widely used scale consisting of items assessing dimensions of personality: extraversion, neuroticism and psychoticism, and containing a Lie Scale. The EPQ has established reliability and validity.

2 *The Rosenberg Self-Esteem Scale* (Rosenberg, 1967). This scale measures the extent to which one values oneself (i.e., one's self-worth).

3 *The revised Self-Monitoring and Concern for Appropriateness Scales* (Lennox & Wolfe, 1984). The former scale measures sensitivity to the expressive behaviour of others, and an individual's ability to modify the way he or she presents him or herself. The latter scale measures two variables that are directly associated with social anxiety - cross-situational variability of behaviour and attention to social comparison information.

4 *The Marlowe-Crowne Social Desirability Scale* (Crowne & Marlowe, 1960). This scale measures an individual's need to respond in culturally sanctioned (i.e., socially desirable) ways;

5 *The Self-Consciousness Scale* (Fenigstein, Scheier & Buss, 1975). This scale

measures two major components of self-consciousness: private self-consciousness (which is concerned with attending to one's inner thoughts and feelings) and public self-consciousness (which is defined by a general awareness of the self as a social object that has an effect on others). A third related factor, social anxiety (which refers to a feeling of discomfort in the presence of others) is also assessed by the scale.

6 *The Shyness and Sociability Scale* (Cheek & Buss, 1981). This scale measures two distinct personality dimensions: shyness (which is the discomfort and inhibition that may occur in the presence of others) and sociability (which refers to a preference or need to be with people).

Within the questionnaires there are 15 variables. These are extraversion, neuroticism, psychoticism and lie score (EPQ); social desirability (Marlowe-Crowne Social Desirability Scale); self-esteem (Rosenberg's Self-Esteem Scale); ability to modify self-presentation, and sensitivity to the expressive behaviour of others (Revised Self-Monitoring Scale); cross-situational variability and attention to social comparison information (Concern for Appropriateness Scale); public self-consciousness, private self-consciousness and social anxiety (Self-Consciousness Scale); and shyness and sociability (Shyness and Sociability Scale).

The questionnaires were distributed to each of the subjects by post after they had agreed to participate in the study. Subjects were instructed to allow themselves 20-30 minutes (maximum) to complete them. When completed, the questionnaires were returned by post (pre-paid).

Results

The mean scores and standard deviations for the three groups on each of the 15 variables can be seen in Table 1.

The mean scores of the amateur actors lie between those of the professional actors and those of the non-actors on a number of variables (i.e., neuroticism, psychoticism, lie, social desirability, self-esteem, cross-situational, private self-consciousness, social anxiety and shyness).

On the remaining variables, the mean score of the amateur actors are either marginally higher than the mean scores of the professional actors and the non-actors (i.e., on extraversion, ability to modify self-presentation, public self-consciousness and sociability), or there is very little difference in the mean scores of the three groups (i.e. on sociability).

To identify the best discriminating composite of variables between the professional actors and the amateur actors, the amateur actors and the non-actors, and the professional actors and the non-actors, 3 Multiple Discriminant Analyses were performed for each of these pairs of groups

Table 1. Group mean scores (and standard deviations).

	PROFESSIONALS	AMATEURS	NON-ACTORS
Extraversion	14.0 (4.4)	14.7 (4.6)	12.3 (5.2)
Neuroticism	13.6 (4.7)	12.6 (4.9)	11.3 (5.7)
Psychoticism	4.2 (2.3)	3.2 (3.2)	2.8 (1.8)
Lie	7.1 (3.5)	7.6 (3.6)	10.1 (4.0)
Social Desirability	14.0 (4.7)	14.4 (5.0)	17.5 (4.0)
Self-Esteem	20.8 (3.7)	20.8 (4.5)	20.6 (4.9)
Ability to modify self-presentation	23.0 (5.2)	24.3 (4.3)	21.8 (4.8)
Sensitivity to the expressive behaviour of others	21.6 (3.5)	19.8 (4.1)	19.9 (3.7)
Cross-situational variability	20.2 (5.5)	20.1 (6.5)	18.3 (6.3)
Attention to social comparison information	30.3 (9.0)	33.6 (7.4)	34.4 (8.4)
Private Self-Consciousness	25.7 (5.7)	23.5 (6.2)	20.7 (4.9)
Public Self-Consciousness	17.7 (4.3)	17.7 (4.7)	16.8 (5.0)
Social Anxiety	10.1 (4.6)	11.0 (4.4)	12.9 (4.7)
Shyness	12.5 (5.1)	13.4 (5.7)	16.7 (5.7)
Sociability	13.7 (3.2)	13.9 (3.5)	12.2 (2.7)

using a step-wise procedure. Wilk's Lambda was used as the step-wise criterion and in each analysis only one function was extracted.

In the first discriminant analysis which compared the professional actors and the amateur actors, 3 variables which had the highest correlation with the group function mean were: ability to modify self-presentation (0.68), attention to social comparison information (0.68) and sensitivity to the expressive behaviour of others (-0.60). Thus, the amateur actors perceive themselves as being more able to alter the way they present themselves, as paying more attention to external information by which they can compare themselves, and as being less sensitive to the expressive behaviour of other people than do the professional actors.

In the second discriminant analysis which compared the amateur actors and the non-actors, the variable which showed the highest correlation with the group function mean was shyness (0.54). Thus, it would appear that the amateur actors perceive themselves as being less shy than do the non-actors.

The canonical discriminant function coefficients of the third discriminant analysis with the composite of variables which best discriminate between the professional actors and the non-actors can be seen in Table 2.

Table 2. Dicriminant analysis: Professional actors & non-actors.

Canonical discriminant functions

CANONICAL : CORRELATION:	AFTER FUNCTION	WILKS' LAMBDA	CHI-SQUARED	D.F.	SIGNIF.
0.70	0	0.49	69.31	9	0.00

Standardized canonical discriminant function coefficients:

Variable	*Function 1*
PRIVATE SELF-CONSCIOUSNESS	-0.82
ATTENTION TO SOCIAL COMPARISON INFORMATION	0.52
LIE	0.48
SOCIAL ANXIETY	0.46
SHYNESS	0.38
SELF-ESTEEM	-0.37
SOCIABILITY	0.32
SENSITIVITY TO THE EXPRESSIVE BEHAVIOUR OF OTHERS	0.25
NEUROTICISM	-0.18

In the order of their degree of correlation with the group function mean, the variables are private self-consciousness, attention to social comparison information, lie, social anxiety, shyness, self-esteem, sociability, sensitivity to the expressive behaviour of others and neuroticism.

If the mean scores (Table 1) of the professional actors and the non-actors on these variables are examined, it appears that the professional actors perceive themselves as being more privately self-conscious, less attentive to social comparison information, more honest, less socially anxious, less shy, more sociable, more sensitive to the expressive behaviour of other people and marginally more neurotic than do the non-actors. As far as self-esteem is concerned, there is only a minimal difference between the two groups (the non-actors possess slightly higher self-esteem), with both displaying a moderately high self-esteem score (on a scale range of 10 = high self-esteem, 40 = low self-esteem).

Discussion

From the findings of the present study, it is clear that there are personality dimensions which distinguish professional actors from non-actors. However, the differences which have emerged do not support the negative stereotype of professional actors previously put forward (e.g., Henry & Sims, 1970; Barr et al., 1972; Fisher & Fisher, 1981). Rather, they reflect theoretical assumptions which suggest that by the very nature of their profession (i.e., involving public performance), professional actors are less likely to be socially anxious and shy, and will be more sociable than non-actors. Furthermore, the continual change of roles played, the portrayal of "other characters", and the exploration of the psyche and behaviour (inherent aspects of both the acting profession and acting process), may also explain why professional actors are more privately self-conscious and display greater sensitivity to the expressive behaviour of others than do non-actors.

It would be incorrect, however, to suggest that an actor personality type *per se* exists. While the present study has revealed a number of variables which appear to distinguish professional actors from non-actors, on several of them (e.g., attention to social comparison information, and private self-consciousness), the standard deviations are large, indicating that within the acting profession itself, the personality of individuals and their self-perception lie within a broad band.

Of course, whether the dimensions of personality examined by the present study are developed within professional actors through the process of acting, or whether individuals become actors because of their personality characteristics remains unclear. In view of the similarities between professional actors and amateur actors on a number of personality dimensions, the latter would appear a more viable conclusion - that both professional actors and amateur actors seem to feel a need to express aspects of their personality through the adoption of dramatic roles.

However, considering that within the acting profession itself the personality of individuals and their self-perception vary markedly on particular personality dimensions, pathological factors alone would not appear to provide an adequate explanation. It is for future research to take a more phenomenological approach and to investigate whether (and, if so, the extent to which) the acting process, and the playing of dramatic roles affect the actor's personality and self-perception.

References

Barr, H.L., R.J. Langs, R.R. Holt, L. Goldberger & G.S. Klein (1972) *LSD: Personality and Experience.* New York: Wiley

Bates, B. (1986) *The Way of the Actor.* London: Century

Cheek, J.M. & A.H. Buss (1981) 'Shyness and sociability'. *Journal of Personality and Social Psychology,* Vol. 41, No. 2, 330-339

Crowne, D.P. & D. Marlowe (1960) 'A new scale of social desirability independent of psychopathology.' *Journal of Consulting Psychology,* Vol. 24, 349-354

Eysenck, H.J. & S.B. Eysenck (1975) *Manual of the EPQ* San Diego: Educational & Industrial Testing Service

Fenigstein, A., M.F. Scheier & A.H. Buss (1975) 'Public and private self-consciousness.' *Journal of Consulting and Clinical Psychology,* Vol. 43, No. 4, 522-527

Fisher, S. & R.L. Fisher (1981) *Pretend the World is Funny and Forever: A psychological analysis of comedians, clowns and actors.* Hillsdale: New Jersey: Erlbaum

Goffman, E. (1959) *The Presentation of Self in Everyday Life.* Harmondsworth: Penguin

Hammond, J. & R.J. Edelmann (1989) 'Behind the Mask: An exploratory psychological study of the professional actor.' Paper given at the London Conference of the British Psychological Society 20/12/1989

Henry, W.E. & J.H. Sims (1970) 'Actors' search for self.' *Transaction, 7,* 57-62

Layder, D. (1981) *Structure, Interaction and Social Theory.* London: Routledge and Kegan Paul

Lennox, R.D. & R.N. Wolfe (1984) 'Revision of the self-monitoring scale.' *Journal of Personality and Social Psychology,* Vol. 46, No. 6, 1349-1364

Meehl, P.E. & S.R. Hathaway (1946) 'The K factor as a suppressor variable in the MMPI.' *Journal of Applied Psychology, 30,* 525-564

Rosenberg, M. (1979) *Conceiving the Self.* New York: Basic Books

Snyder, M. (1974) 'The self-monitoring of expressive behaviour.' *Journal of Personality and Social Psychology,* Vol. 30, 526-537

Acting as an insecure occupation - The flip side of stardom

Estelle M. Phillips

Birbeck College, University of London

The aim of this study was (a) to discover more about the under-researched occupation of acting and (b) to provide an insight into the behaviours and attitudes of people who have chosen an insecure lifestyle which may help the unemployed, who have not chosen an insecure lifestyle, to cope with joblessness and the uncertainty in which they find themselves.

As it was important not to rely on people's reconstructions of their lives from their current vantage point at the top, this study involved only 'conspicuously unsuccessful actors' to use the terminology of one of my interviewees. The study is unusual in that it does not rely on the information provided by actors who are well-known and therefore have to think back to how it had been for them many years ago.

Recently, Charles Handy (1989), a respected management consultant, said that people should think increasingly of work in terms of having a portfolio of skills and activities, some for sale, some as gifts. The portfolio might include wage or fee work, from cleaning to conveyancing, homework and child rearing, gift work done voluntarily and study work, training or preparing for a new skill. In this research I am using the acting profession as a model for 'portfolio work' from which people in uncertain job situations might learn.

First, a few basic statistics given by Peter Pluvier, the General Secretary of Equity (the actors' union) during an LBC interview on the A.M. programme during February 1989: Equity now has 41,000 members compared with 10,000 in 1960; 50% actors earn under £5000 p.a.; 72% actors earn under £10,000 p.a.. All the actors in my sample were earning below £10,000 p.a. and many of them were below £5000 p.a. at the time of interview.

The study I have undertaken considers the lifestyle of unknown actors whose very existence is based on job insecurity and, as such, may make a contribution to our knowledge of how it feels to have to cope with ever present uncertainties and constant flexibility.

Method

In order to discover more about the lives of actors whose names are not household words I conducted semi-structured interviews with 12 men and women, whose ages ranged from 24 to 65 years.

Recruiting my sample was not easy as I did not know any actors. However, they move in an extensive network and so once having gained entry, access to many more is almost automatic. But actually gaining entry is fraught with difficulties. It took several months from conception of the idea to being in a position to undertake it. Eventually, I received permission to put a notice on the board at the Actors' Centre and from then on my phone did not stop ringing.

While this can hardly be called a random sample, my interviewees are a self-selected group who may be typical of actors who have had only limited success in their chosen profession. They do not include those at the very bottom - they could not afford even the £12 p.a. it costs to join the centre nor would they have their Equity card which is a requirement of membership - or those who have been very successful; the stars and household names of the business.

Each interview lasted a minimum of onc and a half hours and some lasted twice as long as this. Participants promised not to talk about the interview to their friends - thus guarantees of confidentiality were given on both sides. This approach gave me information on such things as breaking into the profession and getting an equity card; flexible alternative work; the role of the agent; how it feels when they get a part and then how they cope with the break-up of the group at the end of the run; actors' co-operatives (managing their own careers and being each other's agents) and what happens when they or one of their close friends finally 'makes it'.

Results

The actors in the sample talked frankly about their expectations and the realities of their chosen profession. Some of them had worked almost non-stop since they started and some had hardly been employed since they left drama school. The accounts are from people who have chosen an insecure occupation and reveal how they manage socially, emotionally and financially.

a Beginnings

All the people interviewed spoke of difficulties in gaining information about how to get started in an acting career. This was partly due to the embarrassment of saying 'I want to be an actor' and partly to the general lack of publicity given to drama schools and theatrical publications such as *The Stage* and *Contacts.* It is almost a "catch 22" situation in that you have to be in touch with the profession in order to learn how it operates. One woman described the frustrations of her early years thus:

> I always had a secret desire to be an actress. I didn't know how to go about it and had so little confidence that I kept completely quiet about it. Then I thought about modelling. I was about 11 years old when I wrote to the careers office. The reply was opened by the headmistress of my boarding school and her reaction was one of shocked horror. I told her I wasn't serious. After that I didn't do anything for some years. I just had no way of finding out how to get into acting. There was nobody to talk to.

The interviews reveal that there are a variety of ways of breaking into the profession and that it could happen at almost any age. The following two extracts are taken from people who started unusually early and unusually late. One man told me:

> I always wanted to be an actor - well since I was about 12 years old. I went to see a James Bond film and decided I wanted to be a spy. But when I thought about it I realized he wasn't a spy at all; he was an actor. I sent a letter to Equity and they replied saying I should go to drama school. Meanwhile, there was a local amateur group I heard of and I arranged to go after school and just sat out front watching. An 18 year old in the group asked me to his birthday party where I met a 16 year old girl who was a member of a youth theatre. She told me that that's where I should be. I went along immediately and got totally involved. I was about 14 or 15 by then."

A different introduction is described by another actor:

> I was never in a theatre before my early 20's. I was in a career-type job and was reasonably successful. I played in a group in my spare time for some years but that never came to anything. I was in my early 30's before I did any acting. I just heard about a professional theatre group in the East End and joined them on an unpaid, part-time basis. While I was with them I heard of another local theatre group who were looking for people with some musical experience for a production of *Hair*. I went along and had my first audition. They took me. This meant that I was working with real professionals. It felt fantastic, like being given birth. I did other shows with that company and went from the chorus to leading roles. I was 35.

These descriptions show the importance of being in contact with people who are in a position to give information and, possibly, help to aspiring beginners. It is clear that, at least from the point of view of the actors, careers officers are not very useful. It seems they have no literature to give out and little or no information regarding drama schools. In general there was considerable bitterness about the possibility of getting started depending on whether or not your parents knew people 'in the business' and some people complained about nepotism in the profession.

b Attitudes to agents

Many negative attitudes to Equity were expressed but these are not covered here. Suffice to say that the only thing that actors like less than their union are their agents. The following comments are typical:

"I've had three agents in all. All despicable. Parasites."

"I've had an agent for two and a half years. Really bad relationship."

"Overall I've had about six agents. I leave them because they don't get you work."

"I've never ever had a job through an agent but had to pay them commission for work I got myself."

"Actors' co-operatives began because actors weren't satisfied with their relationship with agents. We employ them but they have the power and we have to crawl. Co-ops give us more control and also act as a support group."

"I used to go to interviews scared and treated people like gods. The co-op helped here. I spoke as an agent, not a young actor. It rubbed off when I went for an interview. They were just agents too, like I was for other people."

More and more of these jobbing actors are joining actors' co-operatives in order to get round the problem of having to engage an agent. A question that needs to be investigated is whether there is a relationship between amount of success in an actor's career and degree of liking (or dislike) of the actor's agent.

c Coping with rejection and refusing work

Although jobbing actors are forever putting themselves in the position of having to compete for work they still suffer from the pain of being passed over:

"A stab in the guts every time it happens."

"It's hell and results in raging depression."

"I've had some really big disappointments; I prefer to go off and cry on my own."

But they have developed some defences that help them to think a little differently about themselves as people and themselves as actors suitable for the part on offer:

"It can be very hurtful. It's only in the last two years that I've come to terms with it. It's not *me* as a person, or my ability as an actor, it's to do with what they're looking for in the part."

"It feels like it's you but really it's that you're too tall or you look like someone else who's already been cast."

"I realize it isn't *me* that's being rejected. More likely the agent was bored because I was the nth person or I'm too small for the girl they've already cast."

"When I don't get parts I just think they're stupid; I *know* it isn't to do with talent."

Nevertheless, they are still not as immune as might have been thought:

"Failing auditions is not as bad as not getting called to audition. Failing auditions means 'are you right for the job?' that means, looks, height, etc. Not getting asked is *really* rejection."

"Intellectually I know there are lots of reasons for not getting work but emotionally I feel it's me and it's just terrible."

Despite all this there are times when even these people refuse work that has been offered to them:

"We're aware of our influence on others and take that as a responsibility."

"Commercials are as acceptable as the RSC so long as the product is OK."

"You follow your instinct. If it feels right you do it even if you don't get paid, also if it feels bad no matter what they're tempting you with you turn it down."

"Some companies it would be a slur to work for, you wouldn't get good jobs afterwards."

"I started as an army entertainer during the war. When I was demobbed I did some rep and then my agent offered me Germany. I said 'no'."

"I turned down a job where I'd have had to wangle a green card (USA) and it all sounded very shady. They had accepted me on the spot so I didn't trust it very much."

"I turned down paid work out of London to take an unpaid job *in* London in case I might be seen. Ho! Ho!"

The only kind of career development that exists in acting is the opportunity to choose what you do and what you don't do. The more successful actors become the more they are able to select their own roles. Even at this level their responsibilities to the public and their rights to determine the path of their own career are important considerations to them.

d Alternative work

It is vital for these people that their secondary employment is totally flexible in order to enable them to be free for interviews and auditions at short notice. As a result it is noticeable that the range of jobs undertaken by actors when they were not working in their chosen profession was extensive and considerable ingenuity was apparent in the type of jobs they did. These included supply teaching, cleaning, being a disc jockey, selling shore excursion tickets on a cruise ship, telephone weather information service, driving for a commercial advertising agency, runner for a film company, stocktaking in a pharmacy, waiting on table, bartender, modelling, cashier in a nightclub, usherette, night telephone operator, newspaper shop, chambermaid and DIY on a flat in order to sell it at a profit.

Versatile though they were there was no doubt that first and foremost they were actors, regardless of whether or not they were currently working or even how long it had been since their last acting job.

"Acting is a vocation; no decision to be made."

"I'm totally committed to it as a career - I *am* an actor."

"It's like being Jewish - no matter *what* you're always a Jew."

"At its best it includes every part of you. *All* your energy, nothing else does that."

"You're only as good as your last TV job - leads to type casting."

"There's nothing like it. The attention, adulation without responsibility, applause; it's exciting - the perfect fusion of mind and body."

But when they felt depressed about their way of life there were times when they might, fleetingly, think of changing it, but that would mean having to admit to themselves that they had failed:

"Sometimes you think you'll give up and do something else but you always come back to it in the end."

"Unemployment and then working in worse circumstances than I'd started in. What have I achieved? Nothing!"

"Every time I feel I can't go on any longer something turns up and so it goes on - but that's a terrible pattern. How long can I continue?"

"All the time I applied for jobs but forgot lines. I cried every day."

"I started to write for radio - sold the first play in 1954. I write under the spur of extreme necessity but sell it ages later when I don't really need it."

"I sometimes did dry-cleaning deliveries for my aunt but never seriously considered alternative employment."

"If I gave up I'd go and work on the land - do something creative."

"The change from working to going back to cleaning is difficult to cope with but at least I don't have to teach. Nothing's worse than that."

e Self Concept and Self-Esteem

It is clear that they had a very strong sense of professional identity and always defined themselves as an 'actor' no matter how long it was since their last acting job or what work they were doing currently.

When asked about how they would describe themselves if they were asked at a party what they did they said such things as:

"When people ask what I do and I say 'I'm an actress' there's a sense of panic. I tell them what work I've done and there's a worse panic. Then I become apologetic, 'it's only the fringe', 'I'm still trying for my Equity card', etc."

But when asked how they would describe themselves to themselves they were more positive:

"I see myself as a leading actress, not a jobbing actress. I'm not a supporting actress."

Parallel to this was a sense of waste, of achieving nothing because the talent and ability which they were convinced they had were not being utilized. Even when they had experienced success in another arena they perceived this as merely a stopgap until they could get on with their chosen profession. One woman had a novel published and a play produced on the radio but she insisted "I'm an actress not a writer, that's always true." Another woman had achieved international acclaim as a model in countries as remote as Japan, Australia and America. But the money she made from her modelling (which amounted to around a million dollars in five years) was seen by her only as the means by which she could continue to pursue her acting career. Further research might consider the motivational side of all this. It is clearly not extrinsic, otherwise this woman would have decided that she was, in fact, a model rather than an actor.

There was, of course, another side to all this which is clearly summarized in the following comment:

"For six months after finishing drama school I was *very* depressed. I had my hair cut very short and felt like it was mutilation."

But the final word must go the actor who informed me that in the 'business':

"There is a high incidence of alcohol and drug problems but the lowest rate of suicide of all professionals."

f Networking

The actors had a highly developed system and strategy for keeping themselves within a network both of peers and of job hunting. Most of the people interviewed engaged in a systematic programme of letter writing which served both to structure their time and to help them feel part of 'the business' even though postage was a very expensive item from their meagre budgets. *Spotlight*, which comes out twice a year and lists all actors, was described as 'the actor's bible' and although it costs £65 p.a. to be listed it was a must for all the people in my sample.

Many had friends who were in a similar position and when they went to auditions they met others whom they knew from drama school or rep. These meetings helped them to keep in touch with what was happening elsewhere as information concerning further auditions and interviews was passed between them. Most of them said things like:

"You think of yourself first, but if you're not the right type you tell a friend."

When asked what advice they would give to unemployed people of other occupational groups using networks was a high priority.

"It's vital to keep in touch."

"Be prepared to have a go at anything."

"Be aware that you can do other things. Make a list of what you're good at."

"Be confident and project confidence."

"Gather others around you in a similar situation, you need your peers."

"Target groups to write to."

"Don't be ashamed - it doesn't reflect on your worth - and don't give up hope."

Although these actors had very little money, many worked for nothing. This was in order that they might be seen by a casting director who happened to drop by. They believed that being seen was the only route that might lead to their being offered 'real' work. They also arranged contracts with managers that stated a salary, which they then paid to themselves, in order to notch up the required number of weeks of paid work in order to get an Equity card.

g Attitudes to job insecurity

These people had a fear of security and tended to shy away from responsibility. On the whole they seemed to require the excitement of not knowing exactly what would happen next. As one of them put it:

"If I could see the future stretching ahead with achievable goals, I couldn't see the point of going on."

Others said similar things:

"Don't want security, safety. I *need* lots of short-term contracts. What happens when your 14 year long soap ends and you've got the mortgage to pay?"

"The *joy* of never knowing what will happen next. Can't imagine having to work in an office or teach - set hours. I've always lived a life where pleasure and work mingle."

Regardless of their class origins they had few illusions about the lifestyle that went with the occupation they had chosen:

"I came from a steady working class background and I knew the pitfalls - that I'd be out of work for long periods.'

In some cases it seemed that they were almost afraid of success:

"I know someone who was a top soap star for years, opening bazaars, etc. And after the series ends - unemployable. Everyone identifies you with the character."

Nevertheless, they invested heavily in themselves. In addition to unpaid (or 'showcase') work they spent large sums on up-to-date photographs, which they had professionally taken; CVs; and the eternal letter writing.

Discussion

This research has looked at job insecurity in the lives of jobbing actors. The actors were clear that they did not like security but were not so definite regarding their feelings about insecurity. It was not unusual to find that they actually desired the excitement and hope of better things just around the corner that the uncertainty of their job situation brought.

Although they stereotyped success and then rejected it, it may be that the rejection was necessary in order to help them cope with their current situation. A question that might be looked at more closely is whether they actually liked the uncertainty or merely tolerated it.

I commenced the research with the idea that it might be possible to help the unemployed who have *not* chosen an insecure lifestyle to cope with joblessness and the uncertainty in which they find themselves by learning something of the behaviours and attitudes of people who *have* chosen an insecure lifestyle. I believe that, up to a point, this has been achieved. For the actors interviewed, professional journals such as *The Stage* and books such as *Spotlight* have an important part to play in helping them to maintain their links with the profession. Similarly, venues such as the Actors' Centre helped them to retain their identity as well as their skills and kept them within a well-established network of others in a similar position to themselves as well as in contact with more successful members of their profession who ran classes in various aspects of the performing arts in the rehearsal rooms adjoining the main lounge and refectory. These methods of 'keeping in touch' helped the actors to feel that they belonged to a group and made them aware that they were not alone in their unfortunate circumstances.

The study also considered the emotional and psychological aspects of coping with recurring and, in some cases, continuing unemployment. It was clear from my small sample that actors are people who live constantly in the shadow of 'redundancy' and survive on perpetual short-term contracts. It was also clear that all the respondents had a very deep feeling of *being* an actor.

The important point was that membership of a peer group within a working population based on job insecurity helped individuals to maintain their identity as actors, and, to a certain extent, their perception of themselves as skilled and useful people. It appears that group membership and a socially shared set of beliefs about belonging to an insecure profession reduces the negative effect of such insecurity and helps people to cope with the situations in which they find themselves.

References

Handy, C. (1989) *The Age of Unreason*. London: Hutchinson

Love addiction in performers

Carole H. Field

Psychotherapist, North Hollywood

Early on in my clinical practice, which largely consists of actors, dancers and singers, I discovered a curious phenomenon. These performers' lifestyle - dealing with consistent rejection, low self-esteem, victimisation from being the last man on the totem pole and lack of employment - was not the main reason for seeking therapy. Instead, their presenting problems usually clustered around chaotic love relationships with the overwhelming dysfunction being co-dependency or "love addiction".

In reviewing the academic literature, I find the word "co-dependent" used primarily in relation to substance abuse. In this case, it is specifically referred to as the "enabler" of the alcoholic or drug addict. Rarely is it referred to as a pathological condition, an addiction to love, unto itself. The closest technical labelling in the DSMIII-R to co-dependency is Personality Disorder Not Otherwise Specified (301.90). I therefore turned to the myriad of pop literature on love addiction. The following is a synthesis of this literature, plus my observations on the love-addicted performing artists and non-performing artists whom I have treated.

Definitions

The following definitions are fundamental in understanding love addiction. They have been derived from Webster's 1979 second edition New World College Dictionary. Also, for clarification, the word performer shall encompass actor, dancer, singer and stand-up comic.

Depend
Relying on another for support or aid.

Dependent variable
A variable whose value is determined by the value of another variable. This term is from the statistics discipline and I employ it because the extrinsic factor of other-directedness is introduced.

Love (Gothic)
A deep and tender feeling of affection or devotion or attachment to a person or persons. The red flag here, and as a most fitting definition for this paper, is how the word "attachment" is employed in defining love.

Addict
(Latin from addicere) - to give assent, agreement, to give oneself up. The obvious combustible result presents itself when combining "attachment" with "to give oneself up". I might also add to addiction, it is not a chosen seeking of pleasure but rather, an avoidance response. Interestingly, it mimics borderline symptomatology in its never-giving-or-getting-enough insatiability.

Co-dependency
or love addiction. I define this (since no dictionary definition exists) as partners in dependency. It is not a healthy interdependence, it is two people enmeshed. Wegscheider-Cruse (1981) addresses this as "a specific condition that is characterized by pre-occupation and extreme dependence on a person or object". It is being responsible for other people's feelings, thoughts, behaviours and problems, or how you assume they might have felt, thought, will feel, behave, etc. A distortion of boundaries ensues here: my stopping and your starting is blurred.

An example of this is the Anjelica Huston role in the film *Crimes and Misdemeanors*. In this film she pursued Martin Landau vehemently, without boundaries and demanded he fulfil her every need and her deficient sense of self. Their both being involved in her demands created a true co-dependency as he continued to stay married to another, yet succumbed to her narcissistic requirements.

Etiology

Steinglass (1980) refers to this type of interplay as "a disease with an etiology, set of symptoms, typical course and predictable prognosis". This "typical course" is more clearly understood by dividing it into stages.

Stage One - The seed and its blossom.
The seed in this case is the family of origin. This seed "grows" through an interaction of either abuse, neglect, abandonment or engulfment. An extreme example of abuse would be physical abuse. A more subtle example of engulfment would be the stereotypical, overprotective, Jewish mother. On the spectrums of abuse, neglect, engulfment and abandonment we observe families producing over-functioning rescuers or under-functioning rebels. The blossom, then, of this seed either seeks to refill what the family lacked, or seeks to duplicate their family's chaotic styles of interaction.

Brown (1988) says "The alcoholic family organizes around the alcoholism". Likewise, the co-dependent-agenic family organizes around the other, albeit through fusion or distantiation. Whitfield (1987) says, "When the child within is not nurtured or allowed freedom of expression, a false or co-dependent self emerges".

Stage Two - The crucial stage
The love addicts make an insurmountable attempt to obtain from their partner what their family lacked. He/she pours an overabundance of energy into exacting what they "think" they need from the significant other. This depletes them from relating to outside friends and family. Hobbies and even employment responsibilities begin to pale. A type of isolation sets in. Resentments start to mount here because in reaching for the impossible, the love addict's not-good-enough inner messages kick in.

This is exemplified in the autobiographical book/film *Out of Africa*. The writer, Isak Dinesen, constructed a particular portion of her life around the hopeful return of her suitor. As this does not come to pass, she becomes progressively disenchanted with her initial joy at being in Africa.

Stage three - The habitual stage
These resentments pave the way for emotional and/or physical violence. They are habituated by the addict's tenacious need to over-control/change the other. The reality of broken bones is cast aside for some fantasized idyll or reconstructing "frozen" deficits from childhood.

Stage four - The early help seeking stage
The patients here start to face their powerlessness in that their vain attempts

have all backfired. Seeking help is their only alternative.

Stage five - The "Into recovery" stage
A shift occurs here. An organic focus on "self" versus "other" starts to occur. For the first time in their lives, the love addicts start to touch the joys of intrinsic validation. Because of this, their crippling fears of the unknown start to diminish. With this willingness to step out and accept temporary discomfort, therapy and the road to wellness can begin. A successful actress patient recently exclaimed to me, "I just could not let go of my husband. I attempted everything to turn him around. I'm just starting to see how great it feels inside to stop trying".

Permeability into the performer's psyche

Due to the nature of the entertainment industry, actors acquire an external locus of control: they become overly approval-seeking because of always pursuing the next job. Also, the reasons for their getting or not getting the job are rarely made known to them. These reasons, at best, are usually subjective and irrational anyway. This lack of knowledge, nee mirroring, from their potential employers mimics the neglectful or not-good-enough mothering.

Besides constantly living in the victim-like "void" in order to survive, the performer must build in a well-honed denial system. Without this, the waves of rejection and lack of acknowledgement would, in no time, drown the performer. The pathology this creates, however, is a magnification of any depersonalisation already ingrained. It also further splits the less healthy ego.

Finally, in an era without heroes and shamans to get us through, the world has turned to celebrities - a type of identification with the "benevolent and glamorous" aggressor. This adulation, however, deepens what Miller (1981) refers to as the false self.

All of these, an external locus of control from the non-mirroring mother, depersonalisation from core, and the implemented false self, are identical to co-dependent symptomologies. As Schaef (1986) says, "The need to be needed is directly connected to lack of self-esteem". The actor and the love addict, both, *live* to be needed.

A musician patient of mine finally left an extremely destructive co-dependent relationship after he was accepted (needed, validated) into the Los Angeles Philharmonic Orchestra. We had been working on his inability to leave this two year relationship for five months. As soon as his Philharmonic contract came through, he moved out from her apartment and immediately began reviving old relationships and seeking new ones.

Consequently, even if co-dependency is not an original intrapsychic dysfunction in the individual, because of the nature of the entertainment industry, the performer creates the symptoms interpersonally - and is most vulnerable to integrating them into his identity.

Treatment of the love addict

When a love-addicted patient seeks therapy, it is most important for the therapist to avoid colluding with their "HELP. FIX ME YESTERDAY". Their locus of control has been so external, that by "rescuing" in their hour of need, the therapist runs the risk of refuelling that. However, a balancing act comes into play here because the therapist must be firm in expressing the importance of therapy and/or the twelve-step support groups (such as Alcoholics Anonymous, Al-Anon or Co-dependency Anonymous) for them right now. They must be told, existing without support in their vulnerable state would amplify their old chaotic behaviour patterns. They should also hear the word re-education. Re-education, co-dependents firmly believe, in the arena of love relationships, is an impossibility. The therapist, thus far, serves various, delicate functions for these patients. They are re-educating, setting limits, and posing as a good role model against the backdrop of bad family modelling and witch messages. Also, the therapist is presenting messages of realism in relation to loving. This goes counterpoint to both society's and literature's mythological romanticizing of love.

The Rogerian treatment model of accurate empathy, congruence and genuineness is in keeping, particularly for actors. I have heard actor patients repeatedly say , although they feel better than when they came into therapy, they desire to keep coming because of the acceptance, honesty and tranquillity in the room. One recently explained, "I like coming here before an important audition because I kind of get to look at myself". This direct metaphor for mirroring does not exist for this person outside the office setting.

The therapist must express to the patient how recovery must be their first priority. Recovering love addicts ought to re-acquaint themselves with the love of their art, with friends they have avoided while "people pleasing" their significant other, and with themselves. This all helps to dismantle any transitional object usage of the other. As in physics, energy decreases as it distances from the source.

Jung repeatedly maintained that the only recovery mode for addictions is through spirituality. On a formal level, this can imply religious worship, or even an integration of a higher power as in the twelve-step programmes. On a less formal level, this can merely imply a constant reminder by the therapist to the patient, that any loss does not represent total loss.

In terms of relating to others, the co-dependent should be made aware of their manipulative and controlling tendencies. For them, learning to release demanded responses from people and required results from events is akin to acquiring a new language. However, in conjunction with this, the co-dependent must also learn to establish boundaries. Setting boundaries is a novel, yet somewhat intimidating, proposition for the love addict. Their being reminded that they are worthy of asserting limits is in order.

An afflicted actress patient, who is just learning to establish boundaries (although not yet successfully with her boyfriend; she is doing well with her intrusive parents and over-zealous agents) recently queried, "Is it possible that I can tell people what I need, assert myself, and not make them go away with my specifications?"

Boundaries are usually established by asserting your needs and your limits in as few words as possible, with consequent congruent behaviour. This eliminates victimisation, over-functioning and living in false hope versus living in reality.

Finally, in terms of treatment, when the patient is sufficiently ready, I have them compose, for their object of addiction, a blessing. Creative people find the literal writing of this easy. Emotional resistance, however, is the first response. This blessing can be a poem, song, haiku or something they read in the fifth grade. Although the blessing does not have to be mailed, I do encourage it! This produces a cathartic closure for the patient. Also, it takes some heat off the now ex-love object.

But most importantly, it is a re-confirmation to the once victimized patient, that they are the epicentre and creator in their world. *They* can choose to accelerate compulsive behaviour, or acquire the tools of wellness. And from this acknowledgement that they are the primary connection to the higher source, their power is finally restored.

And, in my deepest desire of protecting healthy relationships, creating new ones, and eradicating the need to overfunction in order to obtain a passport to this planet, I conclude with a quote from Shakespeare.

> "Doubt thou the stars are fire;
> Doubt that the sun doth move;
> Doubt truth to be a liar;
> But never doubt I love."
> *Hamlet* Act II, Scene 2

References

Black, C. (1981) *It Will Never Happen to Me.* Denver, Colorado: M.A.C.

Brown, S. (1988) *Treating Adult Children of Alcoholics.* New York: John Wiley & Sons, Inc.

Miller, A. (1981) *Prisoners of Childhood.* New York: Basic Books

Schaef, A.W. (1986) *Co-dependence.* San Francisco: Harper & Row

Steinglass, P. (1980) 'A life history model of the alcoholic family.' *Family Process, 19,* 211-226

Webster's New World Second Edition College Dictionary (1979) USA: Literary Press

Wegschneider-Cruse, S. (1981) *Another Chance: Hope and Help for the Alcoholic Family.* Palo Alto, California: Science and Behavior Books

Whitfield, C. (1987) *Healing the Child Within.* Pompano Beach, Florida: Health Communications

Emotional costs of success in dance

Suzanne T.S. MacDonald

Center for Sports Medicine, San Francisco

The world of dance, most particularly ballet, is very elusive to the outside onlooker. Dance is the only truly addictive sport as it is an athletic discipline performed to music allowing great expression of creativity. "Once a dancer, always a dancer" is true even when a dance career is over. It is forever in the muscles and mind. Dance can be defined as the relationship of movement and physicality to musicality.

The process of becoming a ballet dancer can be quite destructive to the developing female. Dancers traditionally begin training at about eight years old. The body begins moulding itself in the desired dancer image which continues through the adolescent years. The process also changes the minds through a process of criticism (mostly by male teachers beginning at puberty), infantalization and a gradual tuning inward as the world narrows down to just Dance. Formal schooling is frequently abandoned due to dance training and rehearsal schedules. Dancers will often live away from their families in order to attend dance school and apprenticeships. This further removes the level of emotional support and balance necessary for the development of a healthy outlook on life. As a result, many dancers are plagued by feelings of depression, lowered self-esteem, lack of recognition, inappropriate thinking patterns, obsession with weight, perfectionism, few socialisation skills, lack of support systems, little ability to cope with stress and little preparedness for a future after dance.

Cognitive and behavioural therapies are successful therapies for dancers. They respond well to various techniques such as visualisation and imagery, affirmations, goal setting, meditation and relaxation, role play and humour. Quite often they lack skills in daily living, such as budgeting finances and time, dealing with the bureaucratic maze of life and functioning in society at large.

Working with dancers therapeutically requires an understanding not only of dance, but of medical indications, physical therapy and rehabilitation and other modalities used by dancers such as the Pilates Method (Nagrin, 1988).

Therapists should be constantly aware of the need to monitor the dancer's attitude towards competition which can inspire and excite to superb performance or freak them out with negative thinking and inner dialogue (Orlick, 1986). Dancers need to be aware of their bodies and not deny injury. They have a compulsion to allow themselves little rest and to return to dance too quickly thinking that everyone is getting ahead of them.

It is important that dancers begin to consider other career preparation while dancing. Therapists should encourage dancers to realistically assess when they are not dancing to their potential or are not progressing. They can then leave while they are still looking good and work toward new goals from a positive frame of mind. Having to stop dancing due to injury and working through both the injury and career preparation is difficult and time consuming.

Finally, therapists should monitor the dancers' attitudes towards their weight. Dancing is a profession where low weight is required. A realistic attitude towards weight needs to be developed. Screen for factors such as heredity and bone structure, percentage of body fat and lean body mass, encourage a good understanding of nutrition particularly to prevent early onset osteoporosis, mensis history and basal metabolic rate (May & Asken, 1987). Of prime importance is the recognition that low body weight does not necessarily indicate an eating disorder. Frequently our bodies need less than our minds think we deserve.

The joy and delight in dance cannot be measured. The intrinsic rewards are clearly there. The understanding, astute therapist can guide a dancer to an even greater appreciation of her/his unique contribution to society. Dance is a celebration of the mind and body connection in life.

References

May, J.R. & Asken, M.J. (Eds) (1987) *Sport Psychology: The psychological health of the athlete*. New York: PMA Publishing Corporation
Nagrin, D. (1988) *How to Dance Forever*. New York: Morrow/Quill
Orlick, T. (1986) *Psyching for Sport*. Champaign, Illinois: Leisure Press

The effective conductor: A matter of communication and personality

Barbara Pollack

Clinical Psychologist, Denver, Colorado

This is a work in progress on interpersonal communication as it influences the effectiveness of conductors. I began by observing a number of established conductors in rehearsals and performances, and some notions of "communicating and conducting" began to emerge. In addition, I observed a variety of conducting classes in such settings as the Aspen Music Festival, The Juilliard School, Mannes College of Music and a Conductors' Guild Workshop.

It became clear that most of the comments directed to the student conductors specifically focused on *how the conductor communicated* even more than on conducting skills or musical interpretation abilities. Musicians, especially, when asked to provide feedback to these student conductors, overwhelmingly made comments that concerned *how* the conductor communicated.

Furthermore, the comments were verbalized in common and familiar language that was not highly specific to music. For example, musicians said things like, "He was very nice; showed lots of respect for the musicians;

knew his score very well. He was very picky, but nice about it..." "He was having fun, had a good sense of humour, was not overly critical..." "He didn't rub it in when we made a mistake; we know when we make a mistake...".

Additional ongoing interviews with music critics and others involved with the "business" of music, as well as with professional musicians, stressed that how well a conductor performs - how effective he or she is at leading an orchestra to perform a piece of music - depends not just on technical expertise, but, to a very great extent, on the communication ability and personality of the conductor.

Having gathered this information, the challenge has been to focus in on those communication skills that are critical to a conductor's effectiveness. Even more important has been to find a framework for describing the conductor's ability to use these skills as a component of his or her personality. When this can be done, a language exists for working with conductors (specifically, student conductors) to observe their behaviours and give feedback that can lead to improved effectiveness.

The conductor in context

In order to talk about communication between conductor and orchestra, it is necessary to comment on the *relationship* between the conductor and the orchestra, because that relationship provides, for better or worse, the platform for communication - or lack of it.

Historically, the conductor was a time beater, not even mentioned in the programme. But, by the late 1800's the conductor's status was changing and he was described as "... the external factor which holds together a performance, a spiritualizing internal factor." (Galkin, 1988, p. 767). About this time, the conductor became the boss; he was interested in getting a particular sound and did what he felt he needed to do to get it. He did not have to be nice, nor concern himself with the social conventions of "getting along". ("...He may shout and rant and curse and insult his players at rehearsal - as some of our greatest conductors are famous for doing - but if there is love, the conductor and his orchestra will remain knit together through it all and function as one." (Leonard Bernstein, quoted in Galkin, p. 774.)

So, the conductor came to be viewed as a leader, but also a despot - "everything from a priest, rabbi, father-figure, object of derision," according to an internationally-known conductor I interviewed. The relationship was evolving and becoming increasingly complex. As the 20th century progressed, it became more common for conductors to project their own personalities and fantasies onto the orchestra, and the musicians, in turn, projected theirs back onto the conductor.

The initial, very limited relationship between orchestra and conductor became more like any complex interpersonal relationship. As the conductor assumed a greater position of power, he was also imbued with more power, and there was an era in the mid-19th century when the conductor as despot/tyrant flourished. With the musicians essentially having no voice of their own, the "relationship" resembled, in many respects, marriage as it existed in the 1800's, with the orchestra in the role of wife, and the conductor as husband.

Such a role, of course, carries its own burdens. In the past, if the music did not go well during a performance, the perception was that it was the orchestra/musicians' fault, not the conductor's. People did not blame the conductor for being a poor communicator. He might be thought of as not intelligent enough, or perhaps cold and unfeeling, but communication skills were never called into question. Nor was his personality. But with the evolving relationship between orchestra and conductor came the responsibility, placed squarely on the conductor, of communicating effectively so that, at the very least, satisfactory performances were elicited from musicians. Blame shifted, and a poor performance came to be perceived as more the conductor's fault than the musicians', or at least an equal onus.

This brings us to the present, when, my research has shown, those who run the business of music no longer expect a conductor to stay a lifetime with one particular orchestra. Instead, the prevailing point of view these days is that a conductor may be hired for a stint of a few years, but is expected to move on after a certain amount of time. This means, I believe, that it is even more incumbent on conductors to be able to establish a relationship with the orchestra quickly and efficiently. It means that a match of communication skills and personality is critical, if the orchestra and the conductor together are to accomplish their mission of making beautiful music.

Communication and personality

I've been talking about "effective" communication, by which I mean: "How does the conductor get what he or she wants?" And further, how can we put our knowledge of communication and personality into a model of interaction to help the conductor accomplish this goal?

The conductors I've observed and with whom I've worked, both students and professionals, have achieved a certain level of technical expertise. They are knowledgeable about the score, familiar with the method of conducting. Their basic conducting skills are in place. Furthermore, it is not my task here to evaluate what makes for good, much less superb, conductors. Working with the thesis that both "good" communication skills and personality style are critical components of good conducting, I aim to show that there is a way of putting the two components together so that conducting students have a frame of reference - a way of being evaluated and getting personalized, rather than generalized, feedback that will provide a concrete source of information they can use to improve their skills.

To that end, we have to break down the concepts of communication and personality style into manageable components, tease out useful concepts and describe a model, with the result that behaviours and skills can be evaluated, and practical, usable feedback given.

Communication in conducting

Of the two components, communication is relatively easy to address because some literature already exists on the subject. Communication in conducting is noted in several conducting manuals (e.g. Prausnitz, 1983; Rudolf, 1950; Green, 1986). Some of these talk about rehearsal technique: don't talk too much, be positive, don't be overly critical, when to visually cue musicians.

Much of the focus has been on the actual *gestures* - baton technique. In fact, Rudolf coined the phrase, "the relationship between gesture and response", as a means of evaluating whether the conductor is getting the sound desired, not merely as a result of how competent the musicians are, but rather, how clear the gesture is. Research confirms that the conductor has considerable power, through the way he communicates, to elicit the response he wants.

Conductors like to think they *are* good communicators. For example, I observed a guest conductor who did everything in rehearsal he told me afterwards he tells his own students *not* to do: talking too much, being overly critical and negative towards the musicians, singing on and on, interrupting at terrible times, etc. There are conductors who do get what they want, and think it is because they've harangued the musicians. They've bullied them into a good performance and "if it works, who cares what made it work?"

What I've observed, however, is that those conductors who consistently and efficiently get what they want are more interactive in body language and use more eye contact, giving visual clues by looking around often at the musicians at significant moments. There is a very clear and obvious relationship between what the conductor indicates he wants and then getting it. I have observed that a conductor may make several tries at getting a certain response before he changes his behaviour in order to be clearer. But, when he makes the behavioural change, the musicians respond accordingly.

As a case in point, I've observed that young conductors mistakenly believe the orchestra has all the power. ("If they wanted to play well, they would", one commented). Often, there is no awareness that their own behaviour is what primarily affects the musicians, and influences the outcome of their conducting efforts. Time and again, I have observed that the simple act of a conductor's pointing out a section that needs attention results in that section getting better - and the conductor getting what he wants. The conductor has used communication techniques to focus on a particular section: more bodily movements, gestures that may be clearer or even slightly exaggerated and, most important, increased eye contact with musicians, as well as verbalization.

Personality in conducting

Having isolated and confirmed the communication skills a conductor can use to increase effectiveness, the next step is to put these into a framework that is meaningful to the student conductor, that helps him or her apply communications skills in a way that is comfortable and natural to his or her own personality.

As we've discussed, there are some very clear-cut communication techniques conductors can use to enhance the relationship with the orchestra, and it would probably be helpful to make a list of these, hand it over to the young conductor and say "Practice using these over and over, and you'll get better." But saying the same things to all conductors, without regard for their individuality, and what might come more or less naturally to them, is not enough.

For example, if I said, "Use more eye contact", that simple statement can carry a host of meanings, depending on the person hearing the feedback. To one person, eye contact may mean the mere flick of an eyelash; to another it may mean fixing the orchestra with a Rasputin-like glare. The feedback is only useful to the individual in light of his or her own understanding and preferences - his or her personality.

The key to making the feedback meaningful is to give the conductor an understanding of his personality type. What comes naturally to him; what are his usual and comfortable ways of behaving? To address this, I use the Myers-Briggs Personality Type Indicator. This survey, which the conductor fills out on himself, takes about 30 minutes to complete and yields a personality type that provides the framework for giving feedback.

I have used the MBTI successfully with patients in my private practice and with business and non-profit organisations and expect to do the same with conductors. For, just as the personality types break down across the general population, so do they break down across the population of conductors.

Prior to observing a student conductor, I ask him to complete the MBTI. When I have tabulated the results I observe him during a rehearsal session, taking notes on communication strengths and weaknesses in the context of the MBTI results. Then follows a feedback session, during which I help the conductor to understand the MBTI results in terms of his professional behaviours, and what steps he can take to integrate communication techniques in a way that is natural and helpful. The MBTI provides the language the conductor and I use to have a dialogue.

Conclusions

So far, I have only one generalisation to make. There is no "perfect personality style" for a conductor. We are at the point where we can observe what occurs between the conductor and orchestra and analyse the interaction from a typology perspective. We can then consider and report what the pitfalls (and the strengths) will be for various personality types. Here are some of the factors I've looked at and a summary of my findings to date:

- Analytic, critical thinking vs emotional response.
- Attention to detail vs "big picture".
- Trust in intellect only vs searching for an emotional reaction to the sound they're getting.
- Attention to one detail at a time vs attending to several things at once.
- Engage and interact easily with the orchestra vs distancing and giving the orchestra only minimal information and directions.
- Use historical precedent and timeframe vs more instinctual and creative personal experience in present timeframe.

Let's look at some of these more closely:

1. Analytical thinking vs emotional response

It has been reported by a number of the conductors I have interviewed that the critical analysis of the score must be completed prior to the rehearsal; it cannot occur spontaneously. This is, of necessity, primarily a solo activity; the conductor may seek out other sources of data (recordings, historical information, etc.), but his score analysis is not dependent on personal values and feelings. In other words, his emotional response to the score takes a secondary position to his critical analysis at this point. Later, in his interactions with the orchestra, the emotional component enters the equation. Since both analytic and emotional mechanisms seem to go into making for a complete conductor, questions are raised as to how the naturally more analytic conductors handle the emotional component, and vice versa. Furthermore, extroverted conductors - those who are energized by interaction and engagement and, in fact, get many of their creative ideas in this manner - may have difficulty handling the more solitary activity of score analysis. And, there is the implication that those conductors who are naturally more introverted risk being unable to access their emotions.

2. Attention to details vs the "bigger picture"
In some ways this is an on-going dilemma: when to stop a rehearsal to make a correction, when to trust that the detail will correct itself, etc. The danger the detail-oriented conductor faces is that he never gets to the larger meaning because he cannot let go of the details. The threat to the big picture, pie-in-the-sky conductor is this naive expectation that if the musicians would only tune in, get on the same wavelength he is on, then beautiful music will result.

3. Extroverted vs introverted
Extroverts, those who look for interaction and engagement, will tend to want a response - verbal feedback from the orchestra. They may talk a lot but are frequently quite open to suggestions and spontaneous changes. Those conductors who do all of their evaluating and critical thinking internally run the risk of not giving enough feedback to the musicians regarding how they are playing. They give no meaningful response to what they get from the orchestra. It is an irony that the majority of conductors actually are extremely private folks; they are private not only about their personal feelings but also their ideas and how they put them together.

By combining these observations with an individual conductor's MBTI results, which will tell whether he is introverted vs extroverted, for example, or analytical vs emotional, it becomes possible to talk about when it is important to be engaged, or analytical, or interpersonally responsive. *All* of these are necessary functions for the conductor. If one understands one's own preferences for dealing with the world, it becomes much easier to make the needed shifts without feeling that one is acting out of character. It provides an objective perspective for looking at what goes on in the complex interaction of conductor and orchestra, and evaluating what works and what doesn't work.

Appendix: Anecdotes

1. Mark, (a conducting student and participant in a Conductors' Guild Workshop) went over and introduced himself to the flautist prior to starting the rehearsal. He was going to be conducting Debussy's *Afternoon of a Faun*, along with five other conducting students. He did this for himself - knew that he needed a personal connection with a member of this unfamiliar orchestra - and did something that probably worked to relieve some of his anxiety, bolster his confidence and, interestingly, help him focus. He probably will find it fairly easy to observe which musicians seem to appreciate a personal connection and, in fact, function better, and can learn how to incorporate this behaviour into his repertoire.
2. Prior to getting up in front of a student orchestra to be critiqued by a panel, a conducting student was re-reading the score, making the comment, "It is always

the details that escape me; I never seem to learn them as well as I would like." This model might be of use to him. He chose a teacher who is an expert at analytical attention to details. The teacher *could* see this student as flighty, undisciplined. He is, in fact, highly imaginative, intuitive, idea-oriented and has enormous difficulty attending to details unless he knows the purpose of those details. Yet he knows his brilliant insights will amount to naught unless they can be carefully translated into the details of notes, dynamic markings, etc. So, if this teacher can tolerate this student's style and the student can remember *why* he chose this particular mentor, it could be a very creative relationship.

3. There was an incredibly analytic, obviously bright, conducting student who described minute nuances in the score and obviously understood it very well. He had a very clear baton technique. However, there was no facial expression, minimal eye contact and he gave out so little information, except for his baton, that the result was a boring performance. Looking at the videotaped recording of this performance, he still did not attend to anything except the response of the musicians to his baton. When I raised the question, "Who was he looking at in the orchestra and why", it opened up a whole new perspective and he was clearly interested as well as convinced that if he were more extroverted and showed more emotion, he would in fact get a better result.

References

Galkin, E.W. (1988) *A History of Orchestral Conducting.* New York: Pendragon Press

Green, B. (1986) *The Inner Game of Music.* New York: Doubleday

Prausnitz, F. (1983) *Score and Podium: A complete guide to conducting.* New York: W.W. Norton

Rudolf, M. (1950) *The Grammar of Conducting.* New York: Schirmer Books

PART III
Therapy for Performers

From the bard to the board to the consulting room

Simone F. Sternberg

New York Center for Psychoanalytic Training

What has the theatre contributed to psychoanalysis and psychotherapy? First and foremost, theatrical metaphors permeate our clinical theory and practice. It has contributed a goodly number of practitioners, including actors, singers, dancers, directors and playwrights. The theatre has also contributed patients: some famous playwrights, actors and directors have been in analysis and have written about it or incorporated the experience in a play, e.g. *Lady in the Dark* by Moss Hart. Analytic writers often write up cases of actors who were former patients. Performers are not only dramatic and interesting, they're often intelligent and insightful. I have a particular interest in those patients who are not yet fully committed to a career as a performing artist, or the place such a career might have played in the past.

Role theory is pervasive in the literature of psychology and psychoanalysis. Rohrlich (1980) writing about work and narcissism, gives the example of a lawyer arguing his case before a jury "... if we do our homework, if we 'learn our lines', we are surer of being successful. In personal relationships, learning techniques, strategies and playing roles" get us only so far. Erikson (1950) uses the concept of role in discussing the adolescent's concerns with how they appear in the eyes of others in contradistinction to what they feel they are. He poses the problem of how to connect roles and skills earlier cultivated with present requirements. Adolescents artificially appoint "innocent" persons in the role of adversaries. The ensuing integration, in the form of ego identity, "is the accrued experience of the ego's ability to integrate all identifications with the vicissitudes of the libido, with the aptitudes developed out of endowment, and with the opportunities offered in social roles" (p. 261).

Jones (1922) uses theatrical metaphor in his remarks on the latency period. He speaks of a rehearsal of the whole process being performed in the first years of life. Then, at puberty, the person has to start again from the beginning and go through the drama in a more serious and dramatic fashion. Brenner (1982) writes of societal and environmental circumstances as factors setting the stage for the drama of each person's life "... by furnishing material used by each component of conflict that gives rise to compromise formations in psychic life" (p. 224).

Theatrical concepts are often used as metaphor in psychoanalytic writings from Freud to contemporary theorists, notably Joyce McDougall. Her two latest books are entitled *Theaters of the Mind* and *Theaters of the Body* respectively (1985, 1989). McDougall uses a theatrical metaphor for the analyst/analysand relationship in which the analysand is directing the play, peopled with transferential characters from his past. The analyst is cast in, and lends himself to, the role assigned by the patient in a particular session. It is the unconscious part of the mind of the patient in charge of all this activity; directing, playwriting, acting and behind-the-scenes stage crew.

The child therapist and analyst is often trained in these modalities. In play therapy the young patient is both playwright and actor, literally enacting scenarios; sometimes through puppets, sometimes casting the therapist in complementary roles. It is most helpful when the child supplies the dialogue and stage directions for all of the *dramatis personae*. Kernberg (1975) describes how the borderline patient assumes alternating identities within the same session, often alternating and/or exchanging with the analyst the opposite role, through projective identification.

Literature, poetry and plays have long been the wellspring of psychological and psychoanalytic insights. The Bard, Shakespeare, has such profound psychological acumen that one can find in his plays the most vivid, dramatic delineations of character types and the human condition. It is generally accepted that, like dreams, the careful reading of this playwright is an excellent road to learning about the unconscious and human motivation. How aware Shakespeare himself was of his psychological acumen and how much was unconscious is open to question.

[Some even question the true authorship of the plays attributed to him, as did Freud (Holland, 1964)].

Many analysts have been inspired by Shakespeare and have appropriated names of his characters to describe complexes and character types; there are those who have attempted the analysis of Shakespeare's characters and of the Bard himself. Some examples are Ernest Jones' paper, *The Oedipus Complex as an Explanation of Hamlet's Mystery* (1910) and his later published book, *Hamlet and Oedipus* (1949) and *The Amorous Death of Romeo and Juliet* by John Munder Ross (1987).

Freud's fascination with Shakespeare (and with other dramatists) is well known. In *Some Character Types Met With in Psycho-analytic Work* (1916) he uses Richard III, Lady Macbeth and Rebecca West (from *Rosmersholm*, Ibsen, 1866). Freud wrote extensive analyses of Hamlet (as did Jones, 1910), Macbeth and King Lear. In his paper *Psychopathic Characters on the Stage* (1942a) Freud delineates the preconditions for the enjoyment of this character on stage. To this end he used Hamlet, and boasted to a friend: "The conflict in Hamlet is so effectively concealed that it was left to me to unearth it." (Sachs, 1944, p. 105).

Freud believed that the purpose of drama is to reveal the sources of pleasure and enjoyment in our emotional lives. The spectator's enjoyment is based on illusion. Someone other than the spectator is acting and suffering on stage. As it is only make-believe, one's personal security is untrammelled. Hence, drama explores emotional possibilities and gives an enjoyable shape even to suffering and forebodings of misfortune. While Freud was immersed in the plays of Shakespeare, quoting from them liberally and in English, he was loathe to credit the Bard with authorship of the Oeuvre and never abandoned his conviction that they were written by someone else (Holland, 1964). That Freud could have been jealous of Shakespeare, and therefore unwilling to acknowledge his rightful place, is open to speculation.

Freud borrowed from Greek drama for the character and existential dilemma of Oedipus, identifying with the protagonist in his own triangular drama with his parents; love of his mother and wish to do away with his father, discovered in his self-analysis. The ensuing "Oedipus Complex" is perhaps the most famous complex of all. Sophocles' *Oedipus Rex* was his inspiration.

Shakespeare is not the only playwright to fall under scrutiny of the psychoanalytic community. A case in point is the study of Strindberg by Klaf (1963), in which the author analyses the playwright as well as his plays.

A particularly interesting study of a theatre person is that of Philip Weisman, *The Childhood and Legacy of Stanislavski* (1987). In contradistinction to the deprived, narcissistically hungry child who might later seek narcissistic gratification on the stage, Stanislavski had a golden childhood in which acting and putting on plays was encouraged by his parents, and culturally highly syntonic. Plays and entertainments were often staged at home in the families of the nobility and upper mercantile class (his family came from the latter) in Russia. Stanislavski as an adult continued to express his creativity in the theatre, as actor, stage director, theatre manager and finally theoretician. He was reportedly happily married to an actress, fathered a close-knit family and had a life-long love affair with the theatre, which became the outlet for his passion and energy, both libidinal and aggressive. This is an unusual example in that his early family milieu, and later his social and cultural milieus all supported his love of the theatre and his endeavours therein. For many actors and performers this is hardly the case; they often pursue a career in the theatre against tremendous opposition. Few families would encourage the theatre as a career choice for their children, unless they themselves were in the theatre, or particularly enlightened and monied. The effects of often massive negativity on the egos and self-esteem of performers has to be carefully weighed.

Similar to Stanislavski, others in the late nineteenth century particularly, both acted and managed theatres, often giving themselves starring roles. Also, the roles of actor and playwright are not antithetical. We know of actors who have become playwrights, sometimes continuing to act in their own plays. Shakespeare and Pinter come readily to mind. Writing one's own dialogue then becomes, if not primordial, at least as important as being the actor.

The metamorphosis from performer to therapist

Why do performers and playwrights change professions to emerge after arduous training as psychoanalysts and psychotherapists? A compelling reason for the switch is often an economic one. No matter how talented and motivated the performer, the marketplace is so highly competitive that most actors work at other jobs to sustain themselves, or receive unemployment benefits. The rewards of the occasional good part, or any part, might sustain the performer in his chosen endeavour, as intermittent reinforcement. As the performer grows older this precarious existence can become less viable, particularly if one has a mate and/or children to support. A colleague reported that some students from the Theatre Department had transferred to the School of Social Work to become clinicians at her university when they realized the difficulties of making a life and livelihood in the theatre.

Actors, singers and dancers are victims of the usual procedures for selecting performers at casting calls. Performers' egos are often fragile and it is hard not to feel personally rejected if one isn't given the sought-for role. This was a particular blow when recently an actress was told that she brought new dimensions to the role she tried out for, and yet was not cast in that role.

The difficulties overall, including working hours when most other people are resting or socializing, and less suitable and fewer roles as one gets older, the arduous life of being on tour, away from one's family and friends, and a host of others, lead some performers to re-evaluate their career choices. This is particularly true in mid-life, with or without the attendant "mid-life crisis". Some become directors, others teachers of acting, voice coaches, playwrights or enter other careers where they can utilize their performance skills. Parenthetically, playwriting is hardly more secure. Feirstein (1980) describes the production of a play of his and mentions the enormous difficulties in having one's work produced. In one case the producer died and along with him, the production. "I was soon to learn that American theatre would be a crapshoot I'd eventually stop playing." (p. 81).

Still other performers become psychotherapists and psychoanalysts. A colleague who is a musician/analyst continues to enjoy music by performing in a community orchestra and playing with friends. She says that in the role of psychoanalyst one sublimates one's artistic sensibilities in another way, e.g. having an ear for music, she also has an ear for what is being said, and the tonality (Carol Schultz, personal communication).

Playwrights also become therapists and analysts. The National Psychological Association for Psychoanalysis in New York has at least three affiliated playwrights and a theatre director who have become analysts. Other Institutes can count their share as well. The number of actors and other performers who become analysts is greater still. Feirstein (1988), a playwright poet who made the transition, speaks of the symbol-making ability - the preconscious use of symbols to bridge external and internal worlds. Conversely, the depth of experience gained as a psychoanalyst is useful to the playwright and to the writer. The difficulty is in finding the time to write a play or anything else, when one is in practice and often teaching as well. Role and identity conflicts can be engendered by the pursuit of two careers simultaneously, as both are so demanding. Notwithstanding, I know one New York analyst who is a successful novelist and screen-writer and three in France.

The actor into analyst

Aaron (1988) in discussing the transition from actor to analyst, viewed the actor's building of a character as akin to the birth of the ego. The actor determines the inner needs of the character, somewhat like Freud's (1923) delineation of the impulses. The actor's conduit to his own unconscious in realizing his character might sensitize him later as an analyst to the communications of his patients. The kinship between actor and analyst is often discussed in terms of empathy, necessary to both professions. Rowe, (Rowe & MacIsaac, 1989) following a Kohutian model, writes:

> Perhaps more than anyone, the professional actor exemplifies Kohut's idea that training and learning can make a difference. It is well known that a serious actor who really wishes to "get into the shoes" of the character he is to portray - not merely to do an imitation of that character - will spend hours in training workshops to get a sense of what that particular character might experience in certain situations. To enhance this awareness the actor may travel to a particular geographical locale, read biographical works, examine photographs and view films. These efforts help him gain access to a deeper, more accurate experience of how that character might think or feel .... There is a clear directive for the analyst to develop .... the potential for empathy. This is not unlike the responsibility the serious actor assumes in discovering the inner life of a character .... An actor uses the discovery of a character's inner life for artistic purposes .... an analyst uses the awareness of a patient's inner life for scientific purposes; that is, for understanding and explaining in the treatment situation. (p 22)

Reduced to their lowest common denominators, there are two major schools of acting. In one, the externals are most important. The actor depicts the character through make-up, costume, gait, accent; putting on a show of the character to be portrayed. This actor can bring an audience to tears while making his fellow actors laugh on stage. The other, "method" acting, takes its sustenance from the work of Stanislavski and his collaborators (Weissman, 1987). In its most exaggerated form we have the "Dybbuk" model, or the actor possessed. We know of actors who have so merged with the characters they are portraying that they speak in the accent and retain the mannerisms and psychological problems of the character offstage, possibly to the point of a break with reality.

Most good actors work somewhere in between. The actor lends of his own experience, his own past and current sufferings, triumphs and joy to better empathize with the character he is portraying, while retaining his mastery of technique and contact with external reality. This is also a model for the analyst and psychotherapist, who must be well-trained, have a well-honed technique, but also the ability to place himself in the other person's shoes, to feel an empathy for the other and the correspondences within himself.

The former actor, unlike the musician turned analyst, has a harder time keeping his hand in the theatre and often finds himself giving it up altogether. The one exception I know of is that of a psychotherapist who continues to act in her community local theatre. I wasn't privy to the reactions of her patients but am sure they went to see her perform. She had leading roles and is a good actress. Another colleague had a last role in a Broadway play while making the transition to analyst. He analysed his patients' reactions and feelings about this. (I am not discussing here certain "Sullivanian" groups where the theatrical community and the therapeutic community are merged. Nor am I discussing psychodrama, which has its own benefits and pitfalls.)

Most analysts would shun the public exposure of the performer, although many of us sublimate our performance (with its connotations of exhibitionism) wishes by giving talks and teaching. How to sublimate "appropriately" can become a personal issue for the performer turned analyst. One colleague, a former actor, often dreams that he is on stage. When anxious, he dreams that he has forgotten his lines. We as clinicians have to be careful not to vie for centre stage, or to upstage our patient in the analytic dyad.

From mime to psychoanalyst

While preparing this paper I mused on how my background and training as a mime influence and shape my work as an analyst and psychotherapist. We all know of actors and singers as well as dancers who have become therapists. This is not a transition that mimes are apt to make. Perhaps this is a loss to both disciplines.

Recently, I saw again the film of Marcel Carné, *Les Enfants du Paradis*, depicting the life of the French 19th century mime, Dubureau. Carné's father is played by Etienne Decroux, my mime mentor. At a given point, speaking of a ham actor vaunted by the theatre owner as having talent, Decroux as Dubureau's father answers "But he is not a mime". "What is he then?" asks the owner. "An actor" responds Decroux, with a touch of disdain. The superiority of the mime over the speaking, grimacing actor, is clear.

I was trained as a mime in a hothouse atmosphere where the teacher was addressed as "Maitre" (as in art studios, and more commonly in Europe). We students/disciples dedicated a good part of our lives to the study of this art form and if we had vestiges of private life we tried to keep it quiet. We studied intensively, performed wordless improvisations on themes given by the "Master", wore mainly black to highlight the linear qualities of the body, and felt ourselves superior to other species of performers. The object of our study was to express as much as possible, both thought and emotion, through the body without the use of facial expression (easily turning to the grimace) or the spoken word. This renaissance of mime started in a French acting school by Charles Dullin to force actors to feel and think through their bodies, as an acting exercise. Masks were used to similar effect.

La Mandragore, the theatre company I later joined and comprised of fellow mime devotees, presented dialogue plays as well as pure mime, albeit stylistically performed in the manner of the Japanese Noh theatre. Ultimately the deprivation of the word, of language spoken, was too high a price to pay, and not always sufficiently dramatic. Although we felt the necessity to add the spoken word we still felt superior to other actors, having highly trained bodies and more extensive resources. We had been initiated into the deeper mysteries of corporeal expression.

Perhaps as a psychoanalyst/psychotherapist I feel more privileged, having taken the hardest clinical route and undergone a guild training not unlike my mime training. I don't disdain psychotherapists not trained in analysis (like Decroux *a propos* of actors) but feel that the depth of my perspective and the range of my therapeutic tools is a distinct and added advantage.

Having worked at the cusp of language, where the idea behind the word is expressed by the body, I'm in a privileged position to work as an analyst and therapist, despite an apparent contradiction. A major aim of therapy is to make the emotion expressible by the word, the tool of communication between analyst and analysand. "Acting out" is "verboten", or at least to be curtailed and converted to talking out, or talking through. Similarly, the body as the mute actor gives way to the head and body working in concert to allow expression through the spoken word. Certain forms of dance and movement therapy bypass the word, as does primal scream therapy, at least for a time. A potential problem with these therapies is the need for extraordinarily skilled practitioners who are not fostering ventilation for the sake of same.

My mime background also sensitizes me to the posture of the patient, gesture and body dynamics, as well as pre-verbal and non-verbal language. An artifact of my mime training is a certain distrust of language, which makes writing particularly problematic. I think of words as approximations, valorous attempts to express that which is behind. However, there is a process of successive approximations, each attempt coming closer to the underlying meaning. We do the best we can with the tools at our disposal. Gesture alone also has its grave limitations, as cross-cultural studies are quick to show. The same gesture can have completely different meanings in different countries.

The body as the conveyor of the message, or an organ of the body, as in psychosomatic suffering, is a particularly fascinating arena of study. Here the mind has given up and is no longer aware of the message or metaphor corporeally expressed. This is not true of the mime, whose mind is well-honed and very much aware of the action. Here the body as mute and unthinking actor has to make its peace and become a working (and thinking) part of the whole person.

Traditionally the psychoanalyst is more or less silent, a good listener. We also talk (not only to make brilliant interpretations) but we don't talk very much, so that when we do, the effect is ostensibly greater. The ability to listen is part of the armoratorium of any good actor. The mime has to listen even more, attuned to inner voices and sounds as well as to fellow performers. The use of the unconscious and symbolic representation is evident both by the speaking actor and the mime. These are also the stock in trade of the analyst and therapist, as well as the much discussed "empathy" shared by both analyst and actor (Rowe and MacIsaac, 1989). Perhaps the mime has a more interior orientation, is more self-reflective (as was Dubureau in contradistinction to the actor in *Les Enfants du Paradis*). The idea that the unconscious of the analyst is communicating directly with the unconscious of the analysand, as well as communicating on a conscious level, is quite compatible with the practice of mime. The performer and the audience communicate on many levels, both conscious and unconscious. In therapy and analysis we hope to optimize the conscious communication.

Counter-transference considerations

When working with the creative person, and particularly with the performer, many issues surface for the therapist, especially when the latter is or was himself a performer. The subjects of transference and counter-transference are so wide-ranging that I will only briefly touch on counter-transference issues in this paper. A most obvious problem for the former performer working with performers clinically is identification and over-identification. It is crucial that the clinician be well analysed so that he is not working out his own unresolved issues through the patient. The old saw that we can't go further with the patient than we have ourselves gone is very relevant. We can be less than understanding, too impatient with the performer struggling with matters we think we have put behind, not anxious to have old conflicts re-opened for us. Conversely, we can be too attentive and nurturing, in an attempt to help the patient by-pass some of the pain we might in fact have suffered as a performer. We can try to force decisions that come not from the patient but from our own historical past. Finally, the performer patient might be grappling with narcissistic issues which contribute to his appearing overtly needy and demanding, monomaniacal and/or aloof, which make him more of a challenge to work with. The therapist and analyst must carefully monitor his/her reactions to the patient to deal fairly and objectively with the patient's needs (see Kernberg, 1975, for counter-transference issues in working with the narcissistic patient).

A poignant fear of many artists, especially performing artists, is that they will lose their creative gifts and charisma in the shedding or lightening of their neuroses; that they will be rendered colourless and ordinary. The fear might centre on the therapist who is perceived as the potential robber, or at least, as equalizer. The patient might imagine that the analyst/therapist is jealous of him; his gifts, his youth, his possible success. (Counter-transferentially, this is a special problem for those former performers who became therapists because they couldn't "make a go of it" in the theatre).

Contrary to this misperception, analysis and therapy can help the performing artist to realize his/her potential, to shine more truly and brightly both as a person and as a performer.

References

Aaron, S. (1988) NPAP Panel on Lay Analysis, *News & Reviews, 18 (2)* p. 8

Brenner, C. (1982) *The Mind in Conflict.* New York: Int. Univ. Press

Erikson, E. (1950) *Childhood and Society.* New York: Norton

Feirstein, F. (1988) NPAP panel. *News & Reviews,* op. cit.

Feirstein, F. (1990) *Contemporary Authors: Autobiography Series 11* Detroit: Gale Research, p. 81

Freud, S. (1916) 'Some character types met with in psychoanalytic work'. *Standard Edition XIV* (J. Strachey, Ed.) London: Hogarth Press, p 318

Freud, S. (1923) 'The Ego and the Id'. *Standard Edition XIX* London: Hogarth Press

Freud, S. (1942) 'Psychopathic characters on the stage'. *Standard Edition VII* London: Hogarth Press

Holland, N. (1964) *Psychoanalysis and Shakespeare,* New York: McGraw-Hill

Ibsen, H. (1886) *Rosmersholm.* In: *Eleven Plays of Henrik Ibsen.* New York: Modern Library, Random House (1977)

Jones, E. (1910) 'The Oedipus Complex as an explanation of Hamlet's mystery: A study in motive'. *American Journal Psychology XXI,* 73-113. Also in *Hamlet and Oedipus.* New York: Norton, 1949

Jones, E. (1922) 'Some problems of adolescence'. *Collected Papers on Psychoanalysis.* London: Balliere, Tyndall & Cox (1948) pp 389-406

Kernberg, O. (1975) *Borderline Conditions and Pathological Narcissism.* New York: Jason Aronson

Klaf, F.S. (1963) *Strindberg/The Origin of Psychology in Modern Drama.* New York: Citadel Press

McDougall, J. (1985) *Theaters of the Mind.* New York: Basic Books

McDougall, J. (1989) *Theaters of the Body.* New York: Norton

Rohrlich, J. (1980) *Work and Love: the crucial balance.* 196-210 New York: Summit Books

Ross, J.M. (1987) 'The Amorous Death of Romeo and Juliet'. In: *Tales of Love, Sex and Danger* (Ed. with Sudhir Kakar). Cambridge, Ma.: Basil Blackwell

Rowe, C.E. & D.S. MacIsaac (1989) *Empathic Attunement: the technique of psychoanalytic self psychology*. Northvale, New Jersey: Jason Aronson

Sachs, H. (1944) *Freud, Master and Friend.* Cambridge, Ma.: Harvard University Press p. 105

Weissman, P. (1987) 'The childhood and legacy of Stanislavski'. *Psychoanalytic Study of the Child, 12* pp 399-417

Performance as transitional object

Louise DeCosta

Institute for the Performing Artist, New York

The most frequently expressed fear of performing artists presenting themselves for treatment is that "therapy will take away their creativity". The concern for the artist - be it dancer, actor or musician - is that his ability to be in role, in character, or at one with his instrument will be diminished by his therapist's agenda to normalize him. Every performing artist senses his artistry on stage is contingent upon his own ability to live in and convincingly communicate the illusion he is portraying. In so doing he is asking the audience to temporarily suspend their personal realities and join him in his make-believe world.

Clearly, psychotherapists have come to understand that illusion is a psychological need and that, as such, it can be healthily enjoyed in a socially beneficial way or distorted into pathology, just as any need can be. However, psychotherapy within the Freudian tradition has considered artistry in a strictly pejorative sense - viewing the artist's playacting or artistic production as subliminal activity masking unexpressed or unacceptable instinctual wishes. The implication is that acting, dancing, or any creative endeavour represents, at bottom, compensatory phenomena (Fenichel, 1946). For Freud

(1927) illusion is a product of wishful thinking; a defensive maladaptation the ego has formulated against the harsh realities of the world. It is an irony that Freud, who created the way for us to see the developmental interrelation of pathology and health, was not able to apply his own discovery to the creative experience. Freud's view of adaptation to reality as the *sine qua non* of mental health would later be modified with the emergence of D.W. Winnicott's study of transitional phenomena and so the way was prepared for examining the methods by which the psyche necessarily comes to grips with reality.

Winnicott and transitional phenomena

Winnicott's central theoretical breakthrough is his study of how transitional objects are used by the child as a bridge from the child's inner reality to the outer reality of the adult world. For Winnicott, transitional phenomena are located in the psychological space he calls "intermediate space" or "potential space". In successful psychological development, this "space" becomes the location of all cultural experience, including artistry, which he also ties to "good enough mothering": "Here where there is trust and reliability is a potential space, one that can become an infinite area of separation, which the baby, child, adolescent, adult may creatively fill with playing, which in time becomes the enjoyment of the cultural heritage" (Winnicott, 1971 .108).

What then was the pejorative illusion for Freud becomes for Winnicott positive "potential space" or "the location of cultural experience". Winnicott redeems the idea of illusion in psychoanalytic theory and thereby expands the psychodynamic study of the creative artist. Whereas Winnicott fully recognizes pathological illusion, he contents that illusion *per se* is by no means pathological. For Winnicott, although illusion is not real, that does not mean it is untrue or maladaptive: "We are poor indeed if we are only sane" (Winnicott, 1958, p. 150). The psychologically healthy person is one who can use the transitional phenomena in a healthy way.

Winnicott's view of illusion as transitional phenomena - encompassing both pathological and adaptive resolution - represents a central organizing principle in my own treatment of the performing artist. Recognizing the importance of transitional objects of all kinds, be it the child's play or the adult's playacting, the therapist needs to approach the artist patient with curiosity regarding not only underlying resistive factors but the organizing functional aspects inherent in his choice of an illusion-making craft: the world of make-believe.

Three individual performing artists are presented: Adam, a professional actor, used his acting essentially as a transitional object enabling him to defensively deny any experience of himself as empty and uninteresting, a man who must perpetually play act with a woman. Gillian, a ballerina, used her dancing as a transitional object to deny the untenable reality of irrevocable separation from mother. Chantal's violin served as a transitional object in the service of autonomy and independence. Practising and performing permitted her "potential space" to develop the capacity to be alone.

In addition to viewing how each of these artists used their performance as transitional phenomena, the experience of mothering was focused upon historically as well as how it was lived out experientially in the transference. From the beginning of treatment with these three artists, prognosis was contingent upon 1) the therapist's ability to provide a "good enough mothering experience" and 2) the potentiality that their art, as transitional object, could serve increasingly adaptive functions.

Chantal

Request for professional help was received from a New York conservatory on behalf of a young violinist, Chantal. She was described as "sad, withdrawn, having poor appetite, and suffering from insomnia". Within the first ten minutes of our initial meeting Chantal voiced feelings of personal helplessness, a lack of self respect, and continuing depression. She was on the verge of "giving up everything", including music. To me, she was reminiscent of a large-boned, beautiful straw doll that "somehow lost its stuffing", as she slumped listlessly in my office wing chair relating her story in a monochromatic tone.

She and her lover had just "split-up" ... he was leaving her. This man was a violinist as well - a young artist of national prominence considered the logical heir apparent to Maestro X. Chantal was slow to reveal that her lover had suffered a nervous breakdown and their relationship throughout the previous year had been strained to breaking point. As he became increasingly paranoid, his cross-examination of her for alleged indiscretions (i.e. a glance at a stranger, a smile for a colleague) assumed inquisitional proportions. Anything less than a "full confession" from her admitting disloyalty and repentance failed to suffice. She then began to systematically cut off friends, and whenever they were together on the street Chantal kept her eyes downcast, avoiding the possibility of any visual contact with another. Essentially she became the personification of the Middle Eastern woman in purdah. She lived through and for her lover Abdul. Although she had a dim awareness that "something wasn't quite right" about his incessant demands, she took pleasure in his possessiveness: "Imagine me indispensable to this great genius!" She recalled hours and days together, he with his instrument in the living area and she with her violin in the bathroom. She would describe these moments as sheer ecstasy that surpassed even their sexual unions.

Teachers commented on her continued improvement as an artist, citing in particular the increased sensitivity and feeling in her playing. Before Abdul, "I was praised for my conscientious Swiss clock precision" but "because of him I changed and became an impassioned violinist". Chantal then disclosed a "disturbing" drama that occurred near the end of their relationship.

> Four people are carrying this large box that is shaped like a violin case. There was earth in the bottom but *nothing was growing*. One person was at each corner .... moving ever so slowly.

The dream was puzzling to Chantal but a feeling of great sadness enveloped her upon waking. She glanced across the bed towards the sleeping Abdul but decided against telling him about her dream. She expressed curiosity about the "pallbearers". There was a familiarity about them collectively but she couldn't recognize anyone. What startled her was the box, for it was her violin case, enlarged many times but unmistakenly her case. Where was her violin and why was the case so large and empty? Chantal, in an aggrieved tone, stated that the "case would never be empty unless I was playing". She wondered why she was so upset.

She spoke of her violin as an appendage. "If you took away my violin, it would be like cutting off my arm." She couldn't imagine life without playing music. She knew she was "growing" as a violinist - why, then, was the empty case so frightening to her. Chantal and I came to understand that her ghostly presence resided in the violin case (casket) symbolically represented by fallow soil "in which nothing grows". She had sacrificed herself to Abdul and his illness, which was "squeezing the very life from her". The dream was a recognition of her non-existence as an individual. Her reluctance to tell him of the dream was an awareness that he was somehow involved in her demise as a person despite his ability to help her grow as an artist. Paradoxically, as Chantal and I focused upon this nightmare of internal death, she experienced herself as enlivened.

Recently Chantal confided that she wants to understand her reasons for maintaining "such a sick tie". As she increasingly recaptures ambivalent feelings towards Abdul the person and relinquishes the fantasized "Abdul the Great", she has been able to return to her violin with renewed pleasure. She brings her violin to every session, laying the instrument on the couch while she slips into the chair. She teases me that I should consider charging double for there are two present and "both of us are getting better".

Chantal is renewing "lost" friendships and making plans for her own future. Her history permits us to be hopeful. This youngster, more than any artist with whom I have worked, enjoyed a childhood of nurturance and a more or less typical adolescence, including popularity with peers, academic and sports activities, as well as the presence of an attentive, encouraging, father.

However, she entered treatment in a severe regression. Her masochistic cleavage to Abdul sparked the therapist's curiousity about genetic precursors. Further exploration of her relationship with mother revealed an attachment that appears to have some echoing semblance to the dependency formed with Abdul. Chantal has recently expressed guilt about leaving mother.

> In a funny way, my violin took me away from mom. I was kinda glad. Maybe I even made it happen. I could have continued to study at home, but I chose to audition elsewhere.

Interestingly, this suggests a view of her violin as an "instrument of autonomy"; a way in which she might ultimately secure intrapsychic separation from mother. However, Chantal experiences herself in considerable conflict vis-a-vis her mother; the relationship to her instrument demonstrates this conflict vividly. On a number of occasions Chantal would describe longings for the absent mother and turn to her violin for solace.

> My teacher tells me the violin is the most haunting of all musical instruments for it is akin to the cry of the human voice .... Often when I play my violin I hear mother's voice .... Not words, really .... more intonation of her moods .... at times sad .... at times soothing.

On two occasions the therapist saw mother and daughter together and was strikingly aware of how much mother's own security was contingent upon Chantal. During these sessions mother related to her daughter as if she were a much younger child and made a direct plea that Chantal abandon her studies and return home "until the crisis passes". Chantal, however, chose to remain in training and complete the year "no matter how tough it gets". Her decision was reached somewhat apprehensively but relayed to mother with solicitous tenderness: "You know, Mom, I will call you every day".

Winnicott describes the "normal progression" that hopefully evolves between mother and child. At birth the mother enters a selfless co-mingling union with her infant. But then, as the infant emerges into his own, *so does the mother.* The mother must be able to transcend the experience of living in and for this helpless creature and "recover her own self-interest". My speculation, at this point, is that Chantal is more capable of relinquishing the "all embracing union" than is mother.

> When I am playing my violin, I feel as if I am at the centre of the universe. Nothing else exists except the music.

Winnicott suggests the "Capacity to be Alone" (1958) is contingent upon an experience of internalized good-enough mothering. The individual can enjoy solitude and privacy without feeling any loss of relationship. Winnicott further suggests this capacity may be essential for creativity to exist.

Adam

Adam tenaciously projects himself as an indefatigable lady killer. For him, tasting the joys of sexual and emotional closeness with a variety of women is the *sine qua non* of living. From the first day of treatment, Adam would reflect ruefully upon his own helplessness in the midst of a world populated by "Eve's own creatures". He experiences himself as ever vigilant and available for the next interesting woman.

Adam, an actor and a dancer, saw himself as Baryshnikov, "a cat among the corps". "Baryshnikov has screwed as many women as he had danced with." He, like Baryshnikov, was susceptible to the female presence; he, like Baryshnikov, would be immediately attracted to a strong, beautiful woman, only to become bored in time and move on to the next member of the corps. In treatment, however, he experienced himself as Rudolf Nureyev and the therapist as Margot Fonteyn. In reality, there were similarities - the therapist was an older woman whose role was to encourage and direct the younger man's development. As Nureyev came into his power as a dancer during his association with Dame Margot, the therapist assumed that Adam saw therapy as an opportunity for personal enrichment. His association of the therapeutic duo as akin to the theatrical partnership was seen as representing a hopefulness about therapy. Adam, however, was not so optimistic, and informed the therapist that the balletic partnership "was never what it appeared"; Nureyev was gay; Fonteyn was nearly at the end of her career. "It was not the exquisite romantic duo the public and press insisted upon". To Adam, the pas de deux was composed of two individuals cleaved together essentially for personal gain.

For the therapist, who initially enjoyed "the fantasized Fonteyn", there was a bitter countertransferential aftertaste with which to contend. (I did not appreciate my heroine being held in contempt - and me along with her!) However, I was curious about the transference implications within Adam's view of the calculating female partner and began treatment with an uneasy sense of having been forewarned.

Shortly thereafter Adam disclosed that he hated his mother because she never paid any attention to him, never spoke warmly, approvingly, or affectionately to him, never hugged him, and would only speak to him when she had something critical or disparaging to say. He had no memories of being held or kissed by her as a child. Mother was totally absorbed in providing financially for Adam and his older brother. Father abandoned the family when Adam was born.

His memories included being "left to cry himself out" as a child - a desperate loneliness that he would fill with an imaginary companion he created. This companion was a man who could masquerade in many guises. At times Adam became this other character; he felt unreal, but this was preferable to being totally ignored. Consequently, he came to feel that he was not himself. He recalled as a child having nightmares that he was invisible and was often afraid that he would not be seen by others.

As a teenager "I began to get a reputation". He was considered a ringer for James Dean, and he remembers playing the sullen rebel with effectiveness. "Girls really got off on it, for some reason." Thereafter he began a pattern of "hit and run intimacy" that continued throughout his adult years. Initially the therapist focused upon the flamboyant Adam, analysing his Don Juan activity in terms of conflict over wishes for intimacy and attempts to ward off the woman becoming too meaningful or he too dependent. The defensive mechanism was to decathect the object of either loved or hated aspects and maintain her as an anonymous sexual object - always transitory in nature. However, his conflictual wishes regarding relatedness were secondary to the greater imperative; Adam must take flight. Should he remain with a woman for any length of time, there was the danger that she would tire of him. "A woman can become disinterested real fast" i.e. the disinterested "mother" must be avoided at all costs - he can remain only as long as she appears fascinated with him.

Adam experienced himself working too hard in his conquests but was unable to stop soliciting more and more admiring females. Initially he presented himself to the therapist "for admiration" as well. He spoke of his numerous roles, highlighting a litany of professional achievements, both on and off Broadway. His mother had seen him on stage infrequently, claiming he was too far away. Adam was an accomplished Shakespearean actor and often spoke contemptuously of "lesser" colleagues, referring to popular film stars and TV personalities. Then, surprisingly, he auditioned for a prime time soap. He read for the male romantic lead and was hired. Elated, he mentioned with vindictive glee that this was his mother's favourite programme and "now she'll be forced to see me".

Recently Adam expressed interest in "trying the couch" but is "not ready yet" because he needs my face. Adam's sense of vitality comes from the reflecting presence of the female for it has to be experienced affectively from within. Adam the actor uses the audience's enraptured gaze to secure that experience he so desperately craved as a child. Successful playacting represents the closest phenomenal possibility of being seen by the original reflecting presence - mother.

Gillian

Upon meeting Gillian, my first thought was, "how do you treat an illusion?" A waif-like creature, more like a latency-aged child than her stated 18 years, her physical appearance suggested the skeletal shape of the anorexic and the translucent skin of a portrait on canvas rather than a real live flesh and blood person.

From the first moment in treatment Gillian embraced the therapist with a child-like tenacity, on the one hand clinging to each word and gesture; on the other taking the therapist to task for any experienced inattentiveness. Being with Gillian was like being in the middle of a mine field, living from one explosion to the next. She would rage against me, the unempathic therapist, but these diatribes paled in comparison to the venomous abuse heaped upon herself. Her conversation was filled with what her body was or was not. Mostly, it was fat and repulsive (at 90-95lb on a 5'6" frame). Food was discussed in excruciating detail. At times, I felt like therapy resembled nothing more than a culinary seminar. Her obsessive preoccupation with food was often intended to seek out the calorific culprit. Which offending food stuff was responsible for that additional ounce of weight? Did I think it was the sesame cracker, or might it have been the glass of low fat milk? She purchased clothes by the labelled size. The style of the garment was less important than the ticketed "Size 4". She saved these tiny tags in her jewellery box as if verifiable documentation of her svelte figure. The numbers were decreasing. Size 6 gave way to Size 4, and now she was working towards the magical "2". If only she could achieve this degree of petite perfection, life would be wonderful. She would be "just right" for once. Diuretics and self-imposed purges were part of her routine.

Her day-to-day life was filled with 8-10 hours of dancing (classes and rehearsals); her interest in anything beyond herself or her performance on stage was non-existent. It was as if the universe was limited to and resided within her body and its reflected image, be it revealed in the studio mirrors or the audience's applause. The therapist was overwhelmed with the relentless intensity of her self-absorption and the tenacity of the transference attachment, which was nonetheless experienced as being in constant jeopardy.

Initially Gillian sought treatment for a grief reaction in response to an enforced separation from her mother, who was dying of cancer. She complained of depression and a sense of utter meaninglessness. Gillian began describing life with mother and what they shared together. Their lives had evolved around Gillian's professional career. On several occasions mother and she had left the family behind in order to relocate in cities that offered desirable teachers. Mother as a young woman had enjoyed limited success as a chorine; a career that was suspended with marriage and child rearing. Later, she became a "stage mother", accompanying Gillian every step of the way from baby ballerina days to her final audition (and acceptance) into a prestigious dance academy in Europe. Mother devoted herself to Gillian, preparing nutritious meals, mending costumes and leotards, hammering pointe shoes into supple form, massaging aching muscles, trudging between hundreds of dance studios, the perennial "lady in waiting" rewarded during brief interludes whenever the two could snatch moments of communion. Then, when Gillian was 17 years of age, mother received confirming diagnosis of her terminal illness. Both were thrust into an abrupt separation, mother returning to the USA for treatment, Gillian remaining in Europe for her career.

Outwardly, Gillian "kept dancing", inwardly denying this unacceptable loss by devotedly "keeping mother present". Indeed, she portrayed mother's "hovering presence" so convincingly the therapist would find herself half expecting mother to be waiting outside the therapy room for Gillian to emerge. Time and again Gillian referred to herself as "mummy's tutu tot" - a pet name given in early childhood. It was difficult to think of herself other than as a dancer, for after all she and mother had lived exclusively for this end. Any form of mastery, be it balletic technique, new roles or teacher evaluations could be "validated" only in terms of mother's speculated approval. Invariably, Gillian would wonder what mother would say or feel or think. It was as if she existed 1) only as a performer and 2) in relation to mother; and indeed the intensity with which she clung to mother was reminiscent of an introjected pre-Oedipal alliance.

Gillian experienced herself "alive" primarily on stage. Her exhibitionistic needs were understood as her attempt to secure a sense of psychic wholeness. In performance, she and the audience were intertwined in a symbiotic feeding, a corollary relatedness not unlike the intense early mother child dyad.

> Mom and I were inseparable ..... she never missed a performance.

In order for Gillian to ensure her own psychological continuity, she needed to perpetuate the myth of the "living mother" abiding with her. Performing enabled her to do this. For Gillian, performance was the psychological equivalent of the child's teddy bear or blanket - transitional objects associated with the mother that provide solace in her absence. Gillian's symbiotic bond with her mother (based upon a developmental arrest), and the sudden irrevocable rupture of the enforced separation, had not permitted a gradual process of weaning to occur. It became clear that performance was, for Gillian, a transitional imperative. In fantasized union, mother and she shared one artistic triumph upon another, or more precisely, an unbroken bond.

Gillian would speak of the *timelessness* of the performing experience. While dancing she would have a sense of "time in suspension", a kind of psychic time-warp in which she could be "any age". She articulated the power of moments on stage "dancing for mother", to resounding applause, the triumphant rush backstage towards "mother in the wings". And then the cold, empty, reality .... the forced awareness that "Mother was not there". Those moments immediately after curtain calls were for Gillian unmitigated agony.

Mother died in Gillian's 19th year, the year she was accepted into the academy's principal company. Gillian's despair deepened. She saw herself as "the girl in the Red Shoes". Like the ballerina entrapped in magical pointe shoes that never permitted her to cease dancing, "I feel on a collision course". Thematic dreams of ceaseless pirouetting "round and round in never ending circles" led us to talk about her unending cyclical struggle with food. Essentially she maintained a revolving door existence (permitting nutrients to pass through and be expelled as quickly as possible) working towards the precipice of self-destruction. The inner voices compelling her to starve herself (i.e. symbolic joining with mother in death) would give way to self-preservation forces. However, Gillian's tragic compromise was to live continually on the edge of death. Permission to eat (i.e. to be a separate entity from her mother) occurred as attachments to living individuals began to form. Gillian entered into a quasi-masochistic relationship with one of her teachers; her performances were then devoted to him more and to mother less. The transfer of one dependency for another was nonetheless viewed as a developmental advance. The chaotic nature of the transference reactions seemed to decrease in intensity as she experienced us connected and herself more integrated. She was increasingly able to use something of mine, a word, a gesture, to calm and understand herself, resulting in her feeling better. And in the process, she instructed me in the art of becoming a "good-enough mother".

This represented a significant change. Whereas previously, my insistence on *not* attending her performances were viewed as breaches of unforgivable magnitude, later she was able to share verbal post mortems of her performances with me, and these performances were gradually experienced as more her "own" for as Gillian stated

> Mother is still there with me on stage, but I'm no longer afraid when the curtain falls.

Conclusion

This article has presented ways in which three performing artists used performance as transitional phenomena in bridging their inner and outer worlds. Throughout treatment, the author observed how each artist felt compelled to perform and how their performance served various transitional functions. Prognosis for growth depended on the individual capacity to use their musical artistry, acting or dancing in less pathological and increasingly adaptive ways.

Gillian was the most severely disturbed of the three artists presented, for her dancing represented a lifeline, a primitive cleavage to the maternal introject.

Chantal possessed a greater degree of psychic differentiation; nonetheless she entered treatment in a period of severe regression, deeply involved in a masochistically dependent attachment. However, the adult within sought help to recover from this "sick obsession" and "get back" to her music.

Adam performed non-stop. He lived "in role" 24 hours a day and was always "on" for the woman. Performance served primarily defensive needs, denying a deep conviction that he was unacceptable to the original woman - mother.

Having been influenced by Winnicott's work, I appreciate the importance of transitional objects of all kinds - from recreational play to fine arts to religious ritual - but for these individuals, performance was the transitional object of choice. Each performance was symbolically linked to mother and represented attempts to resolve developmental tasks that had been unsuccessfully negotiated within the mother-child dyad.

For Gillian, the symbiotic-like attachment with mother was never threatened until their separation. Mother remained the source of narcissistic sustenance in both life and death. For Adam, however, mother evoked considerable reactive aggression which seemingly fostered separation but in fact represented a spiteful withdrawal. He fled to a score of admiring females in a desperate attempt to secure from them that which he had never received from mother. However, Adam achieved a "false separation" only, for his acting career was often reactively based on a wish to be seen by her with an accompanying wish to punish her for not seeing him. His soap opera role was the vehicle by which he would force his way into his mother's visual path (i.e. mother's awareness). Chantal's autonomous strivings were tenuous at best, her dependent attachment with Abdul indicated difficulties with the self-object boundaries within the mother-child dyad.

All these artists were accomplished technicians in their craft and all had achieved considerable success. Chantal alone had experienced the father as available to her; Adam had never known his father, whereas Gillian's was experienced as emotionally distant. For each of these performers, mother was the significant figure.

Gillian secured psychological safety in merger-like attachments, clearly more sustaining than threatening to her autonomy. Adam sought safety not in merger but in flight. Rage at the unresponsive mother was re-enacted with a succession of women, who could potentially devalue him within an instant. Houdini-like, he was always poised for escape, the only position of psychological safety. Chantal was less firmly entrenched in either of these positions. Emotional security was precariously balanced on a psychic teeter-totter, fluctuating between moments of childlike dependency and joyful experiences of self-possession.

Each of these artists was struggling with issues related to intrapsychic separation from mother. Much of the treatment therefore focused upon the early object attachments. The aim was to provide a "good enough" therapeutic environment within the transferential relationship. In fact, the "transference as cure" represents an experiential illusion par excellence. The curious comingling of mother/therapist, past/present timelessness is itself a suspension of "reality" as we know it. However, we recognize that treatment experienced as positive and nurturing enables the individual to naturally develop transitional objects and ultimately become his own resource for bridging psychological and social worlds.

Are these performers - Adam, Gillian and Chantal - grown-up children who will always require their transitional objects of music, play-acting and dance? If one considers illusion within a pejorative light and chooses to focus upon their performance as primarily defensive resolution - perhaps so. But if one views the need for transitional objects in the way Kohut views man's ongoing need for self objects - as psychological imperatives from the cradle to the grave - then transitional objects are like oxygen we breathe and illusion is integral to our existence.

References

Fenichel, O. (1946) 'On acting.' *The Collected Papers.* New York: Norton, 1954 p. 349-361

Freud, S (1907-1908) 'Creative writers and day dreaming.' *Standard Edition,* Vol. IX pp 141-154

Freud, S. (1927) 'The future of an illusion.' *Standard Edition,* Vol. XXI London: Hogarth Press p. 5-6

Kohut, H. (1977) *The Restoration of the Self.* New York: International Universities Press.

Kohut, H. (1982) 'Introspection, empathy and the semi-circle of mental health.' *International Journal of Psychoanalysis,* **63**, 395-407

Winnicott, D.W. (1958) 'Transitional objects and transitional phenomena' (1951). In: *Through Paediatrics to Psycho-Analysis.* London: Hogarth Press

Winnicott, D.W. (1965) 'The capacity to be alone' (1958). In: *The Maturation*

Process and the Facilitating Environment. New York: International Universities Press
Winnicott, D.W. (1971) *Playing and Reality.* Harmondsworth, Middlesex: Penguin

Dreams, creativity and the problems of performers

Zuleika Robertson

Analytical Psychotherapist, Exeter

Creative expression is a direct link into the unconscious of every individual, uniting the head and the heart, promoting harmony between left and right hemispheres. For me, perhaps because I love pictures and images, the dream and the wisdom contained in its images is the ultimate creative symbol. And so, I would like to start by telling you a dream.

This is a dream that occurred during the course of the analysis of a man whose talents as a singer had been laid waste with the result that his rejected creativity had caused great havoc in his personal and business life.

> I seem to be travelling along some sort of canal in a large, glass-bottomed boat. It has a curved glass roof. I can see everywhere. At first, the canal winds through fields. It is beautiful. Then the canal winds through an exquisite garden with sweetly scented flowers. It is green and leafy. The colours are wonderful. There are some Greek statues. As I pass by, I see my youngest son, Angus, playing by himself at the water's edge. He looks lonely. As I get closer, I can see that he is

> worried. Then I can see that he is desperate. I reach out for him and bring him into the boat and make him safe. Now it is beginning to get dark. Suddenly, a bat appears and lands on the back seat of the boat. Darkness comes and the bat stays. When I look again, I notice that it has transformed into a moth. As I look at it close up, I see that it is a tiger moth. It stays for a while, resting on the glass roof at the back of the boat. Somehow, as daybreak comes, when I look again I see that the moth has become a butterfly. As I watch, the butterfly spreads its wings in the early morning sunshine and begins to fly about inside the boat. The butterfly then changes into a bird and begins to flutter about urgently. I open a window which has magically appeared on the inside of the boat and the bird flies out and begins to sing. The dream ends and I wake with a sense of elation.

This beautiful dream is a Big Dream. That is one in which the dreamer is brought into contact with the Collective Unconscious, the wisdom of the ages; in this case, the ancient Greek world, which produces the transformation symbol of the butterfly. The Greek word for butterfly is 'psyche' which also means 'soul'. The metamorphosis from bat to moth, both creatures of the night, to butterfly then bird, creatures of the day, defines by stages the emergence of the dreamer's art from darkness, that is the unconscious and the Shadow, where it had been repressed, deemed worthless, and therefore unavailable to the personality, into the light of consciousness.

Birds throughout mythology have been seen as carriers of soul and it is appropriately through the symbol of the song-bird that the dreamer's art is symbolically let out and set free so that it may sing. The glass boat is his vehicle in life, his ego; in its shape it is reminiscent of a cocoon. Glass in dreams often denotes problems with feeling, being a man-made substance, a poor conductor of heat, through which one can see but cannot touch or feel. The boat also seems to stand for his ego-defences, the transparent shell through which he could see the world but not be in touch with it: an attempt to return to the womb, a man-made glass uterus, a retort.

In association to the dream, the meaning of the window, which magically appears in the glass, seemed for the dreamer to do with the analytic process which had shown him a way through the cocoon with which he had needed to protect himself against a difficult childhood, but which had now become counter-productive in adult life and was acting as a constraint. One might say that in the work of the analysis, a window has been made for him. As to the symbolism of the child, Angus is his youngest son, a musical, frail, sensitive and somewhat vulnerable child, into whom he had projected his own 'child', that is, his own lost creativity and potential, which had been abandoned and desperate. In the act of bringing Angus into the boat and making him safe, the dreamer is bringing a lost part of himself on board and taking care of it.

The man's story demonstrates just how powerful a force the creative energies are and how destructive they can be if frustrated, or consigned to the Shadow, that is locked away into unconsciousness, because they are deemed to be worthless. He grew up in a macho, working class culture, where to be creative or artistic meant that you were a 'poofta' (i.e. gay). His father, a cinema proprietor, did not value his son's musical gifts; after all, they were not likely to lead to a secure job (his father came from a Fife mining background where there was no time for art - his love of the cinema was perhaps his fantasy of another way - his mother was obsessed with religion and hugely negative in her influence): so that, with the exception of his music master at school, who saw his abilities and gave some encouragement, his parents' failure to value his creativity meant that he could not value it either and he succumbed at fifteen to his father's proposal that he should leave school and become an accountant.

Not surprisingly, he was a dreadful accountant. His career of twenty years was a catalogue of failures - he never retained any job for very long and was chronically in debt. On his father's death he took over the family's thriving cinema business and within two years it went bankrupt. He tried two other businesses and they too failed.

In his personal life things were no better. He married twice, abandoned both wives and four children. Apart from a constant sense of discontent, restlessness and dis-ease, he also suffered from chronic anxiety and was prone to bouts of depression, migraine and 'flu-like' somatic symptoms. By this time he was so desperate that when a friend suggested he have a Jungian analysis, he agreed, feeling he had nothing more to lose.

Gradually he began to sing again, taking part in local competitions and doing rather well. He had begun to take some lessons. The dream greatly enabled him in the process of laying claim to his neglected creativity and beginning to live it out. In doing so he had to face great fear, but it was in his nature to sing and therefore, although late in the day, he did surprisingly well. As his confidence increased, his symptoms gradually abated and a sense of well-being began to grow. Of course, by the time he was beginning to sing semi-professionally, which he did with some success, it was too late to enjoy the full career he might otherwise have had, and this was a loss he had to mourn and come to terms with. However, in the end, he found that what was possible for him to accomplish was enough, for the most important thing for him was the rediscovery of the joy of singing.

It is this joy in the execution of their art that has very often been lost by the time a performer consults someone like me with their performance problem. Soul has deserted the performer and he is overwhelmed by the primordial terrors of the unconscious, which is another way of describing stage-fright. Many eminent performers have their rituals for containing stage-fright. For instance, Pavarotti is never to be seen on stage without his handkerchief, like Linus with his blanket, and there always has to be a bent nail in the boards to bring him luck. He won't go on without either. Acute stage fright is really the flight-fight response gone into overdrive and often links back to early unconscious fears or experience of rejection; there is usually a shaky mother somewhere at the bottom of the problem. We have to remember that for all performers, our first audience is our parents, and the degree of affirmation we have received from our parents will very much determine our expectations of applause from our audiences of later life and the degree of our need of it.

A 31-year-old viola player in a national orchestra told me of a hand tremor which had troubled him for a number of years. In recent months the problem had worsened to such an extent that he feared he might soon be unable to contain it and would have to give up his job. The tremor was likely to be induced by the playing of a long, slow note, particularly in powerful, melancholic compositions where the melody line built by degrees, breaking off, dissolving and rebuilding again, gradually increasing the emotional tension, and finally arriving at an extended and almost unbearably poignant resolution of the harmonies. When asked if any particular piece sprang to mind, he replied immediately "The Brahms Piano Concerto". His face became contorted with emotion and I thought he might break down. Instead he told me how he had first heard the piece. It was on a school trip to hear a concert given by the Berlin Philharmonic Orchestra. He was ten. The music moved him deeply, but it was in the end too much; he began to feel sick and claustrophobic and finally had to rush from the hall. He sobbed outside by himself until a teacher found him.

I think it was Michael Tippett who observed that music is the quintessential expression of human feeling. The Brahms spoke for the heart of this ten-year-old boy, so perfectly encapsulating his longing and his sadness that at the time it was too painful to bear and he could not stay to listen. However, these feelings, which he was obliged to repress at that time in order to survive were still there now and beginning to fester away inside him. His body, through the hand tremor, was speaking for the sadness in his soul that badly needed to be addressed. Until he was able to do this, the hand tremor would continue to trouble him. The unconscious frequently speaks via bodily symptoms.

He came from an emotionally inhibited English musical family, where the only vehicle for feeling was music. Interestingly, issues concerning freedom were the commonest subject of contention between children and parents. He saw himself as a conformist child who lacked confidence. He was bullied at school. Music, he said, was "the only thing I was good at". His over-protective, rather anxious mother was at the root of shaky internal resources and negative Anima. His critical, repressive father who made his son carry all his own unfulfilled ambitions, was behind his constant fear of failure, feelings of worthlessness and consequent lack of confidence, especially amongst other males.

Ten years ago, he had begun his career as a professional musician and it was then that the first symptoms appeared. In other words, when he was required by the world to pass through the initiation gate into adulthood, by becoming an active, income-generating male, his unhealed wounds from childhood prevented him from accomplishing this task. He was still stuck at this psychological point a decade hence. There is an interesting anniversary effect here. He was ten when he first heard the Brahms. He was twenty when he developed the hand tremor. It was at thirty that the symptoms became so pressing that he was obliged to seek help.

The symbolism of the tremor of the hand is also interesting. The hero warrior needs a steady hand to slay the mythical monsters of the parental complexes that prevent his emergence into adulthood. If his hand trembles, he risks being devoured by the demons of unconsciousness and he is threatened by spiritual death. In the analytic work, the turning to face his internal demons and do battle with them was the task that lay before him.

I have one other case that I would like to share with you which is that of a soprano in her forties who suffered from an annoying tightness in the throat which was liable to be most troublesome in an audition situation and particularly when singing operatic roles. Unlike the viola player, whose symptoms so far remained manageable, this poor woman's singing career had been severely curtailed by hers. In one instance, when auditioning for the role of Despina in *Cosi Fan Tutti*, the tightness had taken a grip, interfering with her high notes, throwing her voice completely off pitch, and she had been obliged, most embarrassingly, to withdraw from the audition. The performer's nightmare had become real and so badly affected her confidence that, terrified it would happen again, she had given up operatic work and taken on more teaching to make ends meet.

We did some active imagination with a recurring dream about the nightmarish Cosi audition which she brought to one of our sessions to see if we could discover something about the throat tightness. We conjured up her panel of judges. We named them and we imagined them sitting around the room, waiting expectantly for her to begin the aria she had chosen. In her imagination she stood ready to sing. I had asked her to monitor her sensations and emotions as the scene unfolded and she now said she could feel the tightness beginning. She became distressed. She tried to sing but found she could not make her vocal chords respond. She could not get into the role. Some feeling was interfering as she tried.

In the past she had always tried to over-ride this interference, but now I asked her to do the opposite, to allow the feeling to come. She said, "I've realized, I'm terribly angry!" Her voice felt positively clogged with the mucus of anger and blocked tears that prevented her singing. As the imaginary drama advanced, memories flooded back of being in the living room of her parents' house, dressed in her pink party dress with the frill around the bottom. She would have to wear white socks and black patent leather shoes, the kind with a strap across the front that buttoned at the side. "I would have to sing for them when they had people in, visitors. I hated it, really hated it", she said bitterly. "They didn't accept ME. Oh, yes, they wanted my sweet little child's voice, they liked to bathe in the reflected glory of their talented little daughter. But when it was all over I just went back to being Silly Nelly, who always makes a mess of things.

In her perception, that is how it was. While she starred as the family's pet nightingale she got indirect approval from her parents - but offstage in her ordinariness she was rejected. In order to grow up whole, we need to have all of us, not just the starry bits, accepted by our parents. If they will not accept everything about us and love us unconditionally, helping us to transform our weakness and frailty into adult strengths, by their firm but loving guidance and support, we grow up carrying a repressed core of unacceptability in Shadow, which we are always terrified someone will see and reject, just as our parents did. It was this internal child/parent drama that got projected into the audition situation and it was onto the judges that she displaced all the stored up feelings towards her parents.

As with any neurosis, before it can be healed, we have first to understand it. We have to say to ourselves, what is the meaning of this or that symptom? Why is he or she getting it? They are clearly not making it up. There has to be a reason. In Jung's words, "If man doesn't pay attention to these symbolic warnings of his body, he pays in other ways. A neurosis is merely the body's taking control, regardless of the conscious mind."

I have to say that I have found analytic work with performers extremely difficult, for, particularly in the early stages, there are huge initial resistances to be overcome. These are the performer's projections into the instrument and the audience which may have become compensations for the parental affirmation, which never came, or was inadequate, thus making his whole relationship to both instrument and audience obsessive and compulsive. Obsessive behaviour is a response to something having been lost in the unconscious. In an analysis, the analyst must persuade the performer to withdraw these projections back from the external world and work with them as originating from the Self. To the performer, this feels as if he is being asked to give up his only means of receiving acceptance and love and is being effectively consigned to the abyss of his insecurities. This is a lot to ask of an analysand; sometimes it is too much and the patient does not stay the course.

The analyst must therefore build a secure and trusting relationship with his patient which is strong enough to hold the performer in the pain and distress to which he will be exposed when he realizes that his art is his best and only defence against rejection. However, if the performer has the courage and sufficient affirmation and support from the analyst to pass through this phase, far from his inspiration drying up, as many performers fear, if his talents are genuine, his performance will only improve, for he will be free of the obsessive need for applause. In other words, the artist will be able to relax and spontaneously and fluidly enjoy the making of his art, less troubled by interference, inhibition, self-doubt and fearfulness arising out of unhealed wounds of soul.

The performer, the father and me

Catherine Butler

Counsellor, Guildhall School of Music and Drama

In my work as a counsellor of music students I have identified two common peculiarities (1) a difficulty in separating their intellectual and emotional processes. Because of the nature of the relationship between themselves, their instruments and the music, there is no room for the observing self. (2) the internalized Father is frequently used not only as role model, but also as a regulator of their self-esteem.

I will explain my theory in psychodynamic terms. In the psyche of the performing or creative artist, the creative aspect of the unconscious formerly known as the id, or child (the emotional part of the psyche) and the ego (or intellect) seem to be *one unit*. This phenomenon subtly affects their relationship with the superego or conscience. The latter seems to have two parts. One has the usual parental characteristics, and the other is an artistic conscience, affecting the creative aspect of the unconscious. This has the effect of making the ego unusually vulnerable and dependent on the superego, and the process of healthy separation from the parents in adolescence is thus complicated.

In the development of baby and child, it is the mother who is experienced as the most influential parent. But I find that, in adolescence, women's lib has not yet permeated the unconscious of the music student, and whatever her career status, the mother is seen as the carer at home. The young artist's primary need is for a father who gives unqualified love, confident admiration, praise and understanding to his child. Without this, the adolescent artist is forced to take the risk of performing under unbearable stress, carrying a crippling burden of anger, guilt and fear.

Research method

The evidence for this theory was provided by the results of my research project completed in 1986. I studied a group of 13 self-selected students who formed a Performance Anxiety Group that met once weekly during the Autumn term, 1985.

One month after the sixth session, I interviewed each student individually for one hour and asked them 20 questions designed to discover how much had been "emotionally digested" (Table 1). I did another check in a group situation in May 1986, and again in December. These interviews gave me an opportunity to look at each student's individual problem and to give them some counselling. I also elicited eleven constructs about their life in general and performing in particular, which were placed within a Personal Construct Situation Grid. Fifteen elements were provided, covering different life situations. Eight were performing situations (e.g. playing to an audience, waiting to go on the platform), the others were social or familiar in character (e.g. being at a pub with friends, being alone at night). The students took away the Grids to rate the constructs on a 1-9 scale in relation to each situation element. The purpose of using mixed situations was to ensure that performance anxiety was placed in the context of the whole life experience, not just a musical one.

The comparison consisted of 23 musicians teaching at the College. Ten were the professors of the student Group members; the other 13 were chosen because (i) they were considered successful in their profession; (ii) between them they represented all the remaining sections of the modern symphony orchestra, early music and jazz; (iii) they were chamber musicians or soloists and thus might experience a higher level of anxiety than rank and file members of an orchestra or choir.

The questionnaire for the Musicians was an abbreviated form of Table 1, designed to elicit constructs about self, background and attitudes to performance anxiety, and their role as a teacher. They completed the same Situation Grid as the students, and all 36 Grids were analysed using a "GAB

Table 1. Questionnaire for the Students

1. What did your parents feel about you choosing to become a musician?
2. What kind of job does your father do?
   What kind of job does your mother do?
3. How do you think they see you as a person?
4. Why did you choose to be a musician?
5. Was the choice affected by your parents' feelings?
6. What would your alternative choice of career be?
7. What is music for - why do people go to concerts?
8. What does music do for you?
9. How did you feel about performing before you came to the Group?
10. How did you feel about performing a month after the Group ended?
    a) physically b) emotionally c) mentally
11. Has your view of your family changed at all?
12. Has your experience as a performer altered?
13. What do you think of your audience now?
14. How is your concentration in performance?
15. Can you accept your feelings of excitement?
16. Do you feel you know and like yourself more?
17. How do you feel about other students?
18. Have you been able to clarify your technical needs in performance?
19. Did you find the following helpful?: Being in the Group
    Self-characterisation
    Self-hypnosis
    Fantasy journey
20. Any suggestions or criticisms for future groups?

Flexigrid" programme which yielded correlations among the constructs and elements.

Results

My first discovery was that the occupation of the father, and expectations of the family was apparently related to performers' professional success. Of the 23 successful performing professors interviewed, no less than 17 had fathers who were either the bosses of industrial or professional organisations or self-employed professionals, skilled tradesmen or craftsmen. It would seem that they had imbued their children with the unspoken family message that life was a challenge, teaching them to value and develop independence, courage, self-reliance and self-confidence. The result was that their musician children had sufficient inner security to withstand relatively high levels of anxiety. Their most frequently shared construct or attitude to performance was "exciting-boring". They seemed to need the excitement of challenge and uncertainty in order to feel really alive. In several cases, boredom was equated with sleep or death.

The remaining six professors who had working-class or unskilled fathers, had a much tougher time. They were pioneers, and they experienced greater stress in trying to cope with the economic insecurity and endless competition. Three of the six had breakdowns in mid-life. The five males had married strong mother/wives from a more privileged background and only one had risked the responsibility of producing a child. The sixth, a woman, had produced two children but never played without taking beta blockers. Their shared constructs about playing were to do with fulfilling a need and expressing themselves; the opposite pole was again boredom. These people said they felt socially disorientated unless they were with other musicians. However, they suffered the dilemma Freud (1950) described: "It seemed that the essence of success was to have got further than one's one father and yet to excel one's father were something forbidden."

The implications seems to be that students with this kind of background need special care and attention while studying at College to prepare them for their future careers. Winnicott (1971) recognized this when he wrote "Artists, best of all people, remind us that the struggle between our impulses and the sense of security (both of which are vital to us), is an eternal struggle and one that goes on inside each one of us as long as our life lasts".

Performers' problems

My music student clients, only about 15-20% of whom will survive to work full time in their profession, are usually of above average intelligence and tend in Jungian terms to be "sensation-intuitive" types. However, they often have tunnel vision, suffer from envy and have a rigid and narrow view of themselves and their world. The exceptions are those who have already been to a university or have an alternative skill or occupational qualification. This was verified in my research by the seven professors who possessed degrees or a craft skill. They felt they had a more relaxed and broader view of life than many of their colleagues.

Artistic children, even when they grow up, never stop playing with the transitional object, the instrument. It is the link between the creative aspect of their unconscious and the creative part of the superego. Like the mother/baby relationship it is all-absorbing, satisfying and interesting. Above all, it is exciting to respond to the artistic superego's urging towards artistic perfection. Musicians have all the characteristics of the obsessional personality and thus are prone, when depressed or anxious, to promiscuity, somatic illness, drug and alcohol abuse. Poverty prevents most of my clients from using alcohol or drugs as a defence against anxiety, but they are frequently attracted to beta blockers. This pill prevents the physical symptoms of performance anxiety by immobilizing the adrenal gland. The performance is dull but accurate, the performer feels guilt about cheating and avoiding the challenge, he loses his much needed excitement and feels ashamed at not using his own natural resources.

A large element in creating good self-esteem in the performer is his relationship with his Professor, who usually shares the same kind of personality traits. This one-to-one relationship is very intense, parental in character, and the pivot of the student's college life. He or she is the musical parent, and often the recipient of his pupil's projected feelings about his real father or mother.

I'm inclined to feel that the performer's ego/creative aspect of the unconscious is one unit because my clients seem only to see themselves in relation to their instrument or voice - I'm a singer, trumpeter, etc. So much of the self is projected onto the instrument or voice that they cannot validate their existence without it. If the instrument is lost or damaged, the musician experiences massive feelings of loss similar to those of a broken love affair or bereavement, and if they cannot play due to injury or illness they suffer loss of identity, and deep depression. They frequently project onto the limb or throat their internal feelings of hurt or inadequacy. They then genuinely feel artistically dead, they have lost their raison d'etre. If they don't or can't practice every day, because of laziness or emotional disturbance they feel physically uncomfortable.

The internalized father

According to Storr (1960), "Most authorities who have studied creative people agree that one of their most notable characteristics is independence." If the musician is independent, and in some ways he is, why is it that sometimes he finds it so hard to separate from the parent? Why does he so badly need to be as John Donne (1967) put it, 'The Apple of the Father's Eye'?"

A paradox indeed. Let us look at why the father is used by the musical child to symbolize his superego, and how the critical internalized father can cause performance anxiety within the performer.

In the unconscious, the Father represents the masculine qualities of strength, both protective and aggressive, courage and daring. He goes out of the home into the unknown world to hunt, to take risks and overcome difficulties, in order to bring home the bacon. His skill and bravery demand pride, love and respect from his family.

In primitive tribes all over the world, adolescent boys go off with their fathers and uncles for months or years, to learn how to be a man. In most civilisations the tradition is that the son, especially the eldest, is apprenticed to his father to learn his craft. This is a powerful element in explaining the importance of the Father in the unconscious development of his child. He is seen as the Teacher, the Master Craftsman, the Wise Old King. The fairy story "The Three Languages" illustrates this beautifully (Bettelheim, 1976). In order to individuate, to find himself, the adolescent must become the Hero, demonstrate his courage and skill, slay the dragon and only then can he become an adult and win the hand of the Princess and inherit half the kingdom. This also applies to girls, who must use their masculine side in order to perform. The feminine qualities of sensitivity and delicate feeling are also shared between the sexes.

"A concert is like a bull fight - the moment of truth" said the great pianist Artur Rubenstein, and it's certainly true that in moments of high stress we are thrown back on our core constructs about ourselves, and our bodies react as if we were going into battle.

Anxiety is not in itself harmful, it creates heightened awareness, physical energy and the excitement which is necessary to communicate the emotion in the music to the audience. It is only when the level of anxiety becomes too high that it interferes with mental and physical control.

In the performing situation it is vital that the musician has really good self-esteem. If his father has given confidently admiring love, appearing in no way fearful about his son or daughter's desire and ability to succeed, the child's ego/creative aspect of the unconscious feels protected and confident. It is enabled to use its healthy aggression in the performance, without fear of retaliation from the parental part of the superego. The artistic aspect is working in concert with it, urging on the creative child to play. The artist is freed to take up his challenge and enjoyable fulfil himself. The Father has freed the child to go forth and become a separate adult.

Research confirms that having parents who enjoy listening to or playing music, gives the child a definite advantage, as they provide encouragement, finance for lessons and discipline for regular practice (Shuter, 1968; Hutterer, 1980). The young musician whose internalized father is seen as critical, envious, uncaring or absent, has low self-esteem, little self-confidence or assertion. He is too frightened of retaliation to express his anger. Life is seen as full of threat and performing is hell. The absent father can induce the guilt of Oedipal triumph. As the student begins to play, the ego/creative aspect of his unconscious projects the critical father onto the audience, which is seen as waiting for him to go wrong. His artistic superego is urging him to play as well as possible, while his parental superego is making him feel inadequate, guilty, frightened and angry. The combined ego/creative aspect of the unconscious experiences massive disorientation as a result of these mixed messages from the superego, chaos ensues and he cannot play. Like the Chinese Emperor's nightingale in the fairy tale, the independent artist can only sing when he is free. He cannot sing or play if he is gagged and tied forever to the internalized disapproving father, who haunts his unconscious like the Commendatore in Mozart's *Don Giovanni*, and who will eventually drag him down to hell. He will be punished for making love and playing with the forbidden muse - music.

This problem is eloquently described by Jacques (1970), who maintains that artists of all kinds who did not enjoy the approval of their fathers become victims of their upbringing during the mid-life crisis. They either suffer depression, breakdown, creative block or death at this period. The psyche seems unable to work through the realisation of the inevitability of death and also cope with the problems of long-held guilt and anger. It is unable to go on developing, so it expires.

Usually the quality of a composer's works and a performer's interpretation improves with age and experience. If he can weather the mid-life crisis, his music grows in depth and spiritual awareness. Virtuosi such as Mozart, Chopin and Mendelssohn show us in their letters, and evidence provided by their biographies, that they never gained their father's uncritical confident admiring love. They suffered recurrent depression and an inability to express their anger, except in their compositions, which, of course, come directly from the creative aspect of the unconscious. Before the mid-life crisis, this seems to enjoy some protection by its artistic superego against its critical parental side. Perhaps this is because composition does not involve the same kind of active physical and mental skills as are used in performance. At mid-life, Rossini went into depression and did not compose for twenty years. Berlioz did not write a note during the two years following the death of his father, who had wanted Hector to become a doctor like himself, and although he adored his son, could not accept his need to be a musician. When Berlioz was elected to the Academy, the greatest artistic honour a Frenchman can receive, his father refused to attend the ceremony. Berlioz wrote this pathetic letter to his sister, Adele:

> I am utterly dejected. I feel as if my life no longer has an object. Instinctively all my efforts had always been directed towards *him*. I wanted him to show that he approved of them. I hoped he would be proud of what I did.

In my research, five of the 23 Guildhall professors had disapproving, anxious or absent fathers. These musicians had suffered severe stress symptoms and breakdown during mid-life. Three had been helped by analysis or psychotherapy, and all said that if they had had the self-awareness gained through therapy when they were students, their lives would have been completely different.

Sexual implications

Much of the evidence I have presented has sexual implications. The instrument can symbolize the phallus and disapproval by the father implies castration and can cause a fear of impotence. The instrument as the symbol of music, the food of the artist's soul, can be seen as the good breast, the mother, and the loss can be felt as starvation. (When on holiday without her instrument one of my clients eats chocolate to comfort herself). The merging of the musician with his instrument is like the original harmonious oneness with the mother, and so the father's approval and support are needed the same way in adolescence as they were at birth. Two of my clients, whose fathers withheld their interest and approval, like the performer/composer Percy Grainger, actually changed their surnames.

For a girl, the same applies, but is shown by a fear of sex, and guilt about using her masculine side if her father shows ambivalent reactions to her assertion as a performer. She feels unsure about her sexual attractiveness; she is expected to be passive, seen, to adorn the background, but definitely not be heard. Most frequently these daughters feel their gifts are not valued, their achievements not recognized by their father. They don't really exist in his reality.

Spiritual fulfilment

The music student's gift cannot be acquired, it is given before birth, but must be paid for. The artistic superego demands that it be constantly exercised, used, practised and perfected. It is a fate the artist cannot escape. What is his reward for this activity, apart from the pleasure of using his skills? Musicians spend many hours alone, concentrating extremely hard on the here and now, which is the only reality, in pursuit of an artistic ideal. There is a strong similarity to the religious mystics who spend their lives in rigorous mental and spiritual exercises and physical deprivation in order to achieve the now, an ideal, the loss of self in the Creator of many names, God, Allah, Buddha.

The musician, who has had a similar discipline to the mystic, who has unconsciously been urged by the artistic aspect of the superego to achieve artistic perfection, has a similar reward. In a great performance he experiences a loss of self in an indescribable bliss - and this usually happens between eight to ten times in his career, it is always longed for, but never spoken about.

I believe that the artistic part of the superego is a representation of the

Father, the Creator, within the collective unconscious. He who gave the gift, rewards the child by revealing the mystery to him. It is through the musician's art that he keeps in touch with the real source of life, and when he is prevented from doing so he feels dead.

In my research all 23 Professors had experienced this phenomenon. In the interviews even the most cynical, had tears in his eyes, and I too, when remembering what was described as "a unique experience - spiritual expansion - into feelings that don't need explaining - fearful with joy - magic elation - happiness not like orgasm - forget myself, we're all together".

Before he can lose himself in the spiritual reality, a man must first find himself. All religions agree on this. This is what I hope to help my clients to do, so that they too may achieve their goal and receive their reward.

A couple of years ago I visited the Casa Verdi, the home for retired musicians and singers founded by the great operatic composer in central Milan. Walking into the courtyard, I was greeted by a tremendous noise coming from rooms on every floor. The residents were doing their daily practice. I was moved to tears. Everyone who could hold an instrument or could open their mouth to sing was, like the birds in morning chorus, singing and playing. For what? Never again would they take the risk of performing before an audience, but these elderly people could not resist the urge of the artistic superego to fulfil their task, to perfect their precious gift, to experience the joy of expressing their feelings. The child was still passionately involved in play within the withered body. These people were in touch with life and they were content. As Winnicott (1971) said, "Artists enable us to keep alive, when the experiences of real life often threaten to destroy our *sense* of being alive and real in a living way.

References

Bettleheim, B. (1976) *The Uses of Enchantment.* London: Thames & Hudson

Berlioz, H. (1969) *Memoires.* London: Gollancz

Donne, J. (1967) *Sermons: Selected Prose.* London: Clarendon

Freud, S. (1950) 'Disturbance of memory on the Acropolis.' *Standard Edition,* Vol. V London: Hogarth Press

Hutterer, J. (1980) 'Structural analysis of the performance anxiety syndrome as experienced among solo musicians.' PhD thesis, City University of New York

Jacques, E. (1970) *Work, Creativity and Social Justice.* London: Heinemann

Shuter, R. (1968) *The Psychology of Musical Ability.* London: Methuen

Storr, A. (1960) *The Integrity of the Personality.* London: Heinemann

Storr, A. (1972) *The Dynamics of Creation.* London: Secker & Warburg

Winnicott, D.W. (1971) *Playing and Reality.* London: Tavistock Publishers

PART IV
Performance Anxiety

Witches, demons and devils: The enemies of auditions and how performing artists make friends with these saboteurs

Martin Lloyd-Elliot

Arts Psychology Consultants, London

I would like to offer a model, a concept, which I use with performers who have specific problems around auditions, with particular reference to their internal voices. Others have referred to the inner voice as the superego. There are any number of labels you can use, but they all mean much the same.

Many performers use their internal voice to useful purpose. Monitoring a performance is necessary during rehearsal and practice, and can serve a valid function. But it is easy for the internal voice to reap destruction upon us and destroy a perfectly learned piece of music, dance or prose in a mere second, on occasion to sabotage five months of practice in a five minute performance.

I think of the saboteurs as being like witches, and the phrases they use to do us in, like spells. The power of this model relates both to the archetypal images it invokes in the client and the direct link with the child in all of us. Also, when therapy works, it is like magic.

This particular model is based upon Transactional Analysis (Campos,

1970) and specifically the concept of Life Scripts: the ongoing programme for our life drama which we follow, out of awareness, having had the original script handed to us like a tablet of stone by the parental figures of our early life. Script ways of being are maintained by messages we replay to ourselves in the privacy of the internal world. Their consequences are acted out in our observable behaviour.

Scripts with a curse are not uncommon. For example a typical script message from a parent might be: "If they gave a prize for being stupid you'd get it". The message may be overt or covert. What matters is the inference that the child makes for itself. On being continually told not to express or show sadness a young child will infer that it is bad to show feelings or express any emotions. This theme links many of the performers I work with, be they actors or musicians (especially singers).

In this paper I will outline a possible explanation of failing auditions, give examples of spells that performers have encountered, and demonstrate how these witches' curses can be lifted, liberating the performer to perform more effectively.

Stage fright at auditions is seen as shameful and degrading and yet paradoxically is accepted as normal and to be expected (Havas, 1973). I also think that auditions themselves can be shameful and degrading. The audition is charged with emotion. The whole setting is so judgemental, so authoritative. One trumpeter I worked with had previously been in the army. Every time he had an audition he immediately saw the audition panel as a collection of stony-faced Generals. This was followed by fantasies of firing squads. Others talk about the "jury" in hushed tones. The very name makes one think of judges, and punishment.

Many performers approach the audition with the unconscious assumption that they will fail. This is a "set up". They write the script before they even start. "I knew my first piece would go fine, but the main text was bound to be a disaster .... and it was." And they sound surprised.

Sometimes this failure prophecy protects against disappointment. It is a classical defence mechanism. Other times, more interestingly, it protects against success. In my experience many performers have a "Don't Succeed" script.

How does the fail script develop? Most performers have early memories of their craft: dancers who first danced the day after they learned to walk; actors who, when aged three, dressed up and stood on chairs for grandma and recited a poem; musicians who have sung for as long as they could remember. The growth of a performance art is truly integrated with physical development. These early recollections are characterized by the simultaneous development of our belief systems about good and bad, and our internal locus of control.

With the child performer there is a freedom and freshness of expression whose loss as adults we mourn. It is a tragedy that so many young people are subjected to the careless comments of adults, whose words are granted such power by children. The cruelty of harsh criticism, especially when unjust or misinformed, cannot be over-emphasized. We have all heard tales of terrible teachers. And some of us have suffered at their hands. As a child, I was rapped continuously over the back of the hands for inaccurate sight reading and as a result gave up the piano for seven years. But it is not teachers who give the worst venom, the harshest spells. It is parents, siblings, friends and, especially in maturity, our musical colleagues.

The biggest culprit of them all is often our own imagination. Children have a magical way of thinking. It is what Bettleheim (1976) calls animistic thinking, in which there is no clear line separating objects from living things. A child believes that it is true that a witch can turn a frog into a prince, and back again. So it is that children project onto adults around them magical powers and properties. Children also believe in good fairies and evil demons, and tend to polarize people into good and bad.

If a spell is cast by a bad figure, its power can be discounted and countered by the forces of good. But when a spell is cast by a good figure, or worse, upon oneself from within, this results in a double bind and internal conflict.

Why is it that some children are more prone to the attraction of spells than others? Why do we unconsciously make friends with these destructive inner powers? Bettleheim (1976) writes, "Evil is not without its attractions - symbolized by the mighty giant or dragon, the power of the witch, the cunning Queen in Snow White - and often is temporarily in the ascendancy. In many fairy tales a usurper succeeds for a time in seizing the place which rightfully belongs to the hero, as the wicked sisters do in Cinderella." It seems to me that some children particularly identify with these dark forces.

Here are some examples of spells that have been cast by outsiders. What matters is the way the words are heard and interpreted by the child.

A mother turns to her five-year-old, whose father is bedridden. "Don't sing dear, it makes your father sick".

An elder brother to his young chorister sibling: "Boys like you who sing are really little girls. Soon they'll cut your balls off." The child's sexual beliefs are often worth exploring as the development of a performing skill, and particularly the voice, is so directly integrated with sexual development and maturity.

Some spells are overheard. A drama teacher speaking to a colleague: "Of course the poor girl is hopeless, can't project to save her life; and her interpretation is terrible".

And this, to a girl, whose beautiful voice was developing and growing ahead of all her classmates: "Sophie, you're singing too loud". Or, more viciously still, "Mark, have you ever thought that chemistry might suit you better than the clarinet?"

Some children seem quite unaffected by these spells and go on to untroubled careers as performers. Others have no problems except at auditions. And others still internalize these negative sayings and slowly build up a whole repertoire of self-denigrating phrases. This mucky witches' cauldron is always happy to receive new additions. And as we develop intellectually so we build an inventive extension to this pot - a production house; now we can generate our own spells.

Society generates stereotypical, ignorant prejudices which we can feed on too: "All actors are neurotic and temperamental". This can be revamped intrapsychically as "I am an actor. Therefore I am neurotic and temperamental". There are also numerous college myths, handed down from one generation to the next. "You've got Mrs X auditioning you. You poor thing. She hates blonds. You haven't got a hope."

As adults, we have access to the internal critics at all times. "The internal voice talks to us largely in terms of the past and looming future, it loves to predict failures" (Green, 1986). As a result we begin doubting ability, become afraid of losing control, convince ourselves that we haven't practiced enough, and so on.

These spells we cast upon ourselves, based on our early experiences of adults speaking to us or about us as musicians, get nastier and nastier. For example, on making one mistake in a Shakespeare recital a young student instantly switched on a psychic tape recorder saying, "If you can't remember that, you might as well give up". You may have noticed that some spells are spoken in the first person singular and others in the third. This often gives a clue as to the origin of the spell.

As we mature, we develop a new repetoire of these spells that are specific to performing at auditions. Under stress we become more vulnerable and what can be more stressful than an audition? One is expected to perform at one's best. The slave driver demands perfection. We are there to be heard, to be marked, to be assessed. The down side of striving for excellence. One member of the panel frowns and the actress says to herself, "They hate my face. I might as well walk out."

Sometimes the spells become almost life threatening. On failing an audition: "You failed. Just like your Mum told you would" and "You're no good at anything else. You're doomed" and the really dangerous, "I am my violin. If I cannot play then I am nothing - I should be dead".

I help clients to identify and catalogue their own internal repertoire of spells which are characterized by being so judgemental.

People are exceptionally adept at discounting progress too. A typical discount one dancer gave me on passing an audition for the first time after previous failures was this: "I didn't really deserve it. It was luck." This alerted me to the fact that the witch was still at work.

Transactional Analysis provides a simple and quickly understood framework for clients to conceptualize their inner processes. I find that the Parent/Adult/Child/Ego State model is especially pertinent to musicians, who quickly associate the 'Critical Parent'; state with their witch, and the 'Adapted Child' state with the scared, powerless, tearful person they turn into just prior to auditions.

Most important of all is the rebellious child ego state. There is a limit to the degree to which an Adapted Child will bow down to the authority figure commands handed out by the Critical Parent. The Critical Parent is often based on a real life ambitious musical parent. What better way to exert independence and control than for the rebellious child to hurt the parent by sabotaging the music.

So within the TA model the saboteur at auditions can either be the Rebellious Child or the Critical Parent. Both are destructive, but both can be usurped. Through awareness of the two principal destructive figures the transformation can begin. The performer rediscovers the Free Child within: that spontaneous, fun-loving, improvising, joyful, performer whose temporary loss they mourn. Simultaneously, they revive their artistic Nurturing Parent, who reassures, comforts, protects and guides.

Eric Berne also described strokes. A "stroke" is a unit of recognition, and can be positive or negative. Many of us actively collect negative strokes and deflect positive strokes about our singing. One opera singer I work with described this process to me.

> "I am halfway through an aria during an audition. There is a panel of three. One looks at his watch. I know at once that he is bored. I think to myself, he hates my voice. I'm singing terribly. I've failed the audition. I struggle on to the bitter end. It is awful. I leave the room shaking like a leaf. I feel sick. I am so ashamed. One of the two other singers waiting to go in comes over to me and says, 'That was really beautiful. I was so moved'. I just couldn't hear what he was saying. It was all lies. All I wanted to hear was someone saying 'That was terrible' and I would have been happy."

No matter how bad it is, if it fits the script, it feels right. There is a paradoxical comfort in a familiar feeling of misery.

On further exploring this theme, this singer realized he had never believed anything positive that someone else had to say about his performance. Previously out of awareness, he had determined that he had a terrible voice and no amount of evidence to the contrary would alter this opinion. To sabotage his performance was therefore to fulfil the prophecy. He had written himself a script. A story with a clear beginning, middle and end. It went like this: "You have the ability to make other people think you have a lovely voice, when in fact it is ugly and nasty. Whenever you sing, they tell you it's lovely, but you know better. You're a fraud. And sooner or later you're going to get found out. One day you're going to go into an audition. These are people who can see through your fraud. They will say, 'This man doesn't fool us. He's got no voice. He cannot sing. Take him away.' This won't happen until the last round. So you almost make it every time. But you'll never pass the audition." And so it was that his history of failing auditions repeated itself again and again. It became a learned response. In this case the treatment plan is to change the conditioned response by positively reinforcing alternative thoughts, thereby changing the witchy script.

Teaching performers to accept strokes can have significant benefits. Positive affirmations made in front of a mirror can also be powerful. For a singer who has an active saboteur to say again and again "I love my voice" can be almost impossible. They will rationalize their reluctance to try it, saying, "It's so self-indulgent, it's immodest". But persistence pays off.

Affirmations are like incantations: "I love music" said again and again, can lead to tears, shaking and ultimately great relief. "I love acting. My voice is strong, fine, clear. My voice has power. I am well and my voice is well. I am an actor." If done whilst standing in front of a mirror, this is even more powerful.

The performer learns that there are allies to be called upon to help at auditions. I say to musicians and dancers: "Befriend the accompanist. He is your ally. You're in this together. Use someone you know and trust. And the board are not the monsters they at first appear. They are there because they too are musicians. They love music, they want to share the experience of what you have to offer them. You have a gift. Your performance is the most precious gift you can give to them. In summary, the stages of change are:

1 Identifying the spells and their origin.
2 Enabling the client to be consciously aware of the bewitching process.
3 A detailed behavioural analysis of auditions, identifying thc point at which the spells begin.
4 Challenging the myths about auditions.
5 Challenging the fail script and offering alternatives.
6 Writing and then absorbing the new positive succeed script into unconscious behaviour and reinforcing the new responses.
7 Aiming all the time for a clear tangible goal, where the performance is characterized by a freedom from negative interferences, and ultimately, from all interference.

The principle is simple, the practical application more complex. But over time, it really does enable clients to change, especially in their performance. Problems at auditions are often multi-faceted and the therapist may find it appropriate to work with a combination of approaches, ranging from behaviour modifications to cognitive re-structuring. I have found an eclectic approach to performance anxiety at auditions most useful, but offer the above model as the starting point for the client.

References

Bettleheim, B. (1976) *The Uses of Enchantment.* Harmondsworth: Penguin

Campos, L.P. (1970) 'Transactional Analysis of Witch Messages', *TA Bulletin,* Vol. 9, No. 34 (April)

Green, B. (1986) *The Inner Game of Music.* London: Pan

Havas, K. (1973) *Stage Fright: Its causes and cures with special reference to violin playing.* London: Bosworth

Stress inoculation techniques and musical performance anxiety

Paul Salmon

The Genesis Center, Louisville, Kentucky

Musical performance anxiety (MPA) is a problem shared by many musicians, professional and amateur alike. It has recently been defined (Salmon, 1990) as the experience of persisting, distressful apprehension about, and/or actual impairment of, performance skills in a public context, to a degree unwarranted given the individual's musical aptitude, training and level of preparation. The treatment of MPA has received increasing attention in recent years, and although relatively few outcome studies have been conducted to date, available evidence suggests that techniques broadly on the Cognitive Behavioural Therapy (CBT) model (see, for example, Meichenbaum, 1977; Clark and Beck, 1988) hold considerable promise.

Cognitive Behavioural Therapy is based on the premise that emotional problems, including anxiety, stem from faulty ways of interpreting experience as the result of distorted thoughts and beliefs about oneself and the world (Goldenson, 1984). Stress Innoculation Training (SIT) is a form of CBT which focuses primarily on the events (Meichenbaum, 1985). It is the purpose of this paper to discuss applications of Stress Innoculation Training in the treatment of Musical Performance Anxiety.

The term 'stress' has been defined as a dynamic, bi-directional relationship between the person and the environment (Meichenbaum, 1985, p. 3). Stress has been conceived of in both positive and negative terms, depending on how adaptively one responds to it. The concept of 'coping' refers to efforts made by the person to come to terms with the demands of stressful circumstances (Lazarus & Folkman, 1984). In regard to coping with the stresses associated with performing, both short- and long-term strategies have been described. Coping responses to confront the stress of an imminent performance vary considerably. Ritualistic and superstitious behaviours have been described by many performers, including a gifted soprano who insisted that swallowing a raw egg before going onstage was the only way she could relax. "Self-talk", another common coping response, is used by many performers to "psych themselves" up for a performance, though not always with success. The cellist Piatigorsky, for instance, suffered from pre-performance "nerves", and reportedly told a friend, "... Before a concert, I say to myself, 'Grischa, don't be nervous. You are the great Piatigorsky!" The friend asked, "And does it help?" "No. I don't believe myself" (Beach, 1977, p. 61). Some coping behaviours have a regressive quality, as discussed by Aaron (1986), who describes various aggressive, sadistic and erotic back-stage antics of actors coping with pre-performance jitters. It is reported that Sir Laurence Olivier used to stand waiting in the wings, repeatedly muttering "You bastards" at the audience. In a related manner, Burgess Meredith once described the audience as "... the dragon to be slain..." (Little and Cantor, 1970, p 90).

These examples of coping behaviours associated with imminent performances are idiosyncratic and often seem amusing, but they serve the important purpose of helping to harness the powerful, and often threatening, sensations of heightened physiological arousal and disconcerting thoughts and images which frequently precede a performance. Indeed, Epstein (1983) described a process termed "graded stress inoculation" (GSI) through which we grapple in a proactive fashion with anticipatory mental representations of stressful events. "Inoculation" is used in a manner analogous to its medical meaning, in which controlled exposure to weakened pathogens stimulates immune responses which then become capable of withstanding a full-fledged attack. Used in a clinical sense, it refers to a process of a) anticipating the nature and impact of a stressor; b) learning appropriate coping responses; and c) initial implementation of coping responses via controlled exposure to low-intensity variants of the anticipated stressor (Meichenbaum, 1985).

Many individuals in stressful occupations appear to evolve coping responses reflective of GSI without therapeutic intervention. In a series of studies conducted on sport parachutists (Fenz & Epstein, 1967), for example, it was found that relatively experienced jumpers reported highest ratings of anxiety *in advance of*, rather than during, their jumps. These researchers suggested that anticipatory anxiety functions as a signal which stimulates active, preparatory coping responses such as mental rehearsal of the jump sequence, checking one's parachute and the like. In contrast, novice jumpers reported greatest fear within moments of the jump, when it was most likely to seriously interfere with their ability to function, and offered no opportunity to practice anticipatory coping responses. A recent study of pre-performance anxiety in novice and experienced musical performers (Salmon, Schrodt and Wright, 1989) reported similar results. Retrospective rating of anxiety at different time periods leading up to and including a performance revealed that relatively experienced performers report greatest anxiety and fear prior to, rather than during, their performances. It appears that, like their parachutist counterparts, experienced musicians experience feelings of apprehension and anxiety which serve as an adaptive, preparatory "warning signal" which fosters anticipatory coping responses. The components of anxiety reported by such individuals may include thoughts, images and even symptoms of physical arousal, which however, are of lower intensity than those associated with the actual stressor. Responding to these cues by practising, mental rehearsal, guided imagery, are related techniques that can help performers become capable of withstanding the stress associated with the actual event itself.

To a degree, GSI appears to reflect an innate stress coping procedure which many people deploy without conscious deliberation or formal training. A form of psychotherapeutic intervention termed Stress Inoculation Training (SIT) has been developed by Meichenbaum and others to achieve comparable effects in a more systematic manner (Meichenbaum, 1985). Much of the early work in this area focused on people exposed to physical risk, such as soldiers going into battle, or hospital patients facing major surgery. Briefing the person in advance of what to expect, teaching mastery and coping skills, providing a credible rationale for their application, and anticipating problems, insofar as possible, ahead of time are basic components of this model (Meichenbaum & Jaremko, 1983). It is a natural extension of such techniques to apply them in the management of anxiety and stress associated with musical performance.

Practically speaking, anxiety (including MPA) may be conveniently conceived of in terms of three components: cognitive, physiological and behavioural (Lang, Miller & Levin, 1983). The cognitive component of anxiety involves thoughts, beliefs and attitudes associated with a sense of risk and danger. The cognitive component of anxiety involves thoughts, beliefs and attitudes associated with a sense of risk and danger. The cognitive domain also incorporates information processing mechanisms, including attention and memory. Physiological symptoms are related to activation of the autonomic nervous system, and include heightened perceptual vigilance, increased heart rate, altered respiration, increased galvanic skin response (GSR) and related reactions (Papillo, Murphy & Gorman, 1988). Behavioural manifestations of anxiety include both physical reactions, such as shaking and motor tremors, and more generally, responses intended to aid in avoiding the object of one's fears.

All three domains contribute to the experience of anxiety, but the relative proportion of each present in a given individual at a particular time may vary. This is particularly true at relatively low levels of overall anxiety, a condition termed "response desynchrony" (Rachman and Hodgson, 1974). As anxiety increases, the relative intensity of symptoms in each category becomes more highly synchronized. Classes of anxiety measures are least at low overall anxiety levels, and increase as anxiety rises, as in panic states. Manifestations of MPA appear to vary in this manner, and in extreme cases have all the characteristics of a full-blown panic attack, with associated cognitive, physiological and behavioural symptomatology.

How can inoculation techniques help to manage this problem? The basic strategy involves helping performers to: a) come to view the various manifestations of anticipatory anxiety as an *adaptive* response signalling a need for active coping; b) develop appropriate coping responses; and c) implement these responses under circumstances of progressively increasing psychological pressure. Learning to respond to anxiety cues in this manner has two important effects. First, they become less threatening, and may eventually be "reframed" as expectable, and even desirable, reactions. Second, the overall intensity of anxiety tends to diminish as a function of exposure-based habituation. Each of the three components of anxiety; cognitive, physiological and behavioural, can be considered as a target for inoculation-based interventions. We will confine our attention to the first two of these, owing to their particular significance in the treatment of MPA. Treatment of the behavioural component of anxiety, especially pertaining to overt muscular tension, has been extensively discussed elsewhere (see, in particular, Woolfolk and Lehrer, 1984), and will not be considered further here.

Cognitive Inoculation

Performers with MPA are often troubled by worrisome and even catastrophic thoughts associated with performance situations. Fears of memory lapses, failure, physical illness or incapacitation, humiliation, embarrassment, insanity and even death are reported by anxious performers both in advance of, and during, their ordeals. In advance of a performance, such thoughts may evoke repression, denial and avoidance of anything associated with the performance, such as practising. In other words, the anxiety associated with a negative, anticipatory cognitive appraisal of the performance may effectively derail adaptive, preparatory activities, and lead to even greater anxiety in the long run. Appropriate SIT procedures consist of a) helping the performer learn to become aware of, and to monitor, anxiety-provoking thoughts; b) evaluate them realistically in terms of the actual degree of risk which they pose; c) reframe them in light of a more realistic appraisal; and d) use them as a cue for adaptive, preparatory activity.

According to Epstein and others, anticipatory cognitions comprise our principal means of coming to terms with potentially threatening events in advance of their occurrence, allowing us to develop and implement coping strategies. All too often, however, their occurrence invokes maladaptive anxiety, in part because it is the content - not just the occurrence - that is given the most attention. The thought, "I'll never be able to play this piece from memory" may evoke intense anxiety and, in a seemingly paradoxical manner, avoidance of practising altogether, because it is interpreted as a statement of inevitable fact, rather than a thought which is really more like a hypothesis. Anxious thoughts often do warn us about potential dangers, but they don't tell the whole story. In this example, the troublesome thought is an abbreviated, telegraphic summary of a more complete idea, "If I don't practice more systematically between now and the recital, it will be difficult to commit to memory, and I will either have to use a score or play a different piece".

The credibility often accorded these cryptic, telegraphic thoughts can be difficult to understand, because at face value at least, they're not particularly logical. The fact that their occurrence can be difficult to predict may make some performers believe they are accurate insights from the unconscious to be taken at face value, much like dreams with latent, symbolic content. They may have credibility because they've been associated with unpleasant experiences in the past, which we tend to see as predictive of future outcomes. They may reflect long-standing, deep-seated beliefs about ourselves which have continued to affect our behaviour since early childhood. Whatever the reason for their influence, they tend to evoke reflexive, maladaptive responses in many performers. Denial is perhaps the most common reaction to such thoughts, as in, "I don't *allow* myself to think such things". Denial and other defence mechanisms tend to channel mental energy into either patterns of compulsive avoidance *or* practice, as a means of keeping troublesome thoughts at bay.

The goal of inoculation therapy with respect to the cognitive domain of anxiety is to help the performer become more comfortable with, and able to act more adaptively in response to, what may otherwise be extremely disconcerting experiences. Stress is placed on the adaptive significance of the *occurrence* of thoughts, rather than their content, *per se*. The performer is encouraged to learn to accept anxious thoughts as an abbreviated, sometimes cryptic, signal, that something needs to be attended to. This idea draws on the idea of anxiety as a warning signal, which as Hoch pointed out, sometimes "burns down the house", is misconstrued (Beck & Emery, 1985).

Arousal Inoculation

Coming to terms with the sensations associated with physiological arousal can be quite difficult for anxious performers. The arousal state associated with live performances has much in common with that which we associate with anxiety, and indeed, the underlying physiological mechanisms have much in common. It has been traditional to invoke the "Yerkes-Dodson" law, relating task efficiency to arousal level, as a means of relating arousal states to performance. According to this relationship, arousal and efficiency are related as an inverted-U shaped function, suggesting that there is an optimal degree of arousal for the performance of a given task. Despite its persistence, the Yerkes-Dodson relationship has proven difficult to validate empirically, as noted in a recent review article (Neiss, 1988). Nevertheless, it fits well with descriptions by performers of the physical arousal state which they associate with effective performing - neither too high or too low.

Physiological arousal, associated with activation of the autonomic nervous system (ANS), has a mobilizing effect, preparing the person for immediate action. The associated symptoms, including rapid heart rate, shallow breathing, decreased skin resistance, cranial vasodilation, peripheral vasoconstriction and other responses are part of an "alarm system" which have a certain survival value. While they may serve as a warning signal of imminent danger, they may become the object of the individual's attention, with potentially disruptive effects. The likelihood of this appears to be enhanced, moreover, because arousal is associated with hypervigilance, which tends to heighten perceptual acuity. Many performers report feeling that their sensory acuity is enhanced during a performance, that they have clearer perceptions of the music, and they are especially sensitive to very subtle aspects of the music. This effect may carry over to the perception of one's inner, physical state, so that symptoms of even moderate arousal level may be *perceived* with heightened sensory acuity. Self-reports by performers of their physical status often contain gross exaggerations, such as tremors that were *obvious* to the entire audience, a heartbeat that could be heard by everyone, and the like.

To a performer, the state of arousal may thus have two effects: first it may impact directly, either enhancing or degrading performance skills. Second, it may become the object of cognitive appraisal, and a potent distractor which interferes with performing. The detection of arousal symptoms, such as a pounding heart, profuse sweating or shallow breathing, is frequently accompanied by concomitant anxious appraisals of their significance. This is one manifestation of what is termed self-focused attention, which we have recently found to be significantly associated with MPA. It appears to be related as well to the concept of "anxiety sensitivity", which represents a fearful response to symptoms of anxiety (Maller & Reiss, 1987).

Three aspects of arousal: its primary effect of mobilization, the enhancement of perceptual acuity, and the activation of cognitive appraisals, are hypothesized to combine in ways that make the overall subjective impact of this state quite unsettling for many performers. Performance-oriented arousal is associated with a wide range of perceptual and cognitive alterations that led one accomplished performer, an organist, to characterize it as an "altered state of consciousness" (Cramer, 1986). A significant area of investigation concerns the characterization of the performance "state" from a phenomenological standpoint. Indeed, interviews conducted with performers immediately following public performances (Salmon & Walker, 1990) suggest that alterations in time perception, distorted perceptions of body image, and dissociation, are regularly experienced, and frequently prove quite unsettling to the unwary. One organist recently reported that he would mute performance registrations somewhat over what he employed while practising, because, in a heightened state of arousal, fuller registrations sounded excessively harsh.

Clearly, the arousal component of anxiety is a prime candidate for inoculation procedures, the goal of which would be to induce manageable levels of arousal in a context where the performer can learn to tolerate, and eventually, habituate to their impact. There are problems, however, that must be overcome. First, performance-based arousal reflects activation of an innate, protective warning system with a relatively slow rate of habituation. Because of this, exposure-based treatment can be somewhat lengthier than might otherwise be the case. Second, performance-based arousal states can be difficult to otherwise evoke, so that performers don't have many opportunities to become accustomed to the qualities of this "altered state of consciousness". Recollections of performance experiences can change markedly as time passes, and some performers, when interviewed months after a performance, show a tendency to recall the experience as significantly more emotionally intense than they did in its immediate aftermath (Salmon and Walker, 1990). Third, many individuals developed stereotypic ways of responding to stimuli of markedly differing stressful content. This pattern, termed "response stereotypy" has been associated with maladaptive reactions to stress, because it constitutes an "all or none" response of the body to what by objective standards may be minimally stressful events. In contrast to response stereotypy is a more flexible reaction to stress reflecting what has been termed "response differentiation" (Berman & Johnson, 1985).

Despite such problems, graded exposure can, under the right circumstances, bring about significant habituation of arousal states, and at least one study, (Gerew, Romney & LeBoeuf, 1989) has reported that physiological state variables are more amenable to alteration via habituation than are cognitive components of anxiety. Inoculation strategies for dealing with arousal states basically entail inducing arousal in manageable doses while the performer practices active coping skills. The focus here is on "practice performances", with the stated goal of helping the performer become acclimated to the state of consciousness associated with a typical performance.

A state of generalized arousal can be evoked using any of several techniques. Some musicians with MPA find, on reflection, that they are extremely anxious during a lesson, with only the teacher present. Tending to associate their problem with playing before large audiences, they find that the presence of a teacher, or other musically-knowledgeable individual, is sufficient to evoke moderate levels of arousal. To the degree that this occurs, therapeutic intervention can be conducted *in vivo*, under circumstances which the performer identifies as evoking some degree of arousal.

Arousal can be induced in other ways as well, such as by simulating performance conditions. Recently, for instance, we treated a clarinet player who was extremely apprehensive about playing her opening solo notes of a piano concerto, and more generally, about "exposed" solo passages. Her entry occurred near the beginning, and the piece began on a off-beat, which made counting difficult. To make matters worse, the conductor was himself both a clarinetist and a perfectionist, who did not tolerate mistakes well. Rehearsals only seemed to make the problem worse, and she was considering finding a replacement to play the part. We found that exposure to a tape recording consisting of audience noises, the period of silence just prior to the opening notes, and the opening bars of the concerto was sufficient to induce marked arousal and subjective distress. The performer discovered that a number of catastrophic thoughts occurred to her during this period, including anticipated criticism by the conductor, and a conviction that she would be unable to deliver enough air to make a sound. Upon assessing the situation, she was able to identify a critical sequence of steps leading up to the opening notes, which when rehearsed and implemented, markedly reduced her anxious thoughts. The process included a) taking a deep breath and being ready to play prior to the downbeat; b) focusing on the conductor's baton, rather than looking directly at him; c) tapping and counting each beat up to her entry; d) taking a deep breath on the beat before playing; and e) playing the opening phrase. After practising this sequence alone several times, she did so first in conjunction with the tape, and then at the following rehearsal. By this time, having become used to what she had previously described as very unpleasant physical sensations of arousal, she played with substantially more confidence and focused attention, and ultimately handled the performance itself with aplomb.

Much of this treatment programme was developed by the performer herself, in consultation with the therapist. This represents an important aspect of SIT, which places major emphasis on self-oriented processes of self-assessment, skills development and gradual, *in vivo* implementation. Ultimately, the techniques which this performer employed were probably less important than the fact that she had taken an active role in planning and implementing her own treatment. Such an approach runs somewhat counter to what many performers perceive as a need to be told how to deal with anxiety, in a manner similar to the way they expect teachers to tell them how to practice. Since working with performers in this manner, I have noticed how creative, inventive and effective have been many of the solutions they have posed to the problem of dealing with anxiety. One music student, for example, contributed a striking metaphor, comparing performing to "surfing on the waves of anxiety". He used this powerful image to broaden his conceptualization of performing from being risky and dangerous to one that included feelings of exhilaration and excitement as well. Another performer, finding that playing from memory evoked excessive anxiety, experimented with systematically "sampling" the score at selected intervals, closing his eyes or looking away at other times. This evolved into the technique of printing out alternative measure versions of simple scores using a MIDI (Musical Instrument Digital Interface) keyboard, which he used as a transitional cueing system.

The list of potential stress inoculation techniques is virtually endless, and it is not at all clear that any one procedure is inevitably more helpful than another. What does appear to be clear is that the active engagement of the performer in his/her own treatment is an important element in imparting a sense of confidence and mastery of the challenges inherent in performing. Ultimately, the goal of SIT is to free the performer to perform as expressively as possible, unhindered by psychological stressors which complicate what might otherwise be a straightforward task. Perhaps this was said best by J. S. Bach, with respect to playing the organ: "It is quite simple. You have only to put your fingers in the right place at the right time and the instrument plays itself!".

References

Aaron, S. (1986) *Stage Fright.* Chicago: University of Chicago Press

Beach, S. (1977) *Musicdotes.* Berkeley, California: Ten Speed Press

Beck, A.T. & S. Emery (1985) *Anxiety Disorders and Phobias.* New York: Basic Books

Berman, P.S. & H.J. Johnson (1985) 'A psychophysiological assessment battery.' *Biofeedback and self-regulation, 10 (3),* 203-221

Clark, D.M. & A.T. Beck (1988) 'Cognitive approaches.' In: C.G. Last (Ed.) *Handbook of Anxiety Disorders.* Chap. 19, pp 362-385, New York: Pergamon Press

Cramer, C. (1986) Personal communication

Epstein, S. (1967) 'Toward a unified theory of anxiety.' In B.A. Maher (Ed.) *Progress in Experimental Personality Research,* Vol. 4. New York: Academic Press

Epstein, S. (1983) 'Natural healing processes of the mind.' In D. Meichenbaum and M.E. Jaremko (Eds.) *Stress Reduction and Prevention.* Chap. 2 p. 39-66, New York: Plenum Press

Fenz, W.D. & S. Epstein (1967) 'Gradients of psychological arousal of experienced and novice parachutists as a function of an approaching jump.' *Psychosomatic medicine, 29,* 33-51

Gerew, A.B., D.M. Romney & A. LeBoeuf (1989) 'Synchrony and desynchrony in high and low arousal subjects undergoing therapeutic exposure.' *Journal of Behavior Therapy and Experimental Psychiatry, 20,* 41-48

Goldenson, R.M. (1984) *Longman Dictionary of Psychology and Psychiatry.* New York: Longman

Lang, P.J., G.A. Miller & D. Levin (1983) 'Anxiety and fear.' In: R.J. Davidson, G.E. Schwartz and D. Shapiro (Eds.) *Consciousness and Self-Regulation,* Vol. 3, Chap. 4, pp 123-151, New York: Plenum Press

Lazarus, R. & S. Folkman (1984) *Stress, Appraisal and Coping.* New York: Springer

Little, S.W. & A. Cantor (1970) *The Playmakers.* New York: Norton (Cited in Aaron, 1986, p 68)

Maller, R.G. & S. Reiss (1987) 'A behavioural validation of thc Anxiety Sensitivity Index.' *Journal of Anxiety Disorders, 1,* 265-272

Meichenbaum, D. (1977) *Cognitive-behavior modification: An integrative approach.* New York: Plenum Press

Meichenbaum, D. (1985) *Stress Inoculation Training.* New York: Pergamon Press

Meichenbaum, D. & M.E. Jaremko (Eds.) 'The stress literature.' In: D. Meichenbaum and M.E. Jarenko (Eds.) *Stress Reduction and Prevention.* pp 1-4 New York, Plenum Press

Neiss, R. (1988) 'Reconceptualizing arousal: Psychobiological states in motor performance.' *Psychological Bulletin, 103*, 345-366

Papillo, J.F., P.M. Murphy & J.M. Gorman (1988) 'Psychophysiology.' In: C.G. Last (Ed.) *Handbook of Anxiety Disorders*, Chap. 12, p. 217-250, New York: Pergamon Press

Rachman, S.J. & R.I. Hodgson (1974) 'Synchrony and desynchrony in fear avoidance.' *Behavior Research and Therapy, 12*, 311-318

Salmon, P. (1990) 'A psychological perspective on musical performance anxiety: A review of the literature.' *Medical Problems of Performing Artists, 5(1)*, 2-11

Salmon, P. & J. Walker (1990) 'Immediate and long-term recollections of stressful musical performances.' Unpublished manuscript, University of Louisville

Woolfolk, R.L. & P.M. Lehrer (1984) *Principles and Practice of Stress Management.* New York: Guilford

Attention allocation and motivation in music performance anxiety

Daniel T. Wolverton and Paul Salmon

University of Louisville, Kentucky

Research suggests that we have a limited amount of attention to allocate in a given circumstance (Duval & Wicklund, 1972) and that the focus of our attention shifts over time (Kahneman, 1973). For example, during the course of a performance a musician's attention may shift periodically from the music, to the audience, to his or her own bodily tensions, depending on what is most salient at a given moment. During technically demanding passages, the performer may "bear down" and focus on the stream of notes. During more lyrical, slow-moving segments, he or she may become absorbed in emotions which the music arouses. A memory slip or an error may bring the image of a critical audience into clear focus. Moreover, as any one of these aspects of the performance becomes the focus of attention, the other aspects tend to fade in awareness. If attention is limited, then the question arises as to how it can be most adaptively allocated. Answers to this question in the domain of music performance could have useful implications for teachers, therapists and performers.

The primary purpose of this study was to see how musicians' patterns of attention allocation during a performance - the degree to which they focused on the audience, themselves, or the music - related to their experience of music performance anxiety (MPA). For instance, a pianist who *typically* spends a great deal of time during a recital attending to the expressions on an adjudicator's face, or to the tensions in her arms and hands, might be more prone to anxiety than a guitarist who typically spends the majority of the time absorbed in the sound and expression of the music. This possibility is consistent with findings in test anxiety research which indicate that "task-irrelevant" cognitions are associated with high levels of anxiety and poor performance (Sarason, 1986). Worry about negative evaluation and preoccupation with somatic tension are examples of task-irrelevant cognitions. "Task-*relevant*" cognitions, by contrast, are those cognitions which focus on the content and requirements of the task itself. Related to the notion of task-irrelevant cognition, Barlow (1988) has posited that "self-focused" attention is correlated with anxiety in performance situations. To the degree that a performer focuses on concerns of the self, attention to the performance task is diminished, and high anxiety and poor performance result. Our intention was to see if these findings would extend to the realm of music performance.

Motivation, attention and MPA

In a book on stage fright for violinists, Havas (1973) suggests that a useful way to help music students maintain an adaptive attentional focus while performing is to help them change their *motivation* for performing. Specifically, she recommends that they alter their motivational set while performing from one emphasizing concerns with audience evaluation to one emphasizing the broader goal of becoming involved in, and communicating, the music itself.

To clarify, motivation is a broad term for the processes which initiate, direct and maintain physical and psychological activities. It is said to embody persistent and "organized patterns of action" which move the individual "toward relevant goals" (Zimbardo, 1985). With this in mind, it is reasonable to assume that attention allocation is one of the activities affected by motivation. The way a person allocates attention may vary depending on his or her "relevant goals". For instance, if a musician is driven by a desire to impress the audience, then audience cues - facial expressions, applause or its lack - may become more salient. This is because they are integrally related to the performance goal: gaining audience approval. On the other hand, if the performer is driven primarily by a desire to lose him- or herself in the music, then audience cues become less relevant and the sonic properties of the piece may command attention. Presumably, in the latter case, the performer will engage in less self-focused, task-irrelevant attention and will experience less anxiety. In effect, a different motivational set will account for lower levels of MPA. With this in mind, a second purpose of the study was to see if musicians' motives for performing - e.g. to gain audience approval, to live up to their own standards of performance, or to become involved with the music itself - would predict how they focused their attention during the performance, and, additionally, whether they would experience MPA.

In summary, the first part of the study attempted to identify maladaptive patterns of attention allocation. The second part attempted to shed light on factors which could account for maladaptive attention allocation and MPA in terms of motivational differences. Specific hypotheses were (1) that self-focused and audience-focused attention would be positively correlated with high levels of MPA, while music-focused attention would be negatively correlated with it; and (2) that performers who were motivated primarily by a desire for audience approval would experience higher levels of MPA than those who were not. The latter hypothesis, it was predicted, could be accounted for, in part, in terms of differences in patterns of attention allocation.

Method

Subjects

Subjects were 36 popular and classical musicians (25 male and 11 female) performing on a variety of instruments - the modal instruments being guitar/vocal and keyboards. They were recruited by means of public announcements, through contact with a university music school and through contact with a local songwriter's organisation. They were generally experienced performers, having played for an average of 11.31 years. They moreover perceived themselves as proficient, based on self-report measures of technical skills.

Procedure

Upon contacting the experimenter, subjects were asked to prepare a short piece to play from memory before a small audience. Performances were conducted and recorded on videotape in a large practice studio, which contained a piano, a video monitor and videotape recording equipment. In order to induce moderate levels of anxiety, subjects were told upon arrival at the studio that the videotapes of their performances would be reviewed and rated by music department faculty members and skilled musicians. In addition, the experimenter was present during performances and triggered subtle audio and visual distractions. Subjects filled out questionnaires before and after their performances.

Measures

Self-report measures of anxiety were obtained via the State Trait-Anxiety Inventory (STAI) (Spielberger, 1983). The STAI makes a distinction between "state" anxiety - anxiety which occurs in a particular context - and "trait" anxiety - anxiety which is experienced as an enduring disposition *across* contexts. It is the most widely used self-report anxiety measure and has been found to have sound psychometric properties. The instructions of the inventory were altered to make them appropriate to music performance. Two self-report measures were developed for the purposes of this study. The first, the Music Performer's Allocation of Attention Questionnaire (MPAAQ), was designed to assess the degree to which subjects attended to the various aspects of the performance situation. The questionnaire involves 24 items to which subjects respond by circling numbers on five-point Likert scales to indicate how much they "thought about, considered, were absorbed in, were distracted by, or paid attention to" each item. The questionnaire is divided into four *a priori* categories - self, audience, music and other - involving six items each. A score ranging from zero to 24 is possible for each sub-scale.

A second measure, the Motivation for Performing Questionnaire (MPFQ) was designed to assess subjects' motivational set as they approached a performance. It involved six items, or sentence stems, each followed by three responses, which subjects were to rank in terms of how typical the responses would be of them. Based on these responses, subjects were placed into one of three categories: "external" - motivated primarily by a desire for audience approval; "internal" - motivated primarily by a desire to live up to one's own performance standards; or "music-oriented" - motivated primarily by a desire to become involved with the music itself. (Copies of the questionnaires are available from the first author on request.)

Results

Attention Allocation and MPA

Subjects were divided into low, medium and high-anxious groups based on STAI-state scores. Analysis of Variancc (ANOVA) revealed a significant effect for self-focused attention at different levels of MPA, $F(1,33) = 5.80, p < .03$. As predicted, high-anxious subjects scored significantly higher than low-anxious subjects on the "self" subscale of the MPAAQ $F\ (1,33) = 4.18,\ p < .03$. A significant effect was also found for music-focused attention at the different levels of MPA, $F\ (2,33) = 3.53,\ p < .05$. As predicted, high-anxious subjects scored lower than low-anxious subjects on the "music" subscale of the MPAAQ, $F,\ (1,33) = 5.25,\ p < .03$. Figure 1 graphs the apparently reciprocal relationship between self-focused and music-focused attention over the different levels of MPA. No differences were found between the groups on the "audience" subscale of the MPAAQ, $F(2,33) = 1.43$, NS.

Motivation and Anxiety

A significant effect was evident for *trait* MPA across the different motivational types $F(2,33) = 5.15$, $p < .02$. Externals reported significantly higher levels of trait anxiety on the STAI-T than did both Internals, $F(2,33) = 5.85$, $p < .03$, and Music-oriented types, $F(1,33) = 9.74$, $p < .005$. Though trends were evident, no significant effect was obtained on the measure of *state* MPA, the STAI-S, which was used to measure the anxiety subjects experienced during the actual experiment, $F(2,33) = 2.24$, NS. Figure 2 plots the scores for the three groups on the STAI-trait and state versions.

Contrary to expectation, the three groups did not differ in terms of attention allocation. Effects for self-focused attention, $F(2,33) = 1.43$, audience-focused attention, $F(2,33) = 3.23$, and music-focused attention, $F(2,33) = .17$, were all non-significant.

Discussion

Consistent with findings in other performance domains, self-focused attention was associated with high levels of performance anxiety. Barlow (1988) has suggested that self-focus fosters heightened physiological arousal, which sets into motion a spiralling rise in anxiety. This physiological arousal may be particularly damning during a musical performance because it may interfere with the fine motor movement and co-ordination required to play many musical instruments. A pianist whose fingers "lock up" during a run will pay an even greater 'price' for his or her arousal than a test-taker who has shaky handwriting. Also consistent with Barlow's discussion, self-focused attention appeared to vary reciprocally with the amount of attention paid to the task of playing and being involved in the music itself.

Contrary to expectation, audience-focused attention, which included preoccupation with evaluative concern, was not associated with high levels of MPA. This may have been due to the artificiality of the induction and to the fact that the 'live' audience was extremely small.

As predicted, those subjects who were motivated primarily by a desire for audience approval reported higher levels of MPA than those who were not. The fact that the trend was significant for trait and not state MPA may also have been due to differences between the experimental induction and a typical performance. The mechanisms for the overall finding, it should be noted, could not be accounted for in terms of attentional variables as Havas (1973) and Fogel (1982) have intimated. Further research may shed light on the factors which account for the apparent relationship between motivation and MPA.

Figure 1. Amount of self-focused and music-focused attention at different levels of music performance anxiety.

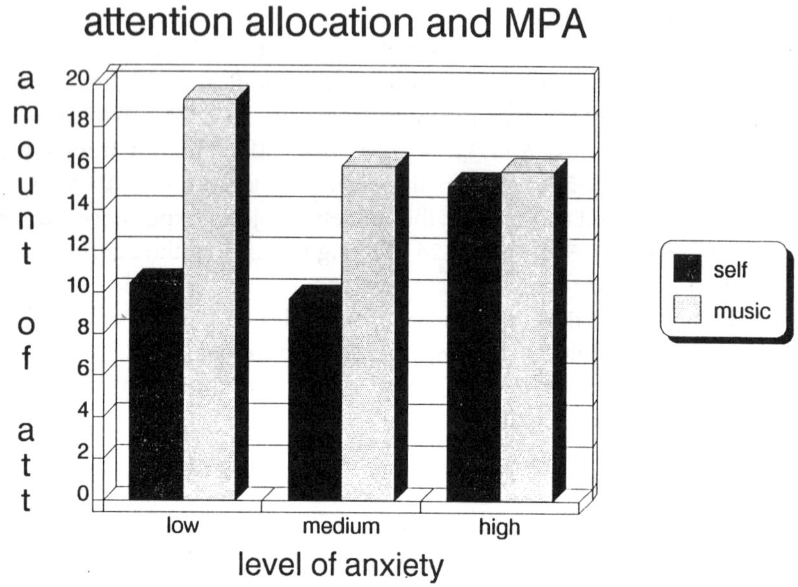

Figure 2. Levels of trait and state music performance anxiety reported by different motivational types.

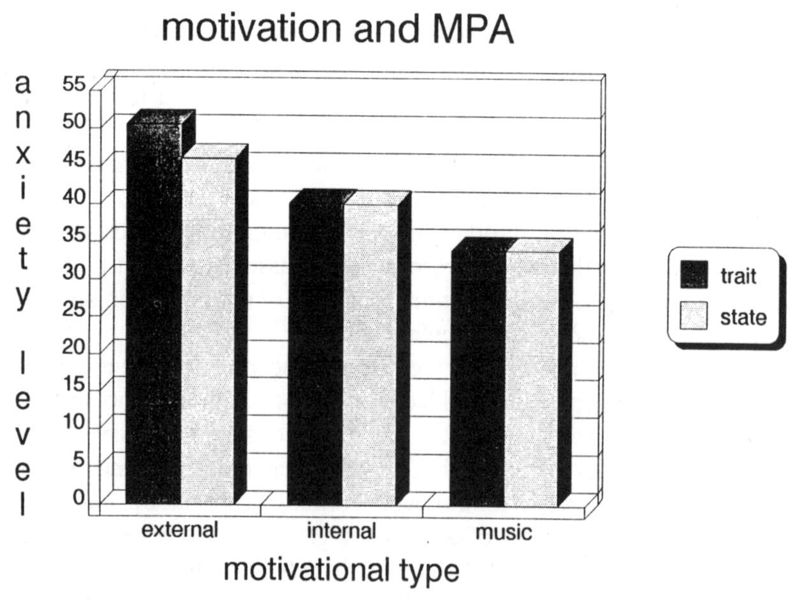

If the findings in the study hold up in replications, they may have interesting pedagogical and therapeutic implications. The Motivation for Performing Questionnaire (MFPQ) might be used as an assessment device to locate performers "at risk" for MPA. Additionally, cognitive restructuring techniques might be developed to help performers alter their performance goals and 'motivational set' as they approach a performance. Finally, attention-refocusing procedures such as those described by Meichenbaum (1972) in treating test-anxious subjects might be designed with the distinctive needs of musicians in mind.

References

Barlow, D.H. (1988) *Anxiety and its Disorders: The nature and treatment of anxiety and panic.* New York: Guilford

Duval, S. & R.A. Wicklund (1972) *A Theory of Objective Self-Awareness.* New York: Academic Press

Fogel, D.O. (1982) 'Toward effective treatment for music performance anxiety.' *Psychotherapy Theory, Research and Practice, 19,* 368-375

Havas, K. (1973) *Stage Fright: Its causes and cures.* London: Bosworth

Kahneman, D. (1973) *Attention and effort.* Englewood Cliffs, New Jersey: Prentice-Hall

Meichenbaum, D.H. (1972) 'Cognitive modification of test-anxious college students.' *Journal of Consulting and Clinical Psychology, 39,* 370-380

Sarason, I.G. (1986) 'Test anxiety, worry, and cognitive interference.' In R. Schwarzer (Ed.) *Self-related Cognitions in Motivation and Anxiety* (p. 19-23), Hillsdale, New Jersey: Erlbaum

Spielberger, C.D. (1983) *Manual for the State-Trait Anxiety Inventory (STAI, Form Y).* Palo Alto, California: Consulting Psychologists' Press

Zimbardo, P. (1985) *Psychology and Life.* Glenview, Illinois: Scott, Foresman & Co.

Alexander technique for musicians: Research to date

Elizabeth R. Valentine

Royal Holloway and Bedford New College, University of London

Frederick Matthias Alexander was born in Tasmania in 1869 and died in London in 1955. At an early age he became a 'reciter of dramatic and humorous pieces' and aspired to become a Shakespearean actor. However, his career was jeopardized by periodic attacks of loss of voice, particularly when under stress. On receiving no satisfaction from the medical profession and finding that rest did not cure his malady, he turned to his own resources, examining his manner of use by observing himself in a mirror. He noticed that whenever he was on the point of reciting he would pull his head back and down, tighten his neck muscles and suck in air through his mouth. Eventually he managed to train himself to inhibit this maladaptive strategy of anticipatory tensing.

Alexander (1932) considered that the key to efficient control of bodily movement was the relation of the head to the neck and back, the 'primary control' as he called it, a position of mechanical advantage. His view was that in general people develop habitual patterns of misuse, perhaps owing to the failure of instinctive control of the body to keep pace with civilisation in the evolution to upright posture. Typically, the head is pulled back and down, as in the startle reaction, when performing simple acts like sitting down. He believed this was particularly insidious because kinaesthetic feedback is unreliable and misleading. Alexander's aim was to re-educate people kinaesthetically in what he termed good use, a co-ordinated and balanced distribution of muscle tension throughout the body, resulting in an attentive state attainable under stress. Habitual, automatic reactions are inhibited and replaced by consciously controlled, directed actions. An important element is maintaining a state of openness with regard to the eventual act to be performed: thus at the critical moment a decision may be made to inhibit the intended action, to perform an alternative action or to continue with the intended one. Alexander preferred the term 'posture' not to be used: Dart's (1947) 'poise' gives a much better idea of what is intended. Lessons in the technique involve gentle guidance of movements by the teacher and the conditioned association of a new postural model to verbal instructions such as 'direct the head forward and up' or 'lengthen and widen the back', first given overtly by the teacher but subsequently covertly by the pupil. Good use is characterized by economy of effort and a subjective sense of lightness.

The work of eminent scientists such as Coghill, Magnus and Sherrington was invoked in support of Alexander's ideas, though now considered an unjustified extrapolation. Although many eminent people were numbered amongst his admirers, including John Dewey (see McCormack, 1958), Aldous Huxley, George Bernard Shaw and Nikolaas Tinbergen, who devoted much of his Nobel prize-winner's lecture to a discussion of Alexander's work, the theory has remained on the fringe of science and medicine. Amongst psychologists, Alexander's admirers have included Harold Schlosberg and Tony Buzan; amongst musicians Sir Adrian Boult, Sir Colin Davis, Barry Tuckwell and Sting have sung his praises.

In 1937 nineteen doctors writing to the British Medical Journal urged that 'as soon as possible, steps be taken for an investigation of Alexander's work'. Dewey undertook to get support for a scientific investigation from the Rockefeller Foundation but Alexander set up too many requirements and it fell through. In 1949 a grateful student gave $500 for research which was used for a pilot EMG study at Tufts. Then Dewey died and not long afterwards Alexander himself. As recently as 1978 Barlow wrote: "I appreciate only too well that the statistical background which doctors and scientists will eventually need is not very much in evidence" (Barlow, 1978).

Research on the Alexander Technique

Watson and Valentine (1987) administered a number of personality inventories and a questionnaire about the use of complementary medical techniques to sixty members of the London Sinfonietta. Of these fifty per cent returned usable data. The sample consisted of 22 males and 8 females with an age range of 26 to 59 years.

Both sexes scored significantly above the norms for trait anxiety on Spielberger's State-Trait Anxiety Inventory (Spielberger, Gorsuch and Lushene, 1979): the sample mean for males was 41.95 compared with the norm of 34.89 ($t = 2.27$, $df = 20$, $p < 0.03$, two-tailed) and that for females was 44.25 compared with 34.79 ($t = 3.12$, $df = 7$, $p < 0.02$). This is consistent with the work of Kemp (1981) who found that professional performing musicians scored significantly above the norms for anxiety on Cattell's 16 PF, that music students were more anxious than non-music students, and talented musicians more anxious than non-talented.

In our sample scores on the Performance Anxiety Inventory (Nagel et al., 1981) correlated negatively with years of experience as a professional musician ($r = -0.331$, $df = 29$, $p < 0.01$), age ($r = -0.38$, $p < 0.05$) and extraversion ($r = -0.41$, $p < 0.05$), and positively with neuroticism ($r = 0.61$, $p < 0.01$), trait anxiety ($r = 0.62$, $p < 0.01$) and state anxiety ($r = 0.54$, $p < 0.01$). The negative correlation between performance anxiety and experience suggests either that anxiety decreases as a function of experience or that those who suffer intolerable anxiety leave the profession. These results are similar in many respects to those of Steptoe and Fidler (1987) who attempted to disentangle the effects of age and experience by comparing three groups: professional orchestral players, music students and amateur orchestral players. However, the interpretation of their results is equivocal.

Fifty three per cent of our sample reported using anxiety reduction techniques of some kind. The Alexander Technique (AT) was easily the most frequently used technique, with 43 per cent of the sample admitting to its usage. This suggests a minimum usage in the general population of musicians of 20 per cent, allowing for possible sampling bias.

Some of the earliest research on AT was carried out by Dr. Wilfred Barlow (see Barlow, 1990) on army cadets. He suspended a tape measure from the back of their heads, enabling measurement of the distance to the bottom of their necks. The vast majority showed a shortening of this distance by an inch or more as they sat down or stood up, which they were unable to prevent and of which they were unaware. This confirms Alexander's view that kinaesthetic sensations are unreliable.

Physiological studies

Most of the attempts to provide objective evidence of the effect of AT have concentrated on physiological measurements. Frank Pierce Jones (see Jones, 1976, for a review), working at Tufts in the fifties and sixties, measured muscle activity and movement patterns for unguided and guided movements, using electromyography, X-ray and multiple-image photography, and a strain-gauge force platform. The X-ray photographs showed that employing the Alexander principle resulted in increased length of the sternomastoid muscles, increased width of the discs between the neck vertebrae and a forward movement of the centre of gravity of the head. The multiple-image photographs showed that the movements were quicker and more direct. This work has recently been criticized by Stevens (1987 and personal communication) on the grounds of artifacts due to touching the subject in the guided movements, slow sampling rates of the photography which induce various kinds of error, and out-moded anatomical and physiological knowledge. Stevens himself, under the supervision of Dr. Roger Soames at King's College London and in collaboration with Professor Finn Boyson-Møller at the University of Copenhagen, has repeated Jones's work, using more sophisticated electronic apparatus. Their results confirm those of Jones in showing that guided movements, in which habitual postural adjustments of the head and neck are inhibited, require less force, show less muscle activity and are quicker and smoother than habitual movements. Stevens, Boyson-Møller and Soames (1989) showed that guided sit-to-stand movements showed a decrease in head movements, ground reaction forces, and EMG activity in the trapezius, sternomastoid and erector spinae muscles.

Doyle (1984) in a PhD dissertation at Lancaster University applied physiological measurements to musicians. He undertook photographic and electromyographic analysis of the head-neck relationship during violinists' initiation of the act of playing. He claimed that the demonstrated association between neck tonus and the attitudinal response in the player supports Alexander and discusses implications for the pedagogy of violin playing.

Nielsen and Stevens (personal communication, 1987) found that AT effected a fifty per cent reduction in blood pressure before a concert in a group of musicians from the Aarhus orchestra in Denmark. This led Dr. Bent Ostergaard, consultant cardiologist at Aarhus University Hospital, to claim that AT offers a realistic alternative to beta-blockers for the control of stress-induced high blood pressure: it has as great an effect without the side effects.

Behavioral studies

The effect of other therapies for music performance anxiety, notably pharmacological and psychological, have been the subject of an increasing number of studies. For example, James et al. (1978) demonstrated the efficacy of beta-adrenoceptor blocking agents in controlling catecholamine-induced symptoms of music performance anxiety. In a two-way randomized double-blind cross-over trial of recitals staged at the Wigmore Hall, oxprenolol was shown to have a beneficial effect on various aspects of musicianship, notably tremor, as well as on both physiological and experiential components of performance anxiety. However, as a result of subsequent studies, there is now greater caution in recommending the use of beta-blockers. On the other hand, there is an increasing literature on the efficacy of psychological therapies for music performance anxiety. To quote two of the best studies: Kendrick et al. (1982) demonstrated the efficacy of cognitive behaviour therapy (involving self-instruction, attention focusing and replacing negative thoughts with positive) and behaviour rehearsal (practising performing) on cognitive and behavioural manifestations of music performance anxiety, although they had no effect on the self-reported experience of anxiety. Both therapies were equally effective in improving the quality of performance and in reducing negative thoughts. Cognitive behaviour therapy was superior to behavioural rehearsal in improving expectations of self-efficacy and in reducing visible signs of anxiety. Sweeney and Horan (1982) examined the separate and combined effects of cue-controlled relaxation and cognitive restructuring (identifying self-defeating thought patterns and replacing them by positive coping strategies, such as shifting attention from anxiety to the task). Cue-controlled relaxation improved performance competence and self-reported anxiety, whereas cognitive restructuring improved behavioural indices of anxiety; in combination they also reduced the physiological component of anxiety (indexed by heart rate).

Early work on the behavioural effects of AT was undertaken by Barlow (1956), who compared 44 students at the Central School of Speech (CSS) where posture was considered important, who were taught by conventional methods (verbal instructions, manual adjustment and exercises) with 30 students from the Royal College of Music (RCM) who were sent to him for lessons in AT. The students were photographed by an independent experimenter but scored by Barlow for postural faults, e.g. retracted head, dropped shoulders, rotated pelvis, lordosis, or internally rotated knees. He sanguinely remarks, "A given observer soon achieves a uniform pattern of scoring. My average scoring for the first and second year group only varied by 1%, which indicates that the method is accurate" (p. 671). The students were categorized as follows: 1 - excellent posture (0-3 faults), 2 - slight defect (4-5 faults), 3 - moderately severe defects (6-9 faults), 4 - severe defects (10-14 faults) and 5 - very severe defects (over 16 faults). Frequencies in each category are given before and after training for each group (see Table 1). Barlow claimed that the RCM group showed considerable improvement and the CSS group deterioration but no statistical analysis was conducted. Applying Kendall's tau to the results shows that there is indeed significant evidence of improvement in the RCM group ($z = 5.76$, $p < 0.001$) but the

Table 1. Postural fault category frequencies before and after training for RCM (experimental) group and CSS (control) group in Barlow's 1956 study

		Category				
		1	2	3	4	5
RCM	Before	1	0	14	13	2
(n = 30)	After	9	14	7	0	0
CSS	Before	4	5	19	12	4
(n = 44)	After	2	3	16	16	5

deterioration in the CSS group is not statistically significant ($z = 1.46$, $p < 0.05$). However, the difference between the two groups is highly significant ($z = 4.12$, $p < 0.001$). This is consistent with Barlow's conclusion that 'postural re-education will be ineffective unless a new "body schema" is taught, by associating the postural model with an improved postural awareness', but more evidence would be needed to demonstrate that this is indeed the crucial element in Alexander training, not to mention the need for the assessments to be made blind by an independent observer.

Barlow (1955, see also 1978) also reported a study of 50 opera students from a London voice and drama college, who had on average 37 lessons in AT. However, the study was unsystematic (he admits that 'a statistician might like to see it all planned out a little more formally') and the results are incompletely reported. Twenty of the students were subjected to Sheldon somatotype photography (while standing on a turntable nude!). Pictures for a selected five of these before and after re-education appear in the published report. Anthropometric measurements were taken and it is reported that 'all the subjects with one or two exceptions show small but definite increases in standing and sitting height and shoulder width'. Questionnaires were given to some subjects but no details are provided. It is said that personality tests and Rorschachs are being done. We are told merely that 'From my own point of view all the students expressed satisfaction with the procedure'. A report was provided by two professors at the college, which included the following generalizations:

1 In each case there was a marked physical improvement, which was usually reflected vocally and dramatically.
2 In all cases students since re-education were easier to teach. The students seemed to become aware of themselves in a new way.
3 Each student reacted in a different characteristic way. The time it took to

get results varied greatly between one student and another. The utilisation of the approach depended largely on the student.

4 Of eight students who entered a national singing competition in which there were over 100 competitors, six reached the semi-final, which is quite out of proportion to what would be expected.

They concluded that 'In our opinion, this approach is the best means we have yet encountered for solving the artist's problem of communication and should form the basis of his training'.

However, there are a number of obvious criticisms of this study. Subjects were not randomly assigned to the treatment, the sample included problem cases as well as 'normals', there was no real control group, assessments were not free from observer bias and the data are incompletely reported.

Frank Pierce Jones (1972) made recordings of a singer when in the habitual mode and when the balance of the head was altered by the experimenter in accordance with the Alexander principle (however, note the criticism made by Stevens). The subject reported that she sang more easily and with greater resonance and better breath control under the experimental condition. The difference in the quality of singing was confirmed by other musicians who listened to the tape. A spectogram confirmed increased richness of overtones and the virtual disappearance of breathing sounds during the experimental session.

In preliminary work at RHBNC, Rachel Williams, a music student, undertook some studies of the effect of AT on musical performance as part of her undergraduate dissertation. In the first study of performance class recitals, she asked performers to complete pre- and post-performance self-assessment questionnaires. Prior to performance they were asked to rate the adequacy of their preparation and their feelings about the piece and the performance, e.g. whether there were particular passages which caused them anxiety and how confident they felt. Performance was assessed by a qualified member of the music faculty on such things as adequacy of preparation, musical and technical quality and behavioural signs of anxiety. The sample is small with only nine subjects in the control condition and five who were receiving Alexander lessons (subjects practising yoga have been excluded from the present analysis). Statistical comparisons of the five AT subjects revealed only one significant difference and that was in a rather discouraging direction: the effects of anxiety upon performance were judged by the independent assessor to be significantly greater for the AT subjects than for the controls. In answer to the question 'How great do you consider the effects of anxiety on this performance?' the AT group scored a mean of 70.1 on a percentage VAS ranging from 0 (not at all) to 100 (extreme effect) compared with a mean of 45.3 for the control group ($t = 2.42$, $df = 12$ $p = 0.03$, two-tailed probability).

There is also a suggestion that in the opinion of the assessor mistakes were more attributable to performance tension in this group ($t = 2.00$, $p = 0.07$). Since the AT group was self-selected, this suggests that more anxious people seek Alexander lessons, which would not be surprising. In a second study on public recitals, two students receiving Alexander lessons were compared with six control subjects. In this case, Alexander subjects were judged to be significantly better prepared than controls (with a mean of 86.65 compared with 71.32, $t = 3.55$, $p = 0.02$, two-tailed test). Judged musicality of performance also reached borderline significance (a mean of 85.00 for the AT group as against 66.18 for the controls, ($t = 2.37$, $df = 6$, $p = 0.06$). However, it is not certain in this case that the assessor's observations were free from bias. So these results can only be taken as suggestive and need to be replicated on a larger sample, with adequate controls.

Summary and conclusions

The principals of the Alexander Technique have been outlined and research on its efficacy briefly reviewed. Most of the work has concentrated on physiological measurements. While considerable progress has been made on pharmacological and cognitive behavioural therapeutic interventions for the treatment of music performance anxiety, there has been very little systematic investigation of the efficacy of AT on behavioural and experiential manifestations. This is all the more surprising in view of the large number of musicians who use the technique and claim to benefit from it. The studies which have been undertaken to date have lacked adequate controls, viz. random allocation of subjects to treatment and control conditions, avoidance of demand characteristics and expectancy effects, and ratings by independent observers blind to subjects' treatment assignment. A study which will meet these requirements is in the process of being planned. If the efficacy of AT can be demonstrated, the next step would be to analyse the critical components.

References

Alexander, F.M. (1932) *The Use of Self.* New York: Dutton

Barlow, W. (1955) 'Anxiety and muscle tension.' In: D.F. O'Neill (Ed.) *Modern Trends in Psychosomatic Medicine*, p. 285-309. London: Butterworths

Barlow, W. (1956) 'Postural deformity.' *Proceedings of the Royal Society of Medicine, 49*, 670-4

Barlow, W. (1978) 'Research at the Royal College of Music.' In: W. Barlow (Ed.) *More Talk of Alexander.* London: Victor Gollancz

Barlow, W. (1990) *The Alexander Principle.* London: Victor Gollancz

Dart, R. (1947) 'The attainment of poise' *South African Journal, 21*, 764-791

Doyle, G. (1984) 'The task of the violinist: skill, stress and the Alexander Technique.' PhD thesis, University of Lancaster

James, I.M., R.M. Pearson, D.N.W. Griffith & P. Newbury (1978) 'The effect of beta-adrenoceptor blockade on the somatic manifestations of anxiety. A study of stage fright.' *Journal of Psychosomatic Medicine, 22*, 327-337

Jones, F.P. (1972) 'Voice production as a function of head balance in singers.' *Journal of Psychology, 82*, 209-215

Jones, F.P. (1976) *Body Awareness in Action: A study of the Alexander Technique.* New York: Schocken

Kemp, A. (1981) 'The personality structure of musicians.' *Psychology of Music, 9*, 3-14

Kendrick, M.J., K.D. Craig, D.M. Lawson and P.O. Davidson (1982) 'Cognitive and behavioural therapy for musical-performance anxiety.' *Journal of Consulting and Clinical Psychology, 50*, 353-362

McCormack, E.D. (1958) 'Frederick Matthias Alexander and John Dewey: A neglected influence.' Unpublished doctoral dissertation, University of Toronto

Nagel, J., D. Himle & J. Papsdorf (1981) 'A cognitive-behavioural approach to musical performance anxiety.' *Proceedings of the International Conference on Tension in Performance*, Kingston Polytechnic

Spielberger, C.D., R.L. Gorsuch and R.E. Lushene (1979) *Manual for the State-Trait Anxiety Inventory.* Palo Alto, Ca: Consulting Psychologists' Press

Steptoe, A. & H. Fidler (1987) 'Stage fright in orchestral musicians: A study of cognitive and behavioural strategies in performance anxiety.' *British Journal of Psychology, 78*, 241-249

Stevens, C. (1987) *Alexander Technique.* London: MacDonald

Stevens, C, F. Boysen-Møller & R.W. Soames (1989) 'The influence of initial posture on the sit-to-stand movement.' *European Journal of Applied Physiology, 58*, 687-692

Sweeney, G.A. & J.J. Horan (1982) 'Separate and combined effects of cue-controlled relaxation and cognitive restructuring in the treatment of musical performance anxiety.' *Journal of Counseling Psychology, 29*, 486-497

Watson, P. & E. Valentine (1987) 'The practice of complementary medicine and anxiety levels in a population of musicians.' *Journal of the International Society for the Study of Tension in Performance, 4*, 25-30

PART V
Therapeutic Applications of Performance

Dramatherapy and psychological change

Lucilia Valente and David Fontana

School of Education, Univerity of Wales, Cardiff

The starting point for the research to be discussed in part in the present chapter was the conviction that the creative arts carry a powerful potential for psychological change in both the therapeutic and the educational fields. Within the culture of the Western world there has been, from the time of the ancient Greeks onwards, an explicit awareness that creative experience fulfils deep-seated affective and social (and perhaps also cognitive) needs in human beings. Anthropological studies have shown that these needs exist similarly in non-Western cultures, and are met through the use of music, painting and particularly the imaginative re-enactment of myths and rituals. The literature on the subject is too extensive to be fully reviewed here (see for example Landy, 1986; Jennings, 1987), but Robbins (1980) suggests that the reason why the creative arts fulfil these needs is that they provide a bridge between the raw affects of our inner experiences and our more rational, conscious modalities.

Within conscious modalities themselves, the creative arts also enable us to deviate from traditional patterns of thinking, to form a new synthesis of ideas and of visual and auditory experiences, and - whether we experience these arts as performers or simply as observers - to allow for a shift of ego states which open us to new possibilities of being. They give permission for emotional expression, for the communication of feelings and insights, and for the re-formulation of self-concepts, of belief systems and of the aspects of overt behaviour to which these psychological structures give rise.

The use of the creative arts as agents for psychological change is now becoming relatively well-established in the therapeutic field through the medium of music, art and drama therapy, but in view of the extreme youth of these therapies there is much need for a formalization of thinking in relation to them. For example, we need to establish precisely which psychological models underpin the conceptualizations of those active within these therapeutic disciplines, and which writers and authorities have most influence upon them. We need to know how they define their respective practices, how they identify those clients most likely to benefit from these practices, how they recognize desirable therapeutic change, and how they monitor client progress.

Formalization of this kind would also help the use of the creative arts for personal/social development within education. For although the creative arts form part of the curriculum in schools at all ages and all levels of ability and need, there is no clear consensus within education as to the role they can best play in this development. Nor is there consensus on how they can best be used to help those children with particular problems of personality and/or social adjustment to come to terms with their difficulties.

The aim of our research is therefore to build up a comprehensive picture of how creative experience is used therapeutically. Our intention is to derive from this picture both some help towards the formalization of thinking within the creative therapies themselves, and some recommendations on how relevant aspects of this formalization can be used to influence the way the creative arts are offered in education. Although creative arts teachers are not therapists, we take the view that at an appropriate level, which we refer to as the pre-therapeutic level (Fontana & Valente, 1990), they can teach their disciplines in a manner specifically conducive to children's personal and social development.

Our examination of creative experience is restricted to one major creative art, namely drama, chosen by us because of its pivotal nature. Drama can variously employ monologue, movement, mime, dance, costume, music, masks, poetry and - through scenery and props - painting. It is dynamic, interactive, expressive and evocative, and as such not only involves many of the psychological processes and reactions engaged by the other creative arts, but many of the techniques employed by them as well. Researching into the therapeutic use of drama therefore allows us to obtain insight into as broad an area of creative expression as possible.

It is, of course, dramatherapists who have most experience of the therapeutic use of drama, and accordingly it was to them we turned for our research data. The broad questions we sought to answer were:

1 How is dramatherapy defined and conceptualized by dramatherapists? (i.e. What *is* drama as an agent of therapeutic change, and what groups of clients are most likely to benefit from it?)
2 What professional practices are used by dramatherapists, and how is client progress in dramatherapy monitored? (i.e. What do dramatherapists *do*, and how do they assess its effectiveness?)

As a first step in the research, in-depth tape-recorded individual interviews were conducted with a panel of experts consisting of 12 leading British dramatherapists. During the interviews one of us (LV) put to panel members a series of questions we derived from a close study of the literature and designed to elicit information related to the research objectives. In reply to the questions the panel proposed a range of items (in the form of statements and affirmations) relevant to dramatherapy theory and practice. After the tapes were transcribed, these were codified into a 354-strong item bank which was submitted in its entirety to the 12 dramatherapists for refinement and clarification of wording, and for further comment and observation. At the conclusion of this exercise, an analysis of the items showed that they grouped themselves under the following two main headings and 12 sub-headings:

The Theory of Dramatherapy
The nature of dramatherapy
Theoretical influences upon dramatherapy
The uses of dramatherapy
Drama and dramatherapy

The Practice of Dramatherapy
Techniques and skills
The role of the dramatherapist
The process of dramatherapy
Dramatherapy and the client
Client suitability for dramatherapy
The supervision of dramatherapists
Assessment in dramatherapy

Space allows us to choose only one of the sub-sections of the item bank in order to give a flavour of the material advanced to us by our panel, namely *The nature of dramatherapy*. This is an appropriate choice since it particularly deals with the first of the research questions identified above, namely the way in which dramatherapy is defined and conceptualized by dramatherapists.

The nature of dramatherapy

Of immediate interest is the finding that our panel of experts considers that drama *as therapy* is not radically different from *drama as drama*. In their view the distinctions that exist stem from the fact that drama as therapy contains the specific intention to facilitate personal change, whereas drama as drama is about working towards performance, whatever the aims behind that performance may or may not be. Drama as therapy is seen as a way of using the art form of drama in order to help the client find a sense of wholeness, or as one panel member put it, 'the purposeful use of dramatic engagement and creative expression in the service of learning, insight and personal change'.

As such, drama as therapy is not an isolated process which takes clients out of everyday life and puts them into something called therapy. A clear point to emerge from our panel is that dramatherapists do not see drama as divorced from real life, but as essentially an expression of it. As another panel member put it, 'in dramatherapy you don't step out of reality into fantasy, but into another sort of reality'. Dramatic processes, we were assured, are a natural part of psychological functioning, from the play of young children to the social roles adopted by adults, and from the creative use of the imagination to the expression of deep emotions, tensions and conflicts.

Our panel pointed out that an important way in which drama as therapy differs from many other forms of psychotherapy is that it allows clients to express their problems through acting them out rather than through simply talking about them. As Jennings (1990) puts it, dramatherapy is a re-working of experience through play, drama, ritual, theatre, role play, performance - all part of a process which is an intrinsically human propensity to dramatize, enact and re-enact life experiences in different forms, for different audiences at different times in our lives. Dramatherapy takes this essential human process and enables people who are stuck on their journey through life to find some kind of freedom.

Our panel agreed that through this dramatization the client discovers that he or she has the potential to express previously suppressed thoughts and feelings, to manifest psycho-social propensities that previously have been kept hidden, and to operate a different being-in-the-world from that operated hitherto. Through dramatic expression, the client receives permission to behave in apparently uncharacteristic ways, and to experience the self in a direct and insightful manner which leads towards integration and wholeness. This concept of self-discovery is also supported in the literature; e.g. Langley & Langley (1983) say that doing drama in a therapeutic way 'is not a matter of donning a mask and pretending, but of *removing* a mask and revealing' (p. 102).

The nature of this revealing differs from client to client, but staying for a moment with the literature, Grainger (1985) considers that the 'liberating power' of dramatherapy lies in the fact that it includes the 'demonstration that roles can be taken up, laid down, exchanged: that we can be, and in fact are, a great range of people' (p. 42). Grainger further insists that 'Dramatherapy alters the way in which people look at the world, themselves and other people' .... and .... 'far from going out of its way to achieve the kind of structured scenario which will be life-like enough to 'stand-in' for the real thing, prefers to regard social life itself as a kind of play' (p. 42).

The reference to 'play' is of particular interest, as our findings suggest that many dramatherapists also practise as playtherapists, and often distinguish few functional differences between the two sets of therapeutic interventions. One of our panel put it that 'the roots of dramatherapy are very much connected with play', while another identified further links between the non-serious activity of children and dramatherapy when he insisted that 'therapy is intrinsic in child drama' and that 'the improvised play of children is natural therapy'.

These references to children show how potentially fruitful it is to draw comparisons between the nature of dramatherapy as revealed by the present research, and the use of drama to enhance children's psycho-social development within educational settings. Such comparisons are particularly relevant in the light of two of the findings from our panel, namely that dramatherapists consider 'drama teaching is preventative of psychological problems, while dramatherapy is curative', and that 'the skills used in teaching drama and in practising dramatherapy are very similar, differing from each other only in the way in which they are used'.

To summarize this part of our research in the words used by one of our panel of experts, drama when used as therapy 'helps the individual to identify and refine the dramatic processes that go to make up much of everyday life, and to direct them in ways which he or she cannot do unaided'. It is therefore a reflection of society rather than a mimicry. It does not differ from the learning processes available in ordinary everyday life except that the learning it offers 'is specifically to do with personal change', is 'not bound by standards laid down by others' and 'helps to build up the ego' instead of threatening it through social failure, and through enforcing repressions, self-denials and self-rejection.

Questionnaire findings

We next constructed from the item bank a questionnaire designed to assess the views and practices of the whole population of British dramatherapists and dramatherapy associates. Essentially, the purpose of this questionnaire was to gauge the extent of agreement amongst dramatherapists on the issues identified by our panel of experts, and to explore such things as the frequency in their work with which they used those dramatherapeutic strategies nominated as important by our panel. For reasons of length, some of the 12 sub-sections and some of the items in the item bank were amalgamated, leaving a final total of seven sub-sections and 273 questions for inclusion in the questionnaire. Samples of dramatherapists and dramatherapy students were also sought in the USA, Israel and Greece.

Space does not allow us to report results of the full questionnaire, which produced an overall picture embracing, predictably, both consensus and controversy. Here we shall look only at the results in the second of the sub-sections listed earlier, namely the *theoretical influences upon dramatherapy*. This section relates in obvious ways to the *nature of dramatherapy*, and gives us a more rounded picture of dramatherapy as a discipline.

Theoretical influences upon dramatherapy

As indicated earlier, the foundation of dramatherapy is the dramatic act itself. However, since dramatherapy is a therapy, it is also open to influence from other therapeutic activities and systems of thought. Drama dictates the nature of dramatherapy, but in and of itself it cannot, for example, fully identify and categorize the nature of presenting client symptoms, or monitor the psychodynamic and behavioural changes that take place during the therapeutic process, or carry out final assessment strategies. In addition, it is open to influence by wider cultural influences. The drama produced by a society is firmly located within the culture of that society, and is in part a product of the processes yielded by and instrumental within that culture; it follows that dramatherapy is also subject to these cultural influences.

Our panel of experts assured us that the theoretical influences upon dramatherapy, both from within drama and from within other therapies and cultural processes, are indeed extensive, and they nominated 28 such influences embracing systems of thought. They also nominated 18 individuals whom they considered to be particularly important in the theoretical area. A further 16 individuals were nominated in reply to a question asking for those most influential on the actual development of dramatherapy theory and practice. All these influences and influential individuals were duly incorporated into our questionnaire, providing us with three questions, one relating to systems of thought and the other two to named individuals. Respondents were asked to provide ratings of importance for the variables contained in each of these questions (4-point scale, with '1' representing the highest rating).

Circulation of the questionnaire to the population of British dramatherapists and dramatherapy associates (as contained in the membership list of the British Association for Dramatherapists; n = 250) produced a good response rate of 50 per cent (many of the non-responders are currently not working as dramatherapists and therefore did not feel in a position to complete the questionnaire). Mean ratings for each variable were then calculated, and rank orders were obtained for responses to each of the three questions. Table 1 presents the rank order for the theoretical influences upon dramatherapy.

Table 1. Influence of systems of thought upon the theory of dramatherapy.

Variable	*Rank order of means*
1. Group dynamics	1.26
2. Psychotherapy	1.57
3. Theories of play	1.64
4. Theories of creativity	1.79
5. Child development	1.85
6. Client centred therapy	1.95
7. Theories of imagination	2.02
8. Psychodrama	2.02
9. Ritual	2.05
10. Disabilities	2.05
11. Child drama	2.20
12. Theories of theatre	2.27
13. Educational drama	2.28
14. Psychoanalysis	2.29
15. Social Psychology	2.29
16. Object relations play	2.40
17. Gestalt psychology	2.40
18. Anthropology	2.50
19. Analytical psychology	2.61
20. Sociology	2.65
21. Cognitive psychology	2.95
22. Philosophy	2.96
23. Behaviourism	2.98
24. Existentialism	2.99
25. Yoga	3.23
26. Theology	3.23
27. Bioenergetics	3.27
28. Alexander Technique	3.43

Table 1 shows that within the field of theoretical influences *group dynamics* emerged with the highest mean importance rating. This is not surprising considering that dramatherapy is essentially a group exercise. Second in mean importance rating came *psychotherapy*, again a predictable finding. Next came theories of *play*, followed by theories of *creativity*, theories of *child development* and *client-centred therapy*. The prominence assigned to each of these is reassuring, since it indicates how firmly dramatherapy is underpinned by current psychological knowledge.

Also well placed on the list are *psychodrama*, which some dramatherapists now see as a sub-division of dramatherapy (one might in fact have expected it to be placed higher), *ritual*, *child drama*, *theories of theatre* and *educational drama*. *Psychoanalysis* is the third of the therapies to be mentioned, occupying 14th place, with *social psychology* in 15th place and *sociology* in 20th. *Cognitive psychology* is relatively lowly placed at 21st, with *philosophy* at 22nd, *behaviourism* at 23rd and more esoteric disciplines lower still (e.g. existentialism at 24, yoga at 25, bioenergetics at 26 and the Alexander technique at 28). However, the very presence of these items on the list indicates they do have an important role to play.

Turning to the 18 individuals who our panel of experts identified as of particular influence, Jung emerges in first place, followed by Winnicott, Rogers, Stanislavski, Peter Brook, Murray Cox, Freud, Bruno Bettelheim and Bertolt Brecht in that order (Table 2).

Rather surprisingly in view of the prominence as formative influences given to them in the dramatherapy literature, Grotowski occupies only 11th place and Artaud 14th. The presence of Jung in first place is of great interest, reflecting the value to dramatherapists not only of his contributions to psychotherapy but also to the psychological study of myths, rituals and symbols, all of which feature prominently both in drama and in dramatherapy. (In view of Jung's importance the relatively lowly placing of analytical psychology in Table 1 is something of a mystery; the probable explanation however is that many non-psychologists do not readily identify the term with Jung.) Winnicott's high position is also interesting, reflecting particularly his work with children, while names such as Stanislavski, Brook and Brecht indicate the importance to dramatherapists of experimental theatre.

Rogers' high position reflects the relevance to dramatherapy of client-centred therapy, while Bettelheim is there for what he has to say about children and about the psychological role of children's fairy tales and story-telling. Freud's strong showing indicates that dramatherapy has not escaped the enduring fascination of psychoanalytical theory. Indeed, elsewhere we found that psychodynamic concepts - in particular transference, projection and repression - featured strongly in the language of the dramatherapists with

Table 2. Influence of specific individuals upon the theory of dramatherapy.

Variable	*Rank order of means*
1. Carl Jung	1.96
2. D. W. Winnicott	2.03
3. Carl Rogers	2.12
4. Constantin Stanislavski	2.25
5. Peter Brook	2.26
6. Murray Cox	2.32
7. Sigmund Freud	2.32
8. Bruno Bettelheim	2.38
9. Bertold Brecht	2.44
10. Melanie Klein	2.54
11. Jerzy Grotowski	2.59
12. Jean Piaget	2.65
13. Abraham Maslow	2.66
14. Ervin Goffman	2.80
15. Antonin Artaud	2.95
16. Victor Turner	3.05
17. Margaret Lowenfeld	3.12
18. Bruce Wiltshire	3.43

whom we spoke, and these concepts obtained high ratings in our questionnaire returns.

Of the 16 authorities recognized as important in the actual development of dramatherapy theory and practice, Sue Jennings heads the list, followed by Moreno, Heathcote, Sherborne, Courtney, Peter Slade and Robert Landy in that order (Table 3).

When asked to nominate the individual who had been of most influence upon the *personal* practice of respondents, Alida Gersie emerged in first place, followed by Sue Jennings and Jane Puddy.

Conclusion

Space has permitted us to give brief details on only two of the areas of what is in fact a wide-ranging research exercise. We are not yet at the point where we can draw clear implications for the use of drama as a pre-therapeutic exercise within education, but our findings to date make it clear that drama is seen by dramatherapy practioners engaged in its use as a potent therapeutic agent. Drama as therapy is also seen by these practitioners as sensitive to a

Table 3. Influence of specific individuals upon the development of dramatherapy.

Variable	*Rank order of means*
1. Sue Jennings	1.59
2. Jacob Moreno	2.08
3. Dorothy Heathcote	2.22
4. Veronica Sherborne	2.37
5. Richard Courtney	2.41
6. Peter Slade	2.44
7. Robert Landy	2.49
8. Dorothy Langley	2.61
9. Gertrude Schattner	2.64
10. Rudolf Laban	2.76
11. David Read Johnson	2.87
12. Brian Way	2.90
13. Gavin Bolton	2.98
14. Viola Spolin	3.07
15. Marian Lindkvist	3.11
16. Audrey Whethered	3.13

broad spectrum of influences both from other therapies and from psychology itself, which suggests that at both theoretical and practical levels it is likely to be a soundly based and effective exercise.

References

Fontana, D. & L. Valente (1990) 'Drama as pre-therapy: A perspective from psychology and dramatherapy.' *Speech and Drama* (in press)

Grainger, R. (1985) 'Using drama creatively in therapy: What are the advantages of a creative approach to therapy over other methods?' *Dramatherapy, 8 (2)*, 33-46

Jennings, S. (1987) (Ed.) *Dramatherapy: Theory and Practice for Teachers and Clinicians.* London: Croom Helm

Jennings, S. (1990) *Dramatherapy with Families, Groups and Individuals - Waiting in the Wings.* London: Jessica Kingsley

Landy, R.J. (1986) *Drama Therapy: Concepts and Practices.* Springfield, Illinois: Charles C Thomas

Langley, D. & E.L. Langley (1983) *Dramatherapy and Psychiatry.* London: Croom Helm

Schattner, G. & Courtney, R. (1981) *Drama in Therapy.* New York: Drama Book Specialists (2 Vols)

Working creatively with the symbolic proces of the schizophrenic patient in drama therapy

Stephen Snow

Bronx Psychiatric Center, New York

The nature of the drama, with its tolerance for the unreal and the imaginative, entices the inner self of the schizophrenic, which is occupied in fantasy, to reveal some part of itself. The patient finds he can explore with freedom the various fragments of himself while, at the same time, actualizing them for others. In this way, the inner self makes contact with the world, and the individual's fantasies become part of objective existence.

David Read Johnson, Drama Therapist

Shakespeare sums it us beautifully in his famous line, "The lunatic, the lover and the poet, Are of imagination all compact." This oft-quoted verse epitomizes the perennial argument for a meaningful correlation between the symbolic process of the psychotic and that of the creative artist. Although this position is commonly refuted by the prevailing medical model of schizophrenia, I hope, in the following pages, to show how the creative and imaginal capacity of the schizophrenic can be viewed in a new light. It is my thesis that the delusional and fantastic thought systems can be used to therapeutic advantage and that the drama therapist is particularly well-equipped to locate the creative element in the schizophrenic's symbolic process and to exploit it for the patient's benefit.

My thinking is indebted to the psychoanalytic object relations theorists, especially D. W. Winnicott, whose concepts of "transitional object" and "transitional space" have been so frequently cited in other papers. At the beginning of *Playing and Reality,* Winnicott (1971) himself correlates the very necessary illusion-making capacity of the infant and what, in adult life, becomes "the hallmark of madness" (p. 4). In this way, he underscores two psychological premises: firstly, that delusions are a major defensive mechanism for the psychotic and, secondly, that, at least in part, psychosis develops as a result of the dysfunction of the earliest object relations. As Edith Jacobson (1971) points out, it is because of this very early maladaptive experience that the schizophrenic is so predisposed to regress into infant-like fantasy worlds in which ".... normal object relationships and identifications disintegrate and are replaced by pre-oedipal, magic types of identification" (p. 246).

In the following pages, I will delineate the case study of an adult schizophrenic patient who regressed, during a period of profound decompensation, to just such a world of primary process imaginings and magic identifications. During this time, his thinking had a mythological dimension and, undoubtedly, he was overwhelmed by this deluge of images. I will describe how drama therapy was employed to construct a "transitional space" in which the patient could both feel safe and work directly with his powerful imagery. By this method, the raw materials of the psychotic imagination were transformed into a creative, artistic process that eventually aided the patient in his recovery.

Peter

Peter is a 39 year-old, Jewish, male patient, fairly tall and gangly, with a lumbering gait and a slightly slow speech pattern. His most common verbal complaint is of "weakness and fatigue". He has been in and out of psychiatric hospitals for most of the past twenty years. As his diagnosis (DSM-III, Schizoaffective Disorder 295.70) suggests, he experiences a full "affective syndrome" and cycles between periods of severe depression and periods of extreme manic symptomatology. His father was a physician and Peter grew up in Scarsdale, so he has quite a different socio-cultural background as compared to the majority of State Psychiatric Hospital patients. He reports having had a negative relationship with his mother and describes her as having been competitive, critical and hypochondriacal. This is important because, when his mother died of leukaemia in 1970, Peter experienced his first psychotic episode and hospitalization. During this time, he became profoundly hypochondriacal, himself, which would seem to indicate a primitive and negative identification with the mother.

I first began working with Peter in the fall of 1987. He was a member of my first Drama Therapy group on Ward 64. At that time, he was wildly thought-disordered and delusional. I had the opportunity, over several months, to see him become more organized, coherent and self-assured. We worked together consistently during that year and, at one point, Peter showed me a play which he had written when he was experiencing a self-described state of "psychotic fantasy". Around November of 1988, we began to work one-on-one, discussing the possibilities of producing this play. However, in February 1989, Peter underwent a severe decompensation. Within a few days, I witnessed the return of most of the psychotic symptoms he had demonstrated during our first meeting and the manifestation of several "psychotic identifications".

Normal and abnormal identifications

Along with many other psychoanalytic theorists, Edith Jacobson delineates an ideal course of individual development in which the child "advances" to "true object relations" and "true identifications". These characteristics are viewed as the accomplishment of the healthy personality.

> .... the child will be protected from relapses into the world of magic fantasies of fusions and early infantile types of identifications to the extent to which he succeeds in building up true object relations .... (1964, p. 51)
>
> *Jacobson*

The whole course of developing identifications is rooted in the earliest symbiotic stage of life: in the child's desire to merge with the mother. And, as Jacobson points out, conscious fantasies of merging with the love object are normal in the child, up to about three years of age. Imitation of the love object is also a normal precursor of true ego identifications. However, in normal development, the child must move through what Mahler (1979) has defined as the "separation-individuation process". The child must ultimately realize and accept its separateness from the original love object, mother. This is accomplished with great pain and difficulty. So much so, that Mahler states: "Inherent in every new step of independent functioning is a minimal threat of object loss" (p. 120). Here is the psychological Scylla and Charybdis which must be passed through if the child is to develop healthy ego functioning and identity. In regard to identification, Blanck and Blanck (1974) write: "Identification proper is a process of internalization .... identification makes for a greater degree of independence from the object. This is the road to autonomy" (p. 36). The litmus test for the development of healthy individuation is the establishment of object constancy and this is exactly where the psychotic personality comes up short. Because of faulty object relations, the psychotic individual cannot attain "true ego identification" and remains stuck in "preoedipal magic types of identification". Again, as Jacobson (1964) writes:

> .... only by becoming enduring, selective and consistent, can identifications gradually be integrated, become part of the ego, permanently modify its structure, and support the organization and stabilization of the ego's defense system (p. 68).

For those individuals prone to psychosis, these processes of structuralization and stabilization never take place and so, the personality remains constantly vulnerable to the regression to "primitive, narcissistic identifications". This is the case with Peter.

The meaning of grandiosity

On February 26th or 27th, when Peter profoundly decompensated, he began to strut around the ward saying "I am an Israeli general". He also made claims that he had recently proposed to "Blondie" (Deborah Harry) and that, as a "medical specialist" he was discovering the cure for cancer. Meanwhile, he had defecated on the ward floor and was becoming increasingly aggressive toward other patients and staff. He was extremely arrogant and bragged to everyone about his degrees in medicine and law, and the fact that he was also a jet pilot. This kind of behaviour went on for several weeks.

What caused this decompensation? What were the factors involved? Several significant stressors can be pinpointed. Peter's father had recently died in a nursing home in early January 1989. Peter had just found out about this and discovered that he would not receive a large sum of money that he had expected to come to him as his inheritance (how much of this is fantasy is difficult to say). There was also the expectation of Peter's imminent discharge to the "open door" transition ward. It has even been suggested that his psychiatrist was putting too much pressure on him to remain on his present ward. Whatever the cause, during this severe decompensation, he was deluged with psychotic identifications. As Blanck and Blanck write: "The decompensating patient is so overwhelmed that, like the infant, no power to alter the situation is available" (1974, p. 100).

In her essay on "Psychotic Identifications", Jacobson clearly defines the causes of such manic elation and grandiosity as Peter was experiencing. She writes:

> We found that the schizophrenic patient's grandiose, elated states .... were an expression not of conflicts or reconciliation and reunion between superego and self image, but of the processes of total fusions between self and object images within the disintegrating ego-id .... The schizophrenic seems to be predisposed to such processes by his defective ego-superego formation. (1971, p. 260-261)

Because of the disintegration of what is undoubtedly a very weak ego structure to begin with, consciousness is flooded with the kinds of images that are inherent to the magical, mythological perspective of the preoedipal child who is merged with the all-powerful mother. From the primitive mental states of psychosis emerge what Jung called the "archetypal images" and what Freud referred to as "archaic vestiges".

Peter's private mythology

During this period of his decompensation, Peter was living in the world of his own private mythology, with little or no ability for reality testing. What is truly fascinating is that he had portrayed this idiosyncratic, cosmological vision in the play (mentioned above) that he had written during a previous period of decompensation. In it, Peter identified himself as the protagonist, Nelson Neuron, who has the heroic task of proving the Devil's innocence, in a trial located in Hell, over which the Lord God Almighty presides. What is so unique about this dramatic vision is that the Devil is depicted as a woman, Lana Love, who is, in fact, based on the personality of the TV newscaster, Michelle Marsh. Peter had for a long time been obsessed with Ms Marsh. In his story, the female Devil is actually innocent of creating all the evil in the world and his character, Nelson Neuron, successfully defends her in a heated court battle with Bernhardt Goetz, the prosecuting attorney. Certainly, much could be made of all this fantastical imagery by way of interpretation, but the main point, here, is that Peter's grandiose theatrical vision of himself as the Hero-Lawyer who saves the Devil from doom fits perfectly into the pattern for the manifestation of psychotic identifications described by Edith Jacobson:

> .... schizophrenics may show the grandiose belief of being the genius who does not need the world, or of being the omnipotent evil or good

> ruler of mankind who can control, destroy or rescue a doomed world. Their outbursts of panic, their fantasies of *Weltuntergang* arising from an inner perception of their disintegration .... of the breakdown of object relations and ego identifications, reverberate the processes of dissolution, both of the object and of the self-representations. Split up into archaic images, they cease to be entities (1971, p. 261).

In his own process of dissolution, the object of his fantasy and sexual desire, Michelle Marsh, became the Devil for Peter and he, in turn, became the legal genius who would ultimately prove her innocence in the Highest (or Lowest) of Courts.

Treatment: The play's the thing

During the period February to June 1989, I worked regularly with Peter, in conjunction with other staff and two drama therapy interns, in order to actualize the play he had written. At first, I was reluctant to do this. I had never worked with a patient in such a chaotic state of what Jacobson calls "the disintegrating ego-id". However, the Unit Chief and the Ward Psychiatrist coaxed me and, gradually, I began to see the ameliorating effect that our weekly therapy/rehearsal session was having on Peter. This gave me a little more confidence. In this concluding section, I would like to attempt to define how and why drama therapy was an effective modality in this case where the patient was experiencing such extreme psychotic identifications.

Ironically, the regular rehearsal periods for his fantasy/play provided Peter with a kind of much needed "Reality Orientation". The consistent presence, over a period of months, of persons whom he could trust not to be overwhelmed by his aggressive, bizarre, thoughts and behaviours, who could weather the storms of his rapidly shifting affect and ideation, gave Peter a ballast for his chaotic and fragmentary experience of the world. As Blanck and Blanck state: ".... the treatment of the very severely disturbed patient involves the use of the therapist as a real object for the purpose of building object relations" (1974, p. 76). In some small way the members of the cast (staff and interns) served as "real objects" for Peter and, although I was not his primary therapist, I had had a consistent two and a half year relationship with Peter.

The rehearsal space and process served as a kind of "safe haven" for Peter during this critical time. In this play space, he could feel free to improvise on the characters and actions that were set down in the script. Although this was often difficult for the rest of the cast, including one non-psychotic patient, it seemed to help Peter to be able to improvise from his delusions of the moment. The scripted characters would become new characters with whom

Peter, both in and out of the role of Nelson Neuron, insisted upon interacting with. The self-created nature of the script was Peter's anchor; in the rehearsal space he could float, sometimes playfully, sometimes chaotically, but with the assurance that his imagery and actions were safely contained. As others have pointed out, the theatrical space is transitional space *par excellence.* Winnicott demonstrated how the infant's original experience of transitional space is the source of future creative and symbolic process. Drama therapy can provide the patient with the kind of transitional space where he or she can deconstruct and reconstruct in a protected manner. I believe this is how rehearsals of his play functioned for Peter. To cite the words of Peter Giovacchinni (1986): " .... the maladaptions that are characteristic of disturbed primitive mental states can be dealt with in a creative fashion in a psychotherapeutic setting" (p. 360).

Finally, it must be noted that the cast, which included a social worker/treatment team leader, a rehabilitation teacher, two drama therapy interns and a patient from another ward, comprised a tremendous support system for Peter. They saw him through the chaotic beginnings to the final culmination of producing the play for patients, staff, family and friends. They assisted him in accruing the ego strength that made the actualization of his script possible.

To end on a hopeful note. Now, more than a year later, Peter has been discharged to a special residency off the hospital grounds; he has recently had a romantic relationship with a young woman (also a patient); he is considering taking a course in paralegal studies at Lehman College (interesting that the character that he portrayed in the performance of his play was a lawyer and the play, essentially, a courtroom drama); he looks stronger and healthier than ever, and he no longer complains of "weakness and fatigue".

References

Blanck, G. & R. Blanck (1974) *Ego Psychology: Theory and Practice.* New York: Columbia University Press

Giovacchini, P.L. (1986) *Developmental Disorders: The transitional space in mental breakdown and creative imagination.* Northvale, New Jersey: Jason Aronson, Inc.

Jacobson, E. (1964) *The Self and Object World.* New York: International Universities Press

Jacobson, E. (1971) *Depression.* New York: International Universities Press

Johnson, D.R. (1981) 'The Schizophrenic Condition.' In: *Drama Therapy,* Vol. 2, Gertrud Schattner & Richard Courtney (Eds.), 47-64. New York: Drama Book Specialists

Mahler, M.S. (1979) *The Selected Papers of Margaret S. Mahler*, Vol. 2. New York: Jason Aronson, Inc.

Winnicott, D.W. (1971) *Playing and Reality.* New York: Basic Books Inc.

The theatre of human experience: An introduction to psychodrama

Dennis C. Gold

North Eastern Pennsylvania Counselling Center, Kingston

It is unusual for us to feel exclusively one way or the other about things. We deeply love someone but are irritated by their toothpaste habits, choice of friends or dreadful snoring. We love their sensitivity and honesty until they utilize these fine qualities to inform us of our shortcomings. Psychodrama is a method for examining the multitudes of conscious and unconscious stirrings of the human psyche (Blatner, 1973; Wethered, 1973).

The founder of psychodrama, J. L. Moreno, MD, describes its birth as occurring on 1 April 1921 between 7 and 10 p.m. On this April Fools' Day at the "Komoedien Haus", a theatre for drama in Vienna, Dr Moreno stood on the stage before an audience of 1000 people completely unprepared. On stage stood a red, plush armchair with a king's crown upon the seat. Dr. Moreno invited members of the audience, which consisted of quite diverse members of European society, to sit on the throne and act like a king, while the audience assumed the role of jury. According to the Viennese press, the experiment was a dismal failure.

Dr. Moreno also tells of an incident that happened when he was four years old and living near the Danube. His parents went out for the evening and left him with some neighbourhood children to play in the basement. He decided to play "God and his angels". They stacked a bunch of chairs on a big picnic table and helped him assume his lofty niche at the top. They circled him, flapped their "wings" and encouraged him to fly. He broke his arm while simultaneously learning that we are dependent on others and that other little children are also interested in playing God.

Moreno (1946) has defined psychodrama as "the science which explores 'truth' by dramatic methods". It contrasts with classical psychoanalysis which prohibits acting out. Traditionally, when a person was involved in psychoanalysis, she was requested not to make any changes in her life (e.g. not to get married nor divorced nor to change jobs) until the analysis was complete. In psychodrama, the attempt is to act out inner conflicts and to make intrapsychic processes visible through outward manifestations. Therefore, one would not discuss one's ambivalent feelings about one's father. Rather, with the help of others, one would act it out so that it becomes visible and observable.

Each person has a variety of roles to play in life: child, sibling, worker, spouse, community member, good guy, bad guy, friend, mediator or parent. These roles change as we mature and new roles are attempted while others are discarded. The word 'role' has its origins in the Latin word 'rotula'. In ancient Greece and Rome the parts in theatre were written on 'rolls' and read to the actors who were attempting to memorize them. It was not until the middle of the 1600's and the arrival of the modern stage that 'roles' were read from paper text. As actors attempt to fill a role in preparation for a play, each individual is continually trying on different roles to identify who they truly are. This "role-playing" is one of the major building blocks of psychodrama.

Psychodrama was one of the first techniques that moved away from individual therapy toward group therapy. This marked the initiation of putting people in a context and not treating them in isolation. Additionally, verbal treatment was replaced by a more action-oriented treatment. For example, in psychoanalysis we free-associate to our idea of our mother; in psychodrama we act out our perceptions of our mother.

Aristotle's concept of catharsis is an important component of psychodrama. Catharsis for him was a secondary, not a primary goal. In psychodrama, catharsis is one of the goals. Catharsis moves from the stage to the audience several times while the drama is being enacted.

There are five basic instruments to psychodrama: the stage, the subject or protagonist, the director, the auxiliary and alter-egos and the audience. Each instrument is necessary for the drama to take place. I will elaborate on each:

1. The Stage

We need a stage to help us define our space and provide us with a safe environment. People are not going to expose the deepest aspects of their psyche if there aren't some safeguards in place. The stage provides participants with a safe place to explore themselves; it is an extension of life with less restrictions.

2. The Subject or Protagonist

She is asked to be herself on the stage. There is no script to hide behind and no words written by someone else. Everything that happens on the stage is a part of the subject. The purpose of the drama is to make the experience of the protagonist as therapeutic as possible. We leave the verbal and move on to action. We don't discuss the problem, we act it out.

3. The Director

The director is a combination of producer and therapist. She is responsible for making the drama as lifelike as is possible. She has to be in tune with the audience and not let the drama "drift". The major charge of the director is to be sure that the experience is therapeutic for the protagonist. She can modify the instruments necessary to ensure the therapy is effective.

4. Egos

The auxiliary-ego's role is to support the subject in whatever manner is necessary. They have a therapeutic function and are the arms of the director in a fashion. They are also extensions of the patient and are frequently called upon to speak for the latter. The alter-ego acts in a contrary fashion. If the subject is optimistic, the alter-ego warns of impending doom. She always assumes the opposite role on the set of polarities.

5. The Audience

The Audience both helps the subject during the feedback and processing phase and is helped when the subject acts out the drama. We have all been confused, loved, disliked and hurt by others. I am always amazed at how universal psychodramas can be and how much benefit observers can derive from them.

The psychodramatic focus

A psychodrama is always done in a group setting for both practical and theoretical reasons. It is difficult to act out several different roles simultaneously; this becomes quite confusing and dilutes the therapy. The psychodrama group helps the individual understand how universal her problems are and examines the individual in the context of a community or society. It is also possible for more than a single individual to gain benefit at one time.

The process begins with a warm-up. This helps the participants prepare for the psychodrama mentally and emotionally. It enables people to make the transition from the outside world to the safety of the psychodrama group. Psychodrama itself is a powerful experience and the warm-up allows us to set the stage. Warm-ups range from something as simple as a group discussion to complex dances. The purpose is to foster spontaneity which is a crucial element in psychodrama.

The next step is to select a protagonist. This can be accomplished in a variety of ways. The person can volunteer. She can be selected by the director or other members of the group. A sociogram can be enacted which would identify the person in the group with whom most members identify. A spectrogram can be done in which participants go to one side or the other of a room based upon how they feel about a specific issue, while those who are indifferent remain in the centre. A discussion about the issue brings out salient points and can eventually lead to the identification of a protagonist.

Once the protagonist is selected, she is asked to come to the stage and describe the basic elements and individuals that are salient. This serves as an additional warm-up to the psychodrama. She is then asked to choose an auxiliary-ego. Some psychodrama groups have professional auxiliary-egos that have been trained and have a great deal of expertise. An auxiliary-ego is chosen by having the protagonist choose an individual that she feels close to and that she feels understands her. It is explained that if during the course of the drama the protagonist is too upset to continue, the auxiliary-ego will stand in (or "double") for the protagonist until she is able to resume her role. From the moment the auxiliary ego accepts the role, she never leaves the side of the protagonist.

The alter-ego is the next individual chosen by the protagonist. This role is played as a counterpart to the auxiliary-ego. She completes the polarity by remaining contrary. She is constantly pointing out the other aspect of the self. In turn, each of the other characters in the drama are cast by the protagonist with the help of the director. As each individual accepts her part, she joins the others on the stage.

The scene is now set. The director asks the protagonist a series of questions to elicit as much detail as is possible about where the action takes place and how each of the characters behave in real life. Chairs and tables are arranged to resemble real situations. All of the characters have an opportunity to question the protagonist directly about how she perceives their characters and what insights she has into the nature of the conflict.

The psychodrama is now enacted with the director paying careful attention to all of the elements and carefully structuring the events to make the experience as therapeutic as possible for the protagonist. The director usually creates several breaks in the action to ascertain how to guide the drama.

After the scene is completed, the processing phase begins. Here the director sits down with the protagonist (at first) and explores her feelings, insights and struggles with others observing. Then the other members of the cast are invited to share their observations, first about the protagonist and her issues. Then they are invited to share their own personal responses and how the drama related to their own lives. Lastly, the members of the audience are invited to contribute anything they wish to. Processing can be a very time-consuming process when the drama deeply affects people and closely relates to many people's own personal issues. This is probably the most important element of the process because this is where learning is crystallized and integrated into future growth and personal change.

Some techniques of psychodrama

1. Soliloquy

Probably the most basic technique, where the protagonist delivers a monologue about what she is feeling and thinking about. This can be done at any point from setting the action to the final scene. A variation of this technique is "walk and talk" where the director leads the protagonist away from the action where everyone remains "frozen". She then explores the protagonist's feelings with her and determines the intra-psychic process of the protagonist.

2. Role Reversal

In this technique, two individuals simply switch roles for a while. When two people are "stuck" this frequently helps free them up a bit and allows them to gain some insight as to how the other person feels. This technique has been adopted by many different psychotherapeutic approaches from marriage counselling to Gestalt therapy.

3. Double

In doubling, the auxiliary-ego assumes the role of the protagonist for a while. This can be done in many different ways. The protagonist can remain in character and respond to the double. The protagonist can remain silent while the other members of the drama respond. The protagonist can just sit off stage and watch the action. The important part is that doubling allows the protagonist to hear some of the inner dialogue that she thinks and feels but rarely speaks and it allows her to see how someone else perceives her.

Psychodramas themselves are as varied as the protagonists who act them out and the directors who guide them. I have never seen two psychodramas that even closely resemble each other, even with the same protagonist. The instruments always vary and so do moods and elements in the action. I would add that I have never been bored in a psychodrama no matter which role I played.

The tool of psychodrama has several advantages over other forms of therapy. It allows us to understand more about what is frequently left unsaid or censored. It permits us to act out our fears, desires or conflicts within a safe and comfortable milieu. It allows us the opportunity to try on new behaviours that might otherwise have been difficult. Finally, it lets us see how others confront, avoid and dance around the quintessential dramas of life. I have always found that I am richer for the experience.

Please note that this paper is merely an introduction to psychodrama. In order to learn properly how to practice psychodrama, one should study the techniques in depth and receive ongoing supervision by an experienced practitioner. Psychodrama is a highly complex technique that requires serious study to practice effectively.

References

Blatner, H.A. (1973) *Acting In.* New York: Springer Publishing Company

Moreno, J.L. (1946, revised 1964) *Psychodrama,* Vol. 1, Beacon, New York, Beacon House

Wethered, A.G. (1973) *Movement and Drama in Therapy.* Boston: Plays, Inc.

Personal clown – A theatrical exploration of the inner self

Glenys McQueen-Fuentes

Department of Film Studies, Dramatic and Visual Arts,

Brock University, Ontario

Jacques Lecoq, the French theatre pedagogue who developed the idea of Personal Clown as a teaching tool, as well as greatly furthering its renaissance as a performance style, describes Personal Clown as the "authentic, pre-social child inside us all - whom we finally let out to play". It is the truly spontaneous self, acutely aware of his/her level of vulnerability in a world of unknowns and also aware of his/her inability to "know what to do" in the onslaught of daily events that present themselves. Discovering and developing a Personal Clown involves having this inner self confront and accept both the vulnerability and the lack of social "know-how".

The word "child" in Lecoq's description of Personal Clown gives some important clues to the actors. Like a "pre-social" child, the Clown is intelligent and curious, but not "smart". It does not know a lot of "facts", share our adult reasoning system or our naming system for objects. Everything is new and yet to be discovered, named and included in the Clown's personal world. Discovering one's Personal Clown means *reconnecting with wonder*. It means reliving the state of *awe*, surprise and discovery which are such constants in childhood and which, as adults, we often learn to cover or ignore. In fact, when guiding a group of actors through clown work, one of the ways of knowing when an actor is constructing his/her clown, rather than letting it evolve, is by listening to the clown's conversation for "smart" reasoning, second-guessing, one-line quips and one-upmanship. These are all signs of the actor controlling the work, as the clown is totally devoid of such levels of sophistication.

Like the child, the clown experiences everything as an immediate physical/emotional response and as a total involvement in the "here and now", without concern for future or for consequences. A clear example of this would be a child in front of a candy counter who wants one particular candy *now*. For that child, at that moment, there is no other candy and no other time frame. This kind of total involvement/concentration in the here and now, with a highly connected physical/emotional response is the essence of Personal Clown work.

It is also important to explain the Personal Clown in relation to other kinds of clowns. For example, the role of humour is different for the Personal Clown and for the Circus Clown. Whereas the Circus Clown provokes laughter *at* what he does, to whom, when and how, the Personal Clown induces us to laugh *with* him. The Circus Clown is a character separate from us, hence we observe it from a distance. The Personal Clown is so universally a part of each of us that we must share its trials and tribulations. The laughter is from recognizing ourselves in the vulnerability, the struggling and the growing of the Personal Clown.

The irony of this most intimate and vulnerable of theatre styles is that the catalyzing agent - the red nose - is the smallest and most revealing of the theatre masks. The actors are required to delve deep into themselves with only a minimum of protection.

There are several rules which must be dealt with before starting. The enormous amount of physicality released by clown work can be surprising and frightening. At no time is a Clown allowed to touch another Clown - or another Clown's possessions - in anger or frustration. With respect to wearing a mask, because the human face is such a strong symbol of personality, actors are asked to turn away from the audience to put the nose on or take it off. This gives the audience the chance to "erase" the actor's face and to prepare for the appearance of the Clown and vice versa. For the same reason, if the actor has a comment to make, the nose should be taken off (facing away from the audience) before doing so. Here again is a point at which actors who are backing off from the work through fear or insecurity will undermine their Clown image by repeatedly forgetting these rules. And finally, as in other mask work, actors are told that at any point, if they are instructed to take off the nose, they are to do so immediately.

Some of the objectives that Personal Clown should achieve for actors in their training process are as follows:

1 increased confidence in recognizing and trusting personal intuition for acting and improvisation.
2 a re-encounter with and enjoyment of personal spontaneity and increasing use of it in the theatrical process.
3 discover depths of energy capacity and provide opportunities in which the actor must commit and develop it.
4 ability to work comfortably on a much larger physical, emotional and vocal scale.
5 free up and extend imagination.
6 rediscover the importance of personal choice in the acting process.
7 free up constrictions of language associations to objects, actions and attitudes.
8 allow actors to explore personal creative expression through a wide range of activities.
9 deepen ability to use sense memory and emotional memory work in the theatrical process.
10 provide opportunities for the actors to experience the difference between stage honesty and "planned" acting.
11 clarify the actor's personal learning process.

The classes involve three progressive sections:

1. Warm-up

The *warm-up* is the most underestimated and misunderstood of the theatrical processes. It seems to evoke images of aerobic classes, tights and sweat, meant only for those who wish to suffer physical pain. In reality, a *warm-up* should create an atmosphere of openness, readiness and concentration in which the actor integrates his/her physical, emotional and vocal self for the work ahead. This may include some sweat, but not suffering. To this end, I have developed a series of "nonsense" exercises based on movements which I have seen children do when experimenting with the new-found joys of mobility. These exercises should create sensations of joy, delight and play in the adult, just as they do in the child. It is remarkable how strong the re-discovery of these corporal sensations can be. They provide instant links to past experiences of exploration and increasing personal power that occurred in childhood. The actual exercises happen sitting, lying, twirling, rolling, etc. on the floor, since I have found that it is difficult for adults to "play" from a normal standing or sitting-in-a-chair position. I also add a short "emotion-laden" phrase to be spoken loudly during the exercises, such as "Yes, I can!", "No, I won't!", "So what!", "Wait and see!", "Whooppee!" These give a rhythmic chant to the physical work, which allows the actors to automatically increase the size of their movements and the loudness of their voices.

2. Sensory/emotional memory work

This involves the "childhood exercises". Although the actor's Personal Clown is not specifically the child that the actor was, by returning to the details of childhood, the actor can rediscover the state of awe so inherent to the child-like state in which the Personal Clown operates. It also allows the actor to relive the special type of logic, associations and way of classifying reality that is so rich, creative and individual in the childhood experience. This work does not mean that the actors must relive experiences that were unwanted. The aim is for the actor to re-encounter reactions, attitudes, likes and dislikes, preferences, wants, opinions - and to remember what they were like as children, rather than dwell on events that happened to them. I ask the actors to remember rooms, furniture, clothes, textures, colours, smells, tastes, toys, celebrations, presents, trips that they liked or disliked. I also ask them to choose emotional events that they wish to use, such as: a happy moment, an angry one, a mischievous or sneaky event. Childhood photos enrich this work enormously. Although I only continue this section for the first four or five sessions, actors always comment that once they begin to try to remember details from childhood, memories continue to come during the entire Clown process and this strengthens their work.

3. Personal clown – Developmental exercises

The work is multi-layered, with the Clown developing slowly through progressively more complicated encounters. Actors need to be assured that there is no "norm". Each Clown develops at its own speed and cannot be compared at any time with another Clown. The following are the layers I use:

The Individual Clown

The Individual Clown and the Audience. I first run a series of simple exercises in which each Clown is cheered onto and off the performance space, with no expectations put on him/her. This is to emphasize the point that the Clown "can do *no wrong*", that his or her mere presence is sufficient for total acceptance. It also becomes the official introduction to the audience, with whom the Clown will share everything. The high level of physical and emotional energy needed sets the tone for the whole group, as the audience will be closely and actively involved in the development of each Clown. From a purely practical side, it also allows the actors time to become accustomed to wearing the clown nose (which tends to drip perspiration and should not be "adjusted" in public, despite discomfort).

The Individual Clown and the Personal Object. This is an extremely important event, as each Clown has an object with which (s)he will identify totally. Finding the object comes very early and forms the basis upon which the Clown begins to evolve. It also forms the Clown's first relationship. A pile of assorted, varied discarded objects, called the Magic Mountain, is placed in the middle of the performance space. I ask the Clown to rush in, find an object that is waiting for him/her, test it briefly and then to leave quickly. Speed is important to ensure that the actors work intuitively and instinctively. Otherwise, they may begin to "perform" for the audience. In this early, developmental stage, the aim of the process is self-discovery and performance values are not to be brought into play. "Testing" also gives the actors a chance to approach objects in a fresh and non-prescribed way. The fact that the objects are piled as junk frees them from their normal, practical associations and allows the actor to discover them for their inherent qualities of colour, shape, texture, sound, size, etc. It is one of these qualities (or a combination) which will attract the clown and begin to reveal the Clown's set of personal preferences. Surprisingly, but consistently, the qualities which attract the Clown may be very different from those which would interest the actor. In fact, the actor may feel his/her personal preferences trying to overtake or "rationalize with" the Clown's choice. This is another reason for speed - to help the Clown's choices emerge before the actor's (inadvertently) subvert them.

The clown, the MC and the audience – Interviews

Although not "circus" clown, Lecoq used the idea of the ring and the circus MC in developing Personal Clown and it provides an excellent progression. Once the object is chosen, the Clown is invited into the ring (performance space) by the MC (the instructor) and interviewed about the object in such a way as to help the actor create The Story of the object - what it is, where the Clown found it, where it (and the Clown) had been before, why it is important to the Clown, etc. The Clown is to answer whatever comes to mind, no matter how "ludicrous" it may seem in "real life". All the information given, plus how it is given, form part of the tapestry which will become the Clown's biography. The "how" - the body language the Clown uses during the interviews also forms the basis for the Clown's personal physicality.

Once begun, the interview technique is used throughout the development process for helping Clowns define and test costume, attitudes, values, likes, dislikes, etc. Also, once it is clear what type of questioning is necessary to keep the process open, inventive and imaginative for the Clown, interviewing can be opened up to involve the whole audience (the actors who are watching always question as themselves, not as their Clowns). Having the responsibility of questioning also makes the audience more involved and sensitive to the whole process - they are helping the Clown create his/her story (history).

The social clown – Meetings and community

The Clown Meets Another Clown. Very shortly after the Clown's interview about his/her object, I set up an improvisation in which two Clowns appear before the audience. This is astounding for the Clowns, as no Clown has met another up to this point - in fact, the thought that other Clowns might exist has up till now probably not crossed their minds. These meetings are usually combined with interventions from the MC and eventually from the whole audience. The improvisation also usually stipulates that each Clown has been given the same task to complete for the audience (usually dealing with giving the audience information about themselves). How the Clown deals with trying to fulfil the task while dealing with the encounter of a fellow Clown will provide a great deal of information for them.

The Clown Creates a Home (The Hideout). At this point, all the actors work their Clowns simultaneously, so the audience is reduced to the MC (myself). I talk them through the essentials of the following work. As they go about finding and creating a Hideout in the work area, they are not to take other Clowns into account, but are to imagine they are alone. My way of introducing this section is to have the Clowns imagine that they are asleep and that when they wake, they will find themselves alone on a new planet that they've never seen before. They are to explore their surroundings (still ignoring the presence of the other Clowns) and as quickly as possible, create or find a Hideout in which they will sleep. The unknown quality of this new planet is stressed - how long days or nights will be, if matter is stable, etc. This is important to keep the need for spontaneity at the fore. It also helps overcome practical problems such as having to move to a new space, encountering furniture missing between sessions, etc.

The Clown Discovers Neighbours. Once the Hideout is established, it remains as intact as possible throughout the development process (although it may grow and become more decorated). On the first "morning" after finding their Hideout, the Clowns emerge to find they are surrounded by other Clowns in other Hideouts - they are in the middle of a community. This becomes a long, extended session, with almost no intervention from me, except to end the work. The Clowns meet each other, begin to establish relationships with their fellow clowns, form opinions and attitudes about their neighbours, discover the layout of their community in terms of who lives where, etc.

It is important that the mask rules of never touching another Clown (or actor or instructor) in anger, impatience or frustration be repeated before this work begins. This rule also applies to Clowns' personal objects and Hideouts.

It would be too easy and tempting to seek revenge on objects with which the clown identifies so closely. Anger, impatience, frustration, revenge, etc., come up often, and are an absolutely necessary part of every Clown, but they are manifested by the Clowns' acknowledging they are experiencing the feelings and expressing them through sound, words (not swearing, which is the verbal equivalent to physical attack) and personal movement patterns (the Clown temper tantrum).

Developing the Community. Once the initial explorations of people and places has occurred (and this may take a couple of sessions), the Clowns and their Community continue to develop through such events as: having a party, creating a communal ritual or celebration, preparing a parade, forming groups to help specific Clowns with specific problems, going on an exploratory trip (beyond the confines of the theatre work space) to other planets, etc. These activities require some intervention from the MC/instructor.

Parallel Personal Development in the Clown. During the development of the Community, the Clowns also continue their personal development. One important aspect for the Clown is dress. From the first day with the Magic Mountain, the Clown begins to become aware of wanting and needing certain kinds of clothes. Nothing is taken for granted and the final wardrobe is necessary to the final detail for the Clown and reflects taste in colours, textures, shapes, etc. Other ways personal development are continued are through (a) frequent reflection in their Hideouts of just-passed events through any creative media they choose or through a combination of media and (b) continuously returning to the interview pattern, where MC and audience question each Clown about ongoing events, usually integrating the reflections made by the Clowns in their Hideouts and (c) through discussion as actors about their Clown's progress.

Some of the topics which I ask the Clowns to return to their hideouts to reflect on include recording impressions of: the first "day" when the Clowns discovered each other and the community; how they feel about their neighbours; dreams and/or nightmares the Clown has had during nights in the Hideout; how a specific event went; planning the perfect celebration, costume or disguise; planning a "master class" of what the Clown does best; recording the Clown's "golden dream" of what he/she wants to do in the future, etc. The Clowns can record their thoughts and feelings through drawing, sculpting, collage, some form of writing or through a combination of them. They store their materials in their hideouts.

These same topics become the themes for the interview process. I often ask Clowns to bring their pictures, writings, etc. to the interview or to recount an incident as a story, playing all the parts. Another technique I use is to have the Clowns present a specific reaction by translating their drawing or writing into a dance or a song for the interview.

Throughout the process, we usually end each session with a discussion about the work, the progress, what we have learned about the Clowns and about the process.

Personal Clown is a process that can continue throughout a lifetime. As we develop and change, our Clown will be subtly changing too. Even after we stop working directly with it, once we have acknowledged it and let it out to play, it's always there, enriching our inner lives and pulling us back to wonder and awe. It continues to be a secret reference and a consolation which extends beyond the realm of pure theatre to our everyday lives. And it is this fact which I feel makes it worthy of consideration for those working in psychology.

Dance/movement therapy: Inherent value of the creative process in psychotherapy

Jacqueline Blatt

Laban Centre for Movement and Dance, London

In this paper I will discuss the relationship between the therapeutic and creative process. I hope to demonstrate that the creative process facilitates the attainment of therapeutic goals and that dance/movement therapy elicits more directly the primary process, making the creative process more easily accessible.

Creativity is the means by which a client makes himself whole in psychotherapy. The process brings the client to the point where he has fuller access to his sensory, cognitive, emotional and behavioural capabilities.

The British Association for Dance/Movement Therapy defines dance/movement therapy as "the use of expressive movement and dance as a medium through which the individual can engage creativity in a process of personal integration and growth". Dance/movement therapy, as defined by the American Dance Therapy Association is "a psychotherapeutic technique which uses movement as a process to further the emotional, cognitive and physical integration of the individual". Movement is one of the most basic forms of expression. At the earliest levels of development our needs, responses, emotions, learning and interactions are expressed through movement. Understanding and interacting with the world around us is inextricable from our ability to move. Movement is a well-established expressive modality prior to the development of verbal proficiency.

Psychological theorists recognize pre-verbal levels of development and primary process. Also well understood are circumstances where verbal communication with clients is impeded. Society, however, has strongly emphasized the verbal and cognitive expression while virtually ignoring the non-verbal medium. Traditional psychotherapists also continue the preference for the verbal approach, thereby limiting their clinical effectiveness.

Zwerling (1979) states that "nonverbal media employed by creative arts therapists more directly tap emotion rather than cognitive process". Best (1974) postulates a relationship between mental emotional experiences and physical behaviour. He points out that in the specific case of emotions we understand mental experience in a context which includes the object cause of the behaviour.

Reich (Baker, 1967) with his analytical and medical background, was able to demonstrate that psychological processes had corresponding physical manifestation. In some instances psychological defences ("armour" in his terminology) were manifested as muscular contraction which caused a reduction in feeling. Reich concurred with Sigmund Freud's theory that the psychic functions included a primary process which occurs on an unconscious level, for example in dreams and in some mental illnesses, especially psychosis. The secondary process occurs when the mind is awake and employs common sense.

The expression of the sensory experience (oral, auditory, visual, kinaesthetic, tactile) finds its way into our everyday expression in phrases like "I was twitching with anxiety" (enactive mode), "I thought that he was going to burst" (image mode), "I felt slightly apprehensive as I climbed up the ladder" (lexical mode). Dosamantes-Alperson (1983) says "...as human beings we have access to the three ways of representing or symbolizing our experiences, enactive, image and lexical". "Meaning is expressed enactively through muscle tension in action tendency or in incipient body movements .... The meaning provided by the image mode is conveyed through the various sensory modalities" (Horowitz, 1972). ".... In the lexical mode, meaning to communicate through words. Because words are specialized for sequential processing, this "mode facilitates conceptualization, analytical reasoning and abstract generalization making detachment and objectivity possible" (Horowitz, 1972, Dosamantes-Alperson, 1983, p. 264-265).

Walker (Hahnemann University, 1985) said, "We also have to develop new languages because words are the only links between creative people and right brain 'retards' like myself - psychiatrists and psychologists who want to be artistic, who want to be in our bodies, who are desirous, but who are frightened. We need the right metaphors; we need the right kind of courtesy to help bring us into our bodies in a way that is not scary to us. The people in movement also need the right kind of words, curving words, to help them move up the spiral into their heads" (p. 73).

The verbal/cognitive view fails to embody the movement/sensation material without resorting to sensory metaphors. Therefore the listener hearing the words "the floor fell out from under me when I was fired" has immediate access to the feelings of anxiety felt by the speaker. This level of understanding is not made available by the cognitive, lexical mode statement, "I felt anxious when I was fired". Sensory metaphors not only provide a valuable access to the individual's intrapsychic working but also give indications to the therapist as to how to communicate with the individual's preferred sensory mode. By speaking directly to the preferred sensory mode, the therapist enhances the client's ability to explore, comprehend and integrate. Arnheim (1969) wrote that the "cognitive operations called thinking are not the privilege of mental processes above and beyond perception but the essential ingredients of perception itself" (p. 13). Arnheim further argues that the more fundamental problem of the modern man is the split between sense and thought which causes various deficiencies in how a human being thinks. Storr (1972) also perceived man as divided and maintained that the divisions within him hamper his ability to use his imagination to create new syntheses.

Arieti (1976) proposed that one of the characteristics of creativity was that it progressed within the artist in an unstructured, illogical and chaotic manner. The Random House Dictionary further describes the results of creativity as "something that is not made by ordinary process" (Urdangi, 1968, p. 314). Creativity is inherent in psychotherapy; Wallas (1926) identified four stages within the creative process: preparation-incubation-illumination-verification. This is the same structure that is found in the therapeutic process. The *preparation* phase, involves the collection of data, materials, thoughts, the preparation of the workspace. As the preparation phase progresses the creative person also engages in conscious thought. The work of the preparation phase is pre-conscious but can also involve conscious awareness. In therapy, the preparation includes establishing a trusting relationship with the client, learning the structure of the therapy session, experiencing how to move and play with minimal structure, relaxing the secondary process so that the primary process can come forward. The effect is primarily a loading of the unconscious with cognitive, emotional and sensory material to carry into the next phase - incubation. *Incubation* is a stage where specific mechanisms must be inferred as the actual process is not visible to the cognitive portion of the mind. It is a period of varying duration in which the material collected during the preparation phase is sorted, re-organized, elaborated and transformed to emerge into the next phase. The incubation phase can be very frustrating as there is little awareness of progress in a linear or goal-oriented sense. In therapy the incubation stage is characterized by an increase in conflict and anxiety. There is a sense of chaos and randomness. As anxiety increases the client will progress towards the illumination phase.

It is at this point, the *illumination* phase, that the material collected in preparation and altered in incubation emerges as a clear insight or solution to the problem. The unconscious movement and verbal metaphors emerge until the client can synthesize the cognitive, sensory or emotional material. This moment of insight is characterized by a great feeling of accomplishment and relief as the uncomfortable feelings of chaos and anxiety subside. The *verification* phase is the only fully intentional, conscious phase in the creative process. In this phase, the individual consolidates and integrates the insights gained in the illumination phase. This is done through discussion with the therapist, exploration of the new movement or behaviour options that the insight has made available, and integration of the new material into the fabric of the client's personality.

An example of a dance/movement therapy session in which a group member utilized the creative process to gain insight into her behaviour: Through weekly sessions, the group member explored in the *preparation* phase the use of physical weight by grounding herself emotionally when she felt anxious and lost. Relating to other group members she would explore the polarities of her weight by using light, playful movements or exerting herself in excessively aggressive gestures. The latter were usually directed at the leader or other members who had the focus of attention. This is characteristic of the *incubation* phase with its heightened anxiety, conflict, sense of chaos and randomness. The *illuminating* session for this group member occurred when she approached the leader by gently pushing her; the gesture had no conviction behind it and she was able to feel this and say "that doesn't feel quite right". Although she was not conscious at that moment why it did not "feel right", she began to embrace the leader while using a rocking rhythm to get herself grounded, a method she explored during the preparation phase. Gradually she began to take on more of the physical weight until she had completely lifted the leader off the floor. While holding the leader she began to show signs of extreme exertion, sweating profusely and shaking. She was now becoming anxious and fearful, and through this period talked about the upsurging emotions. The leader, noticing her emotional state and physical stress, attempted to "help" her by dropping her leg to the ground to reduce the amount of weight the group member was holding. Immediately, the feeling of anxiety and fear diminished. The leader realized this and let herself be lifted once more and the group member immediately regained her feelings and explored the movement metaphor by taking the full "load" of the leader and all the accompanying heavy responsibilities. By discussing the physical sensation of actually holding the leader, and then translating and bringing in the additional emotional material of the fear and the anxiety, a sudden insight occurred that the issue she was working on was her impending graduation from college and searching for a job. The awareness of old behaviour patterns centred around her inability to take full responsibility. In the next phase, *verification*, this group member will need to explore and assimilate the insight that taking on responsibility is anxiety-provoking for her. In exploring new behaviour options for coping with this reality she will hopefully be able to accept greater responsibility.

In this example, dance/movement therapy was the vehicle which moved the client to a fuller understanding of her problem with responsibility. The creative process was in full use by the client and also by the leader throughout the session. It was the non-verbal nature of dance/movement therapy which allowed the insight to occur on a direct sensory level.

Our society's reliance on the verbal/cognitive has separated us from the direct sensory experience so important to our thinking and creative processes. Dance/movement therapy works with the individual's intrinsic body movements and self-awareness to first integrate the cognitive, physical and emotional self, and later to embark on the difficult struggle towards therapeutic goals. Dance/movement therapy's unique ability of harnessing the creative process by establishing direct communication between the conscious and unconscious self is a powerful tool.

> "Man is a creature inescapably, and often unhappily, divided; and the divisions within him recurrently impel the use of his imagination to make new synthesis. The creative consequences of his imaginative strivings may never make him whole; but they constitute his deepest consolations and his greatest glories" (Storr, 1972 p. 295-296).

References

Arieti, S. (1976) *Creativity, the Magic Synthesis.* New York: Basic Books Inc.

Arnheim, R. (1969) *Visual Thinking.* Berkeley: University of California

Baker, E. (1967) *Man in the Trap.* New York: The Macmillan Company

Best, D. (1974) *Expression in Movement and the Arts: A philosophical enquiry.* London:

Dosmantes-Alperson, E. (1983) 'Experiential Movement Psychotherapy.' *American Journal of Dance Therapy,* 257-289

Horowitz, M.J. (1972) 'Mode of Representation of Thought.' *Journal of the American Psychoanalytic Association*, Vol. 20, 793-819

Storr, A. (1972) *The Dynamics of Creation.* London: Pelican Books

Urdangi, L. (Ed.) (1968) *The Random House Dictionary.* New York: Random House

Wallas, G. (1926) *The Art of Thought.* New York: Harcourt Brace

Zwerling, I. (1979) 'The Creative Arts Therapies as Real Therapies.' *Hospital and Community Psychiatry*, Vol. 30, No. 12., December

'Looking Ahead Planning Together: the Creative Arts in Therapy as an Integral Part of Treatment for the 90's.' Hahnemann University, Philadelphia, 1985, p.184

The use of the movement metaphor in movement therapy

Jude Webster

Laban Centre for Movement and Dance, London

Like the other creative art therapies, movement therapy uses the initiation of the patient to accomplish therapeutic aims. What is different is that it only involves the medium of a person's body and movement (though occasionally props can be used). The movement a person makes is his or her own spontaneous movement, it is not prescribed, nor is it determined by anything externally. This often leaves people feeling awkward or self-conscious initially, not liking their bodies or feeling that they cannot 'dance' well.

Gradually, as they learn that there is no right or wrong way to move in the sessions, the self-conscious feeling subsides. The movement, at the same time, provides a powerful analytical tool. The movement therapist, who is trained to observe, replicate and assess movement, moves with the patient to assist in developing this movement into both verbal and nonverbal expression. Within this relationship, one of the most effective tools is the movement metaphor. By the movement metaphor I mean a movement, with or without a direct verbal association, which may become the theme of a session, e.g. "bushwacking". I do not know what it means for the patient initially, but it may be significant to them. The reason these metaphors are so powerful is that the movement provides direct access to unconscious feelings and can provide a concrete way of practising something within a safe environment, before trying it outside and making changes in one's behaviour, which is the ultimate goal of therapy.

Movement often acts as a form of expression for those patients who cannot verbalize their feelings or perhaps do not know how they are feeling. One of the most striking examples is an autistic child who cannot speak and yet manages, in movement therapy, to express a wide range of feelings.

Another illustration is provided by the case of a highly verbal adult who suffered from depression and was sexually abused as a child. She was very insightful, yet when asked directly how she felt, was unable to identify her feelings, other than in a somatic way. In movement, however, she was able to demonstrate that a certain part of her body, e.g. her stomach or throat hurt. She spent one session identifying different parts of her body as having different temperatures, e.g. her legs were hot, her head cold and her torso empty. When it was acknowledged that she did indeed have many feelings, she grew tearful. Continuing with the images and moving the other painful parts of her body at her own pace, she was able to explore for the first time some powerful feelings about her past abuse. Her verbal responses were initiated by her movement expression.

Movement is also used to corroborate what a patient says, either literally or metaphorically. For example, a high functioning woman suffering from depression, began a session saying she felt low and shaky. When she stood up, she feared she would fall down. The image of falling down became the theme of the session. As the patient and therapist moved and played with what the movement metaphor of falling down meant for her, verbal associations followed. When she was a little girl, her mother fell down one day at the bus stop. When the mother fell, she cried and the girl (patient) responded by laughing. Within the session, she realized that she feared that if she fell, the group would laugh, leaving her feeling rejected. As her story unfolded, the next connection she made was to falling in love with her present husband 12 years ago and consequently being rejected by her family. At this point she wanted to leave her husband, on whom she was very dependent, but feared falling down emotionally and financially. The movement metaphor clarified and strengthened the expression of her feelings.

Patients often contradict in movement what they say verbally, providing both patient and therapist useful material to work with. Contradictions may be as clear as a mother offering a toy to her child while simultaneously holding on to it tightly and even pulling it away slightly. In effect, she is saying "Take it but don't take it" - a double bind. There are also more broadly based contradictions in behaviour. For example, a very quiet child was referred to movement therapy because the teacher was afraid he was withdrawn and would get overlooked in class. However, in the session he was quite active and freely expressed aggressive movements of his own accord, behaviour completely different from that displayed in the classroom.

More subtle contradictions were exhibited by a schoolgirl referred because of difficulties at home and suspected sexual abuse. This child had difficulty playing imaginary games or making up dances. One of the routines that developed in the movement therapy sessions was the making of obstacle courses, over which she had complete control, i.e. where the objects were to be placed, what the rules/directions would be for proceeding through the course, how long it would take etc. She either contradicted her own rules or, more frequently, changed the rules each time the therapist proceeded through the course. The theme of uncertainty and changing rules, wherein children were to know the rules but adults were not, seemed to be her response to the sense of constant change at home. Her parents were often separating and reuniting and the family had moved twice during the year. In therapy, she reversed the roles so that she, the child, could change the rules on the therapist, the adult. Apparently, she was trying to gain some control over her feelings of chaos.

Another example of contradiction in movement was a young male patient in a psychiatric hospital who talked about using his strength, giving examples about how he had been in exercise groups and done things like press-ups to build and demonstrate his strength. At the same time, he did not feel strong, physically or emotionally, for when encouraged to use his strength in group movement he had difficulty doing so.

Another patient said in therapy, "I cannot go forward" yet simultaneously took a step. This contradiciton became a major focus in uncovering her desparate need for control and fear she would lose it. As she stepped forward, I said, "but you just did", which supported her and helped her realize that she, in fact, had strength she didn't know she had.

For patients feeling stuck emotionally or verbally, movement may be helpful in clarifying how they are stuck. By externalizing the stuck feeling, acknowledging it in movement and playing with the "stuck-ness", the patient often can find alternatives for dealing with the blocked feelings. One high-functioning patient used her metaphor of "being stuck and sinking in the mud". She said she felt like her legs could not move, but her arms felt strong and active, freely moving with a wide range. As we talked and moved, she realized she could use her arms to move her legs. This exemplified how her insight and range of coping skills increased during therapy.

Practising alternatives in movement and then, if necessary, applying it to one's own life can be insightful. Often, talking about the movement as a symbol alone, rather than translating and interpreting what it means literally in their lives, is powerful enough. Change can be inspired because the patient has been able to step outside of himself for a few moments.

Movement in any of these roles often sparks a lost memory relevant to psychotherapy, sometimes pleasant and playful, other times more painful or destructive memories which have been blocked. The kinesthetic memory begins at the pre-verbal stage of life, approximately the first two years, and is extremely significant to one's personal development and relationships with the family. Therefore, non-verbal expressions, whether conscious or unconscious, elicit powerful responses from those who use them as well as for the group members who see them. Ultimately, these responses can provide a new way of perceiving the present situation, and therefore may lead to change in the patient's behaviour.

An example of the movement metaphor in a slightly different context, a family therapy session, is as follows. The therapist became the role model for a couple, dealing with issues of closeness and intimacy, using his own proximity as the tool. The therapist modelled intimacy by crouching next to the wife, and as he moved toward her, she moved toward her husband without realizing it, thus increasing emotional contact with him. As the therapist returned to his chair, the wife retreated emotionally from her husband. The therapist instinctively went back to his previous crouching position, and the wife regained emotional closeness to her husband without moving. The therapist discussed with the couple the process that had just occurred. This example shows how closeness (physical and emotional) was initially practiced non-verbally and unconsciously, then integrated verbally and consciously.

Movement metaphors are important because they allow the patient to take a part of himself outside of his body, to look at it and examine it. This part, or this movement, is still himself, but the process of externalizing these feelings through movement makes them safer to explore. The patient can then internalize and begin to integrate these insights in order to make life changes.

Use of theatre as a therapeutic and educational tool within community structures and social service programmes

Victoria Bryan

Stop-Gap, Los Angeles, California

Stop-Gap is a theatre company that uses drama as a therapeutic and educational tool. Our mission statement reads "To effect positive change in individual lives through the use of theatre as a therapeutic and educational tool". While that may seem rather obscure as a description of what we do, it is hard to offer a more concrete short description.

The key word in describing Stop-Gap is diversity. The people we work with range in age from 5 to 95. We include other arts in our drama-based programmes. We work in schools, hospitals and many other community settings as well as regular theatres. Our resident playwright provides us with scripts for the plays that tour into school classrooms, but our therapeutic drama workshops are based on role-playing. We use professional actors in most of our touring plays, but we also use recovering teenage substance abusers in the play about drug abuse prevention. The subjects we cover range from birth (often a subject for scene work with pregnant teens or teen mothers) to death - a topic that we are frequently asked to address in our senior adult programmes - and all stops in between.

We are eligible for arts funding as well as social service and educational grants - and, despite the risk of sounding opportunistic, I can usually ask any potential funding source their specific area of interest, confident that we address that issue in some way.

We have come to believe that there is no issue or problem area in our community that cannot be addressed through some form of therapeutic or educational theatre programme. While we do not claim to "cure all ills", we do seek to be a useful resource which can enhance the work of other social service, therapeutic, health care or educational programmes. We do not limit our methodology to any particular kinds of theatre work, but design programmes that use a variety of techniques to work towards the goals of each group.

Therapeutic drama workshops

Stop-Gap's first area of concentration was in on-going therapeutic drama programmes in community settings. When Don Laffoon and I started Stop-Gap twelve years ago, we did not foresee all of the directions that the work would take. We concentrated on work with senior adults, in a variety of programmes. As with any new programme that Stop-Gap starts, we had no pre-conceived workshop plan, but began by asking questions. We talked to the directors, the staff and the senior participants at each site to find out about their concerns and the issues that they felt affected the quality of life for seniors. Not surprisingly, many of the issues were those we all face, but some were specific to the senior population. The issues included:

- loss of independence
- drug abuse
- loss of health
- isolation and depression
- fear of being victimized by criminals

From that information, we designed weekly programmes that use: scripted scenes, role-playing, discussion, word-games, acting exercises, reading scripts, music, theatre games, guided imagery, artwork, poetry and oral history. After the entertainment value of each workshop engages the interest of the participants, the discussion facilitator is able to promote group interaction, leading to group suggestions for responses or alternative solutions to individual problems.

By using a team of actors and a workshop leader, we are able to begin a workshop with a presentational scene or other introduction. With this non-threatening lead-in to the session, the participant can relax and join the discussion, trusting that he or she will not be forced into acting, or any level of involvement beyond that which feels comfortable. Discussion of the presentation, participant role-playing and group exercises encourage each group member to become involved up to the level of individual ability. Seeing situations acted out, and making suggestions that influence how a scene may end, or be replayed, bring clarity and understanding to situations that group members may have been struggling with alone, such as:

- living with sons and daughters and their families;
- having to leave their home and live in board and care facilities;
- experiencing a shrinking world through losses associated with aging.

These scenes are among those frequently suggested by seniors when the workshop leader requests participants' input to determine the content of the day's programme.

When role-playing or discussion elicits information about serious individual problems, such as thoughts of suicide or elder-abuse, the host facility staff who observe each session are able to follow-up with individual counselling afterwards.

Out of the workshops with the general senior population, we were asked to devise more specialized programmes for senior groups such as stroke victims and frail elderly in senior adult day care programmes. As with all of our programme design, we worked in partnership with the experts in those fields (including facility staff) during the development of the workshop plans.

We expanded our programme to include other age groups and special populations in response to requests, until currently we provide 17 different therapeutic drama workshops each week for groups including:

- battered women and their children (in shelters for victims of domestic violence);
- abused and neglected children (5 age groups, ranging from 7-19 years old);
- recovering women alcoholics;
- recovering teenage substance abusers;
- pregnant teens/teen mothers;
- developmentally disturbed young adults;
- children with life-threatening illnesses;
- frail elderly;
- incarcerated youth.

While the content and format of these workshops varies considerably, certain basic issues surface in almost every programme we serve. Whether we are working with children with cancer, battered women or senior citizens, certain underlying issues are raised repeatedly: dysfunctional family backgrounds, repeated cycles of domestic violence, substance abuse, lack of communication skills and lack of self-esteem are among the most common.

When we give participants the ability to choose which scenes they would either like to see played out or participate in, we seek to empower people who, for the most part, have lost power over their lives. Their suggestions are anonymous, however, written on identical cards offering them the option of using their personal history as well as the choice of whether to claim it publicly as their own. While many "authors" of scenes are ready to own their material, we choose names for our characters other than those of the actors and participants playing them, so that they are not forced to do so.

While the Stop-Gap team can focus on clarification, understanding of available choices, responsibility, breaking cycles of abuse and development of decision-making skills during workshops, we rely on the host facility staff for individual follow-up in situations where abuse and violence are present. Staff can sometimes gain information about programme participants through Stop-Gap workshops which was not available before. An example of this was a 15-year-old girl, placed by the court at the Crittenton residential programme, who reported 7 incidents of molestation and incest during a Stop-Gap presentation about those issues. She had not reported the incidents before because, as she said, "she didn't know what *she* had done to make that keep happening to her".

We have many requests on file for new programmes which we will implement once we secure the necessary funding. These groups include:
- homeless street youth;
- homeless women
- Cambodian teenagers
- emotionally disturbed girls.

Touring plays

Out of one of our on-going therapeutic drama programmes with teen substance abusers at the Phoenix House Recovery Programme, came the material from which Robert Knapp, our resident playwright, created *Under Pressure*, a presentation about drug abuse prevention. This play is different from the other three Stop-Gap plays that currently tour into school classrooms in that it includes three recovering teen substance abusers from the Phoenix House programme as cast members. Before the play begins, the young cast members introduce themselves to the audience, telling their ages (which range from 13 to 17) and their histories of drug use. Following the 25-minute play, they join the facilitator for the discussion, frankly answering any questions that the student (or sometimes parent) audiences have about their reasons for taking drugs and the effects on their lives and relationships. The same format of short play followed by facilitator-led discussion and role-playing is used in our other current school plays:

My Brothers' Keeper, about AIDS education.
When No Means No, about date or acquaintance rape.
Use My Real Name, about ethnic diversity and prejudice.

Although *Under Pressure* was written for ages 12-14, and the other plays target students 14-18, we will perform the plays for varying age groups, at teachers' requests. We do limit the audience size to 50 for each performance in order to encourage free and open participation in the discussion. In the 1989/90 school year we performed the plays approximately 300 times throughout two counties.

As parents and teachers identify priority areas of concern to us, we seek funding to develop new plays to address those areas. We are currently developing a newly-funded presentation to go into elementary schools (for ages 9-12) about alcoholism and its effects on families. We are also seeking funding for new plays on the following subjects:
- prevention of gang involvement (for children 9-14),
- prevention of teen pregnancy, and
- overcoming illiteracy.

General public productions

In addition to these two main areas of work, Stop-Gap also stages general public productions three times a year, allowing us to focus attention on the key issues that we address throughout our therapeutic and educational programmes. These published and original plays have included:
- *Extremities* (about rape)
- *Shadow Box* (about death and dying)
- *When the Bough Breaks* and *Shadow and Song* (both original musicals about the effects of incest, based on our work with residents at Orangewood, the County Shelter for abused and neglected children)
- *Beyond Therapy* (about the lighter side of psychotherapy)
- *Eleemosynary* (about mother/daughter relationships and dysfunctional families). This play, as with previous productions, offers us the opportunity to use theatre in another way with the participants in the weekly therapeutic drama workshops being invited to attend the production and use it as the focus for discussion of the issues as they relate to their own lives.

The schedule is full. Our eight person full-time staff, augmented by part-time staff and volunteers, is busy as we cover days such as this typical Wednesday:

At 10.30 a.m., a team of actors and workshop leader begin a weekly therapeutic drama workshop with recovering women alcoholics at New

Directions in Costa Mesa. At 10.43 a.m., in the city of Orange, another Stop-Gap team start work with children suffering from cancer and cystic fibrosis at the Childrens' Hospital of Orange County. At the same time, fifty miles north, in Los Angeles County, another team is working with young women who live at the Crittenton Center, a residential programme which offers an alternative to incarcerations for young offenders. This programme combines therapeutic drama with rehearsals for their original play to be performed for their staff, peers, probation officers, social workers and families, including their young children who live with them. Just after lunch, an Orange County team moves on to the weekly programme for the frail elderly at Anaheim. This programme is now in its eleventh year, and has become an integral part of the centre's weekly schedule, as have many of our other programmes. Later in the afternoon, a Los Angeles cast of actors and discussion facilitator take three performances of *Use My Real Name* into school classrooms in Long Beach. At 3.00 and 4.00 an Orange County team conducts 2 hour-long therapeutic drama workshops, one with teen boys and the other with teen girls, at Orangewood, the County shelter for abused and neglected children. Following those workshops, certain staff meet the cast and technical crew for an evening rehearsal of a public production.

The issues we deal with have no respect for programme boundaries. We may find that the therapeutic drama workshop planned for women alcoholics has to be instantly revised to meet the needs of that day's participants when staff tell us that 80% of the women in that day's programme are victims of incest. Or the planned session on career choices for teen mothers is scrapped to allow exploration of shared experiences of death and loss when that subject surfaces in a workshop. The format is kept flexible in order to accommodate the participants' needs on that particular day.

Neither are the issues limited to people within social service programmes, schools or hospitals. Stop-Gap also reaches general audiences through worksites and colleges as well as through productions in public theatres and presentations at conferences and seminars.

If this description sounds like everything has fallen neatly into place over the last 12 years, that is more a reflection of the time limitation of this presentation than of the reality of our history. We continue to struggle with difficult issues such as: prioritization of community needs, development of evaluation methods and tools - an area where we have a great deal of work ahead of us. And then there's funding ....

The future

As always, our future looks very exciting.

- The development of new programmes in response to identified community

needs is an on-going goal, with worksite programmes being a particular area of expansion.
- We anticipate formalization of our training programme, which would provide the structure for people to come and learn with us, through both classes and participation in the workshops.
- We look forward to having a permanent home one day - currently we're in donated office space.

Finally, another dream - that the original Stop-Gap may become a model for similar programmes in other communities. We've made that move once already - the original Stop-Gap started in Orange County 12 years ago and two and a half years ago we started a second Stop-Gap in Los Angeles County. Both programmes are running successfully. We believe that one day there will be many others.

Live music in hospitals

Sylvia Lindsay

Council for Music in Hospitals, Surrey

At a recent hospital concert an elderly gentleman in the front row sighed happily and said, "Ah, that beats diamorphine any day!". After another concert a patient told us that this had been the happiest day of her life - "It was like being in a magic world", and again, "I was ill when I came in and now I am well!".

Music has the supreme power to transcend and to overcome communication and other problems, being non-verbal and completely non-threatening, and as Plato says, "has the power to penetrate the innermost recesses of the human soul and to put order upon it".

The *Council for Music in Hospitals* was founded just over 40 years ago by a group of people who took a gramophone and a few records onto the ward of a psychiatric hospital. Almost immediately it was realized that a live performance was infinitely more meaningful than even the finest recording as it enables the patients to cross the line between just hearing something and of actively listening and participating in the music. The visual aspect of the performance, the feeling of being at a "real" concert with all the excitement and glamour of the concert hall, together with the warmth of the performer's personality and the fact that the programme can be tailored to the individual needs of the audience. Through these factors and many more, all those who, because of their age or the nature of their illness have been unable to attend a concert for perhaps 20-30 - even 40 - years, can experience the joy and benefit which music can bring.

The early concerts were given in the vast halls of psychiatric hospitals. Now, over the years, we have learnt to respond to the changing needs within the hospitals. With few exceptions the formal concerts in the halls are gone and we take our music to the patients wherever they may be - the social centre, chapel, tea bar, onto the wards or day rooms, and frequently, of course, to individual bedsides. In this way we feel we can bring the maximum benefit to the greatest number of patients as, for example, when our artists give short concerts on a great many wards in one day so that no patient need be left out or denied the delight of hearing their own special concert. That this policy has proved successful is borne out by the fact that, whereas in the 1970's we were giving less than 200 concerts a year, in 1989 we arranged nearly 2500 performances in England, Wales, Scotland and Northern Ireland. No venue is too small or too remote to have a special concert from the Council for Music in Hospitals, and we now go to every kind of hospital, home, hospice, day centre, training centre, etc.

Over the years we have learnt from our not inconsiderable experience that the success of a concert is in *direct relation* to the ability of the artists to communicate with the most withdrawn and apathetic - to create an informal atmosphere in which the patients can enjoy a professional performance, and which is also very much a shared experience between the artists and their audience.

For this reason we choose our professional musicians with tremendous care. Not only do we require a very high standard of musicianship but, perhaps even more important, is the warmth of their personality, ability to talk on every level about the music, the patients, their problems - together with being able to respond sensitively to the patients' needs. Our artists are expected to play without the barrier of the printed page, so that wherever possible they can move among the audience using all the communications skills - touch, voice, eye contact, thereby making each and every patient feel very special. Considerable experience is necessary to achieve all this, together with a wide repertoire to suit all tastes and the ability and flexibility to adapt this to the needs of the moment.

It is not always easy to give a successful hospital concert - in fact, it is often most tiring and demanding work. The situations are unpredictable, and the artists tell us this can be stressful at times - they seldom know in advance what the patients' musical tastes may be or, indeed, how they will react - or if they will respond at all! They may be working in difficult venues, in the corridor or the garden, or a dreadfully stuffy ward. There may be noises, interruptions, tea, pills being given out, patients going to the toilet, and sometimes excruciating pianos which provide a tremendous challenge! They may have to cope with outbursts of emotion or crying (which may be a good thing) and in the hospices our artists have told us on a number of occasions of patients actually dying during the performance. Throughout all this the musicians must perform with confidence and enthusiasm and even while working individually must have regard to the audience as a whole and for the need of a high quality professional performance. I should note in passing that artists who are successful in this work tell us that they view these concerts as perhaps the most rewarding aspect of their career. As one artist wrote to us after a demanding four-day tour in which she had given nine concerts at venues ranging from large hospitals for the mentally handicapped to a tiny hospice, "Although we were left emotionally and physically drained, our tiredness goes and I count it a privilege to have been given the opportunity to provide moments of happiness. Applause, recognition, money, mean nothing in comparison. Working in hospitals has been, without hesitation, the most important part of my musical career".

The reports which we receive from doctors, staff and artists after each concert have enabled us to assess many of the benefits which music brings to patients in hospitals and of the new avenues which are opened up through the music for patients of every age from infancy to those in terminal care. For example, the patients at Queen Mary's Hospital for Children at Carshalton, Surrey, have music of every kind brought to their wards five or six times a week. This gives these profoundly mentally and physically handicapped youngsters the opportunity to experience - to see and to feel - the music of guitars, accordions, wind and string instruments and even to have fun with castanets, musical clowns or perhaps the hosepipe! The residents with learning difficulties (mental handicap) are among our most exuberant hospital audiences and for those whose intellectual horizons are limited the concerts can give them a chance to benefit from a high quality live performance in which they can actively participate with movements and with singing. This is something they would not otherwise be able to experience, and the music is seen not only to be a socializing influence, of educational and entertainment benefit, but also to have a very deep effect, as when recently a young man became noisy and violent at a hospital concert. The artist went over to his chair, and holding his hands, sang a verse or two very quietly - the change was dramatic and he became almost instantly calm and serene.

For the psychiatric patients who may be lacking in volition, music is a motivating force. A social event of this kind enables them to practice forgotten social skills and staff tell us that, due to the high degree of interaction between artists and patients, they seem to come to life and be like different people, so that they appear in an entirely different light. Also, they are frequently amazed at the concentration span of patients who are normally restless and disturbed. Again, music can be a catharsis for a strong emotion, bringing, through tears and laughter, a great sense of release, as happened, for example, during a concert for mentally ill patients, when a young girl started to scream hysterically. She was led out, but the doctors said this was the emotional breakthrough for which they had been working for months and at last they could start to treat that patient. We hear of many cases like this - of how the music helps the patients to cry, to reveal their fears and to come to terms with their illness. Music as a means of communication can be far more meaningful than words, can become a bridge between the patient and those around him, and the most confused can relate to familiar music. Again, music can stimulate patients with speech difficulties and frequently we hear of people who have spoken for the first time for weeks, or even months, during a concert and this can be a starting point for the speech therapists using melodic intonation therapy.

A great number of the concerts take place on wards or in tiny day rooms with the very frail and elderly. For all those whose outlook is confined to the same four walls, as for all in long-stay care, the music can combat the sense of isolation which is so sadly felt by the patients, confirms their sense of identity and makes them feel special and loved. Of course, the familiar music takes the old people back to a happier time and is a valuable resource in recall and reminiscence therapy. Also, the rhythm can stimulate disused limbs; backs become straighter and eyes brighter, and it is a very moving experience to watch one of our artists perhaps kneeling beside a very old, frail, patient, holding his/her hand and singing together a favourite song. The visual aspect of a concert, the long dresses (one of our artists changes 5/6 times during a performance) are an added benefit and make a talking point for days after the event. The fact that the patients can feel that these super artists really care about them and go to so much trouble is of tremendous importance. In addition, for everyone concerned, the concerts are a most welcome break from hospital routine.

In cancer hospitals, we hear that our concerts help the patients to forget their pain and, by reducing fear and tension, discomfort can become more bearable. After one of our concerts at the Royal Marsden Hospital, the Director of Nursing Services said, "The true value of these concerts lies in the fact that music enables the patients to forget about hospitals, illness and all that involves and it is like a fabulous night out!"

We are asked to perform in hospices all over the country. In these venues, a short concert in the chapel or day room is followed by a great deal of time spent at individual bedsides. These concerts mean that music lovers who never thought they would have the chance to hear live music again can yet have their favourite music played gently and specially for them. Tremendous sensitivity is required, but we find the music is welcomed, not only by the patients, but also by families and staff. The relatives tell us how much it means to them to have something they can share and talk about with their loved ones and we have even been asked to give special concerts for the bereaved.

Quite often we are actually asked to provide music for a dying patient, as at a famous London hospice when the relatives requested that a harpist should play by the bedside. As the music played the patient surfaced from a comatose state and was able to embrace his family and say farewell before he died. This was a profoundly moving experience for the staff and the artist and was *very* greatly appreciated by the relatives. Because music can break down so many barriers, even in the last days it can be a starting point through which people can come to terms with their illness. Patients learn to talk about and to share their problems and can even through music make new beginnings at the deepest spiritual level.

Schumann once said, "The musician's art is to send light into men's hearts". For all those who are locked in a cage of pain, loneliness or fear, music can be the key which will unlock the door and let in happiness and the light of the sun. Perhaps this is the greatest benefit of all, and must always be the aim of all who are involved in working for the Council for Music in Hospitals.

The effects of brief relaxation techniques and sedative music on levels of tension

Louise Schuster

Psychotherapist, Los Angeles, California

Since ancient times, music has been used as a method of tension reduction, often in association with religious meditative practices or ceremonial traditions inherent in many cultures. As early as the second century B.C., chants were used by the Hebrews to induce inner solitude. Tribal ceremonies connected with shamanism have been identified in diverse cultures that include Africa, Japan, North and South America, Indonesia, Siberia, Australia, as well as many islands throughout the South Pacific.

Nearly every culture has reported experiencing the extensive powers of music in relieving tension. Greek mythology assumed a divine origin of music. An essential element of this theory was the belief that music could heal sickness and work miracles in nature. The utilization of music in Greek culture was also based upon the idea that music was connected with the pursuit of truth, and the experiencing of aesthetic pleasures.

In a similar vein, Benson (1975) refers to the early contributions of Eastern religions in using meditation and repetitive sounds as a means of bringing the soul into harmony with the outside world.

It has been generally accepted that a cause and effect relationship exists between music and human behaviour. Until recent times, however, scientific research had not systematically investigated the possible ways in which music affects the physiological and psychological processes of the listener. Helmholtz, the nineteenth century physicist, was the founder of musical aesthetics as a science (Boring, 1950). In addition to meticulously examining the physiology of musical perception, he was first to investigate the relationship between music and individual human response, and the first to measure its influence scientifically. It became generally accepted that music affects people in at least three ways. First, music seems to cause emotional changes in the listener; second, music may cause kinaesthetic change in the muscular system; and third, it appears to have a probable effect upon psychological processes such as memory, learning, cognition and perception.

With regard to exploring stress responses, there have been few attempts to conceptualize music as a relaxation technique (Sears, 1960; Stoudenmire, 1975). Sears' was the first to study the possible sedative influence of music on autonomic functioning.

Researchers such as Jacobson (1964), Wolpe (1958), Selye (1974) and Benson (1975) have theorized extensively regarding efficient methods of stress reduction. Based on Wolpe's theory of reciprocal inhibition, music was conceptualized, for the purposes of the current experiment, as a possible way of interrupting destructive behaviour chains (a response incompatible with tension).

In order to compare the effects of music with other methods of relaxation, the following techniques were included:

1 Progressive Relaxation (PR): a technique developed by Jacobson, and refined by Bernstein and Borkovec (1973).
2 Relaxation Response (RR): a system of autonomic conditioning developed by Benson (1975) as a means of inducing relaxation.
3 Sedative Music (SM): a stimulus condition consisting of four possible types of carefully controlled music judged to be calming. Highly trained judges rated compositions on components that included pitch, rhythm, intensity and tempo.

Relaxation levels of subjects receiving treatment were compared to subjects assigned to a control, non-treatment (silence) condition. Subjects were assessed for changes in electromyographic data, anxiety scores and self-report of relaxation.

It was hypothesized that subjects receiving one of three treatment conditions would respond with greater significant reductions in tension levels compared to those who received no experimental manipulations. It was also hypothesized that subjects with high internal locus of control scores would respond to relaxation to a greater degree than subjects with high external locus of control. Thirdly, it was predicted that sedative music would produce a greater effect than either the traditional relaxation methods or the control condition.

Method

Sixty subjects (28 men, 32 women) were recruited through announcement in the Los Angeles area. The population included students, professionals, business executives and housewives between the ages of 25 and 40 years. Subjects were selected according to age, sex and absence of debilitating physical or psychological distress (such as hearing difficulties, muscular discomfort or self-reported emotional disorders). Four groups of 15 subjects each were used.

A randomized control group pre-test/post-test design, using repeated measures was employed to test the effects of the four treatments. Each subject received just one of the treatment or control conditions. Monitoring was continuous throughout the course of the repeated measures design.

Muscle tension was monitored by recording of frontalis and forearm muscles. Pre- and post-treatment levels of state anxiety were assessed, using the State-Trait Anxiety Inventory (Spielberger, Gorsuch and Lushene, 1969). Change due to treatment was defined as the pre-test minus post-test state anxiety score (Spielberger shift score or SPR-SRO).

A post-study self-report form was included, to give the subjects an opportunity to describe any subjective experience of tension reduction after exposure to the treatments. Each subject was asked to answer brief questions covering such topics as changes in level of tension throughout the procedure, usefulness of the treatment, alternative methods of relaxation previously used, use of drugs or alcohol, and previous experience in psychotherapy or meditation.

Finally, the Rotter Internal-External Locus of Control Scale (1966) was administered. This 29-item test measures personal response to hypothetical situations in an attempt to assess whether they see their life as determined by their own actions or outside forces beyond their control. Rotter Scale scores were referred to as the RIET variable.

Analyses were conducted on possible interactions between previous experience in meditation or psychotherapy, as well as the influence of using stimulants or sedatives on ability to reduce levels of tension. These variables were chosen as part of an exploratory attempt to determine whether or not previous experience in tension-reducing situations might influence individual response to treatment.

Results

To test the assumption of between-group homogeneity, an analysis of variance was used to compare group means in reference to the following variables: 1) Taylor Manifest Anxiety Scale scores 2) Self-Report Arrival scores (derived from the Post-Study Questionnaire) 3) first frontalis EMG measurements 4) first forearm measurements and 5) subject age. The mean age of participants was 25.1 years. Results of the analysis of variance indicated that there were no significant differences between treatment groups on any of the variables listed above, suggesting that the groups contained similar subjects.

Upon completion of the preliminary data analysis, the emergence of an electrode attachment factor (inherent in biofeedback data) suggested an influence on analysis of the integrated scores. Moreover, it was found that reported movement artifacts were interfering with analysis of the integrated scores. Average integrated scores were designated as standardized difference scores, and defined as the average of two pre-test EMG scores minus the average of two post-test EMG scores. Finally, given the wide range of standard deviations, logarithmic transformations were used to assist in stabilizing the variance. This appeared to eliminate negative scores, produce consistent data and reduce the possibility that statistical outliers would significantly alter the distribution. After data transformation, four subjects with recorded movement were deleted from the final data analysis in order to reduce movement artifacts. Sample size was thus brought to $N = 56$.

Analysis of variance and t-tests were used to compare relaxation levels between and within groups. T-tests were used to assess the efficacy of treatments within each group. Table 1 shows results of tests used to assess physiological outcome measures. Logarithmic transformations of standardized difference scores showed highly significant treatment effects within all four groups. However, the frequent occurrence of negative shift scores in the Control Group should be noted.

There were significant differences between the groups on three physiological measures of forearm EMG. ANOVA revealed significant effects as follows: $F(3,52) = .266$ for forearm (FO) 1-5 measurements, $F(3,52) = 3.08$ for FO 1-6 and $F(3,52) = 2.81$ for FO -7 shift scores. Treatment effects were found to be similar between groups on all other variables.

Originally, it was hypothesized that significant reductions in levels of tension experienced by subjects in the control group suggested the possibility of interference from the Rosenthal (1966) effect in experiments of this type. However, what appeared to be a problem in the statistical analysis has since been reported in similar findings by Borgeat (1983), Curtis (1986), Guyer and

Variable	PR	RR	SM	CG	df	F	df	P
1. LG1SDAFO	x: .99 ± 0.05 t: p < .001	x: .98 ± 0.08 t: p < .001	x: .99 ± 0.04 t: p < .001	x: .98 ± 0.03 t: p < .001	14	0,22	3,52	NS
2. LG1SDAFR	x: 1.00 ± 0.02 t: p < .001	x: 1.00 ± 0.00 t: p < .001	x: 1.00 ± 0.01 t: p < .001	x: .99 + 0.03 t: p < .001	14	0.50	3.52	NS
3. LG2SDAFR	x: 1.01 ± 0.02 t: p < .001	x: 1.00 ± 0.02 t: p < .001	x: .99 - 0.01 t: p < .001	x: .99 ± 0.01 t: p < .001	14	1.10	3.52	NS
4. LG2SDAFR	x: 1.00 ± 0.01 t: p < .001	x: 1.00 ± 0.01 t: p < .001	x: 1.00 ± 0.01 t: p < .001	x: 1.00 ± 0.01 t: p < .001	14	0.18	3.52	NS
5. FO1-FO2	x: 42.07 ± 89.95 t: NS	x: 11.08 ± 57.13 t: NS	x: 25.47 ± 95.05 t: NS	x: -15.43 ± 46.26 t: NS	14	2.27	3.52	NS
6. FO1-FO3	x: 78.93 ± 153.17 t: NS	x: 24.69 ± 72.80 t: NS	x: 8.60 ± 31.78 t: NS	x: 39.14 ± 151.81 t: NS	14	2.53	3.52	NS
7. FO1-FO4	x: 52,14 ± 172.24 t: p < .05	x: 12.00 ± 92.43 t: NS	x: 1.13 ± 61.55 t: NS	x: -54.36 ± 145.55 t: NS	14	1.72	3.52	NS
8. FO1-FO5	x: 85.00 ± 145.93 t: NS	x: 4.54 ± 128.55 t: NS	x: 16.67 ± 81.95 t: NS	x: -37.86 ± 130.99 t: NS	14	2.66	3.52	<0.057
9. FO1-FO6	x: 79.50 ± 148.03 t: NS	x: 2.15 ± 100.49 t: NS	x: -2.40 ± 48.56 t: NS	x: -35.14 ± 95.71 t: NS	14	3.08	3.52	<0.04
10. FO1-FO7	x: 78.29 ± 152.32 t: NS	x: 16.08 ± 78.26 t: NS	x: -5.80 ± 67.86 t: NS	x: 34.14 ± 108.94 t: NS	14	2.81	3.52	<0.05
11. FR1-FR2	x: 18.64 ± 74.11 t: NS	x: 2.15 ± 48.15 t: NS	x: 10.33 ± 51.60 t: NS	x: 6.21 ± 80.34 t: Ns	14	0.16	3.52	NS
12. FR1-FR2	x: 10.71 ± 152.15 t: NS	x: 37.38 ± 64.54 t: p <.058	x: 53.27 ± 82.00 t: p <.02 t: NS	x: 23.71 ± 84.25	14	0.47	3.52	NS
13. FR1-FR4	x: -21.07 ± 219.43 t: NS	x: 42.54 ± 40.10 t: p <.01	x: 47.73 ± 80.85 t: p <.04 t: NS	x: 30.71 ± 88.03	14	0.87	3.52	NS
14. FR1-FR5	x: 7.28 ± 120.13 t: NS	x: 33.31 ± 37.85 t: p <.01	x: 46.93 ± 83.55 t: p <.05 t: NS	x: 31.14 ± 93.87	14	0.49	3.52	NS
15. FR1-FR6	x: 22.57 ± 112.14 t: NS	x: 28.46 ± 71.05 t: NS	x: 49.40 ± 81.66 t: p <.03 t: NS	x: 1.86 ± 127.04	14	0.55	3.52	NS
16. FR1-FR7	x: 38.93 ± 134.41 t: NS	x: 41.54 ± 54.74 t: p <.01	x: 29.60 ± 97.10 t: NS	x: 14.21 ± 116.83 t: NS	14	0.19	3.52	NS

Outliers deleted. N = 56. Critical value for p <.05 is .225
Table 1.

	N = 15				N = 60			
Variable	PR	RR	SM	CG	df	F	df	P
ARR-END	1.33 (± 1.11) (p <.001)	1.47 (± .74) (p <.001)	1.53 (± .83) (p <.001)	0.87 (± 1.19) (p <.01)	14	1.39	3,56	NS
AFT I-END	0.60 (± .74) (p <.01)	0.73 (± .88) (p <.01)	1.07 (± .88) (p <.001)	0.33 (± 1.05) (p <.24)	14	1.74	3,56	NS
DURP-END	0.40 (± .51) (p <.01)	0.33 (± .49) (p <.02)	0.40 (± .51) (p <.01)	0.27 (± .88) (p <.26)	14	.16	3,56	NS
AVG-END	0.78 (± .71) (p <.01)	0.84 (± .58) (p <.001)	1.00 (± .60) (p <.001)	0.49 (± .93) (p <.07)	14	1.33	3,56	NS
SPR-SPO	8.67 (± 6.99)	10.13 (± 6.85)	11.60 (± 8.15)	6.73 (± 6.08)	14	1.30	3,56	NS

Chi-Square Tests to Determine Signicant Change in Psychological Outcome Measures, N = 60

Variable	*X*	*df*	*p*	*F*	*df*	*p*
Procedure Useful	9.39	3	<0.02	2.92	3,56	<.04
Reuse Procedure	3.90	3	<0.27	2.00	3,56	NS

Table 2.

Guyer (1984) and Gregoire (1984). In each of the above studies, control groups that were designated as a silence condition yielded treatment effects. Borgeat has suggested that silence may elicit relaxation. Although there were no significant differences between groups on psychological variables, there were highly significant changes within each of the groups on self-report variables, with Control Group means being lower than the treatment conditions (Table 2).

Correlational analysis was used to examine the hypothesized relationship between the levels of relaxation and locus of control. As predicted, subjects with high internal locus of control did manifest increased ability to relax. Pearson r tests also yielded significant relationships between internal locus of control and ability to lower levels of tension. Table 3 shows results for all groups combined but more detailed analysis showed that the effect was due to three groups in particular (PR, RR and CG).

Table 3. Correlation table examining possible relationships between locus of control and outcome measures.

Variable	*Correlation*
LG1SDAFO/RIET*	-.22
LG1SDAFR/RIET	-.10
LG2SDAFO/RIET	-.20
LS2SDAFR/RIET	-.18
FO1-FO2/RIET	-.10
FO1-FO3/RIET	*-.23
FO1-FO4/RIET	*-.26
FO1-FO5/RIET	-.21
FO1-FO6/RIET	*-.28
FO1-FO7/RIET	*-.29
FO2-FO3/RIET	-.19
FO2-FO4/RIET	*-.21
FO2-FO5/RIET	-.20
FO2-FO6/RIET	*-.25
FO2-FO7/RIET	*-.24
FR1-FR2/RIET	.04
FR1-FR3/RIET	-.19
FR1-FR4/RIET	*-.25
FR1-FR5/RIET	-.12
FR1-FR6/RIET	-.18
FR1-FR7/RIET	-.15

FR2-FR3/RIET	*-.24
FR2-FR4/RIET	*-.28
FR2-FR5/RIET	-.15
FR2-FR6/RIET	-.14
FR2/FR7/RIET	-.18
FO3-FO7/RIET	-.08
FO3-FO5/RIET	-.07
FR3-FR7/RIET	.05
FR3-FR5/RIET	.11
FOA12-5/RIET	-.20
FRA12-5/RIET	-.16
FO5-FO7/RIET	-.05
FR5-FR7/RIET	-.12
FOA12-3/RIET	-.21
FOA12-4/RIET	*-.24
FOA12-6/RIET	*-.24
FOA12-7/RIET	*-.24
FRA12-3/RIET	-.21
FRA12-4/RIET	*-.27
FRA12-6/RIET	-.21
FRA-12-7/RIET	-.18
Pre-treatment Spielberger/RIET	.08
Pre-treatment Spielberger minus post-treatment Spielberger/RIET	02
Reuse procedure/RIET	*-.25

A strong trend emerged in the data between treatment and electrode placement. In the PR treatments, both frontalis and forearm measures generated significant differences in physiological variables. However, the ration was weighted toward the stability of the frontalis measure.

Analysis of variance was used to evaluate comparative effectiveness of Sedative Music as a means of lowering levels of tension. Significant differences between groups were evident on three physiological variables (Table 1). These forearm shift scores represented the only treatment effects between groups - probably traceable to the natural relaxation factor affecting the Control Group condition.

T-tests used to assess relative effectiveness of the experimental conditions resulted in highly significant values (see Tables 1 and 2) on both psychological and physiological variables. According to rank order comparisons, Relaxation Response and Sedative Music conditions appeared to induce particularly deep levels of relaxation as measured by EMG scores (Table 4).

Table 4. Sum of Significant Outcome Measures for Each Group.

Variable	Progressive Relaxation	Relaxation Response	Sedative Music	Control Group
Psychological	5	5	5	2
Physiological	12	22	18	9

N = 56

Chi-square tests were used to analyse two self-report variables (Procedure Useful, Reuse Procedure). Frequency tables indicated 92% of the subjects found the procedure useful, regardless of which condition they experienced. Procedure Useful variable was significant x^2 (3) = 9.39, p<.02, regardless of subject by group assignment.

Self-report questionnaires were analysed in an effort to generate ideas for further research. Four variables were examined, using a two-way analysis of variance in an attempt to determine possible relationships involving these variables and relaxation shift scores. The four variables studies were: 1) previous experience in psychotherapy 2) previous experience in meditation 3) use of stimulants and 4) use of sedatives. Both main and interactional effects were reported for variables 1 and 2. Variables 3 and 4 yielded no interactions - probably due to a differential scale used in variables 1 and 2.

Only physiological variables showed trends toward significant interactions involving experience in psychotherapy and physiological response. Both main and interactional effects were found and are reported in Table 5. Of particular interest was the finding that these interactions occurred almost exclusively in forearm measures, pointing to the possibility of an unexplored electrode placement factor. Only physiological variables tended to suggest the influence of previous experience in meditation as a factor in ability to relax. Interaction effects were also calculated for experience in meditation and lowered levels of tension, F(3)52, p < .01 (Table 6.). In contrast to the previous variable (influence of experience in psychotherapy on ability to relax), significant interactions were reported on frontalis variables.

Discussion

The main intention of this research was to assess the usefulness of sedative music as a relaxation technique. Both psychological and physiological measures showed significant shift scores that would seem to suggest the possible value of including carefully controlled musical selections in the

Table 5. Two way analysis of variance comparing the four treatment groups and experience with psychotherapy

Variable	Source	Mean square	F	df	P
FO2-FO4	Group	50431.89	4.34	1	*
	Experience in psychotherapy	54652.89	4.71	1	*
	Interaction	12711.50	1.09	1	NS
	Error	11610.67		26	
FO2-FO5	Group	20752.28	2.29	1	NS
	Experience in psychotherapy	36339.17	4.01	1	*
	Interaction	28757.02	3.17	1	NS
	Error	9060.96		26	
FR3-FR5	Group	81.33	0.08	1	NS
	Experience in psychotherapy	2571.34	2.46	1	NS
	Interaction	7235.19	6.92	1	**
	Error	1045.02		26	
FOA1,2-3	Group	14846.15	1.21	1	NS
	Experience in psychotherapy	65846.13	5.36	1	*
	Interaction	14190.97	1.16	1	NS
	Error	12279.80		26	
FOA1,2-4	Group	22635.70	1.95	1	NS
	Experience in psychotherapy	65718.68	5.68	1	*
	Interaction	17010.80	1.47	1	NS
	Error	11578.49		26	
FOA1,2-5	Group	4891.20	0.50	1	NS
	Experience in psychotherapy	45456.45	4.64	1	*
	Interaction	35065.87	3.58	1	NS
	Error	9788.74		26	
	Group	2667.75	0.20	1	NS
	Experience in psychotherapy	56719.02	4.23	1	*
	Interaction	6019.02	0.45	1	NS
	Error	13405.80		26	

* $p < .05$, ** $p < .01$, NS = Not significant

Table 6. Two way analysis of variance comparing the four treatment groups and experience with meditation.

Variable	Source	Mean square	F	df	P
FR1-FR3	Group	16879.66	2.06	3	NS
	Experience in meditation	2125.09	0.26	1	NS
	Interaction	41687.62	5.08	3	**
	Error	8207.70		52	
FR2-FR3	Group	17204.69	2.32	3	NS
	Experience in meditation	7974.25	1.08	1	NS
	Interaction	25956.75	3.50	3	*
	Error	7409.40		52	
FR3-FR7	Group	14658.33	2.35	3	NS
	Experience in meditation	6417.21	1.03	1	NS
	Interaction	24235.77	3.88	3	**
	Error	7250.10		52	
FR3-FR5	Group	2408.10	0.46	3	NS
	Experience in meditation	6106.30	1.18	1	NS
	Interaction	15309.50	2.95	3	*
	Error	5193.32		52	
	Group	14578.53	0.98	3	NS
	Experience in meditation	7925.57	0.53	1	NS
	Interaction	48164.98	3.25	3	*
	Error	14818.37		52	

* p <.05, ** p <.01, NS = Not significant

repertoire of relaxation techniques. However, the comparative effectiveness of such music cannot be fully evaluated at this time because of methodological difficulties.

A major corollary of this study is that there is a demonstrated lack of appropriate technology with which to assess the impact of various relaxation techniques upon individual levels of tension. In addition to the absence of a proper explanation found in the literature regarding measurement of physiological change in studies of this type, it appears that many procedures used in prior experiments are inconsistent.

Using the findings of this study-notation of movement artifacts, determination of baseline and final measurements, sedative music as a relaxation technique and logarithmic transformation of data - it may be possible to create the kind of standardized methodology necessary to test such hypotheses.

Further research could be initiated to investigate other effects that music might have upon human response. This could include examination of the relationship between music and imagery, the effect(s) of natural sounds upon physiology, or a varied combination of paired stimulus conditions such as Sedative Music and Benson's Relaxation Response. The intriguing issue of a natural (silence-induced) factor also lends itself to further study.

It would seem useful to design carefully controlled studies, using methodologically standardized procedures, with the intention of contributing more efficient and meaningful ways of altering individual response to the effects of stress. Continued systematic investigation of the therapeutic uses of music as a way to relieve tension could be utilized to help individuals develop more adaptive patterns of social interaction, particularly in group settings.

Acknowledgements

Appreciation for assistance in preparing this manuscript is given to Drs. Arthur Kovacs (Michigan State, CSPP), Noel Wheeler and Carol Newton (University of California at Los Angeles) and David Wine, Veterans' Administration, Brentwood, California.

References

Altschuler, I.M. (1944) 'Four years' experience with music as a therapeutic agent.' *American Journal of Psychology, 100*, 792-794

Archer, R.P. (1979) 'Relationships between locus of control and anxiety.' *Journal of Personality Assessment, 43 (6)*, 617-626

Barger, D.A. (1979) 'The effects of music and verbal suggestion on heart rate and self reports.' *Journal of Music Therapy, 15 (4)*, 158-171

Basmajian, J.V. (1974) *Muscles Alive: Their function revealed by electromyography.* Baltimore, Maryland: Williams & Wilkins

Beary, J.F. & H. Benson (1974) 'A simple psychophysiologic technique which elicits the hypometabolic changes of the relaxation response.' *Psychosomatic Medicine, 36*, 115-120

Benson, H. (1975) *The Relaxation Response.* New York: Avon Books

Bernstein, D.A. & T. Borkovec (1973) *Progressive Relaxation Training: A manual for the helping professions.* Champaign, Illinois: Research Press

Borgeat, F. (1983) 'Psychophysiological effects of two different relaxation procedures: Progressive relaxation and subliminal relaxation.' *Psychiatric Journal of the University of Ottawa, 8 (4)*, 181-185

Boring, E.G. (1950) *A History of Experimental Psychology* (2nd Ed.) New York: Appleton-Century-Crofts Inc.

Cox, D.J., A. Freundlich & R. Meyer 'Differential effectiveness of electromyographic feedback, verbal relaxation techniques and medication placebo with tension headaches.' *Journal of Consulting and Clinical Psychology, 43*, 892-898

Curtis, S.L. (1986) 'The effects of music on pain relief and relaxation of the terminally ill.' *Journal of Music Therapy, 23 (1)*, 10-24

Goldfried, M. & C. Trier (1974) 'Effectiveness of relaxation as an active coping skill.' *Journal of Abnormal Psychology, 83*, 348-355

Greenwood, M.M. & H. Benson (1977) 'The efficacy of progressive relaxation in systematic desensitization and a proposal for an alternative competitive response - the relaxation response.' *Behaviour Research and Therapy, 15*, 337-343

Gregoire, M.A. (1984) 'Music as a prior condition to task performance.' *Journal of Music Therapy, 21 (3)*, 133-145

Guyer, N.P. & C.G. Guyer (1984) 'Implementing relaxation training in counselling emotionally healthy adolescents: A comparison of three modes.' *American Mental Health Counselors Association Journal, 6 (2)*, 79-87

Hudson, W.C. (1973) 'Music: A physiologic language.' *Journal of Music Therapy, 10*, 137-140

Husek, T.R. & S. Alexander (1963) 'The effectiveness of the anxiety differential in the examination of stress situations.' *Educational and Psychological Measurement, 23*, 309-318

Jacobson, E. (1964) *Anxiety and Tension Control.* Philadelphia: Lippincott

Lehrer, P.M. (1972) 'Physiological effects of relaxation in a double blind analog of desensitization.' *Behavioral Therapy, 3*, 193-208

Miller, M.P., T.P. Miller & P.J. Murphy 'Comparison of electro-myographic feedback and progressive relaxation training in treating circumscribed anxiety stress reactions.' *Journal of Consulting and Clinical Psychology, 46*, 1291-1298

Miller, R.K. & P.H. Bornstein (1977) 'Thirty minute relaxation: A comparison of some methods.' *Journal of Behavior Therapy and Experimental Psychiatry, 8 (3)*, 291-294

Parker, J.C., G.S. Gilbert & R.W. Thoreson (1978) 'Reduction of autonomic arousal in alcoholics: a comparison of relaxation and meditation techniques.' *Journal of Consulting and Clinical Psychology. 5*, 879-886

Paul, G. & D.T. Shannon (1966) 'Treatment of anxiety through systematic desensitization in therapy groups.' *Journal of Abnormal Psychology, 71*, 124-135

Paul, G.L. (1969) 'Physiological effects of relaxation training and hypnotic suggestion.' *Journal of Abnormal Psychology, 74*, 425-437

Paul, G.L. & R.W. Trimble (1970) 'Recorded vs "live" relaxation training and hypnotic suggestion: comparative effectiveness for reducing physiological arousal and inhibiting stress response.' *Behavior Therapy, 1*, 285-302

Plutchic, R. (1959) 'The effects of high intensity intermittent sound on performance, feelings and physiology.' *Psychological Bulletin, 56*, 113-151

Rachman, S. (1968) 'The role of muscular relaxation in desensitization therapy.' *Behavior Research Therapy, 6*, 159-166

Rosenthal, R. (1966) *Experimenter effects in behavioral research.* New York: Appleton-Century-Crofts

Rotter, J.D. (1966) 'Generalized expectancies for internal vs external control of reinforcement.' *Bulletin Psychological Monograph, 80 (1)*, Whole No. (609)

Schandler, S. & W. Grings (1976) 'An examination for producing relaxation during short-term laboratory sessions.' *Behavior Research and Therapy, 14*, 419-426

Sears, W.W. (1960) 'A study of some effects of music upon muscle tension.' Doctoral dissertation, University of Kansas. L.C. Card No. Mic. 60-2316

Selye, H. (1974) *Stress Without Distress.* New York: Signet

Snow, W.G. (1977) 'The physiological and subjective effects of several brief relaxation training procedures.' Unpublished doctoral dissertation, New York University, Canada

Spielberger, C., R. Gorsuch & R. Lushene (1969) *The State-Trait Anxiety Inventory: Test manual for form X.* Palo Alto, California: Consulting Psychologists' Press

Stoudenmire, J. (1975) 'A comparison of muscle relaxation training and music in the reduction of state and trait anxiety.' *Journal of Clinical Psychology, 34*, 490-492

Talone, J.M., M.J. Diamond & C. Steadman (1975) 'Modifying hypnotic performance by means of brief sensory experiences.' *International Journal of Clinical and Experimental Hypnosis, 23 (3)*, 190-199

Wallace, R. & H. Benson (1972) 'The physiology of meditation.' *Scientific American, 226*, 84-90

Weidenfeller, E. & G. Zimny (1962) 'Effect of music upon GSR of depressives and schizophrenics.' *Journal of Abnormal and Social Psychology, 64*, 307-312

Wolpe, J. (1954) 'Reciprocal inhibition as the main basis of psychotherapeutic effects.' *AMA Archives of Neurological Psychiatry, 72*, 205-226

Wolpe, J. (1958) *Psychotherapy by reciprocal inhibition.* Stanford, California: Stanford University Press

Zimny, G.H. & E.W. Weidenfeller (1963) 'Effects of music upon GSR and heart-rate.' *American Journal of Psychology, 76*, 311-314

Zlutnick, S., W. Mayville & S. Moffat (1975) 'Modification of seizure disorders: the interruption of behavioral chains.' *Journal of Applied Behavior Analysis, 8*, 1-12

List of contributors

Nicholas Arnold, BA, PhD. Head of Theatre and Performance Studies, Leicester Polytechnic, Scraptoft Campus, Scraptoft, Leicester, LE7 9SU, England.

Brian Bates, MA, PhD. Senior Lecturer and Chairperson, Department of Psychology, University of Sussex, Falmer, Brighton, BN1 9QN, England.

Jacqueline Blatt, MCAT, ADTR. Co-ordinator, MA Dance/Movement Therapy Course, Laban Centre for Movement & Dance, Laurie Grove, New Cross, London, SE14 6NH, England.

Victoria Bryan, Director, Stop-Gap, 10779 W. Pico Blvd, Los Angeles, California 90064, USA.

Catherine Butler, LRAM. Student Counsellor, Guildhall School of Music and Drama, Barbican, London, EC2Y 8DT, England.

Fairfid M. Caudle, PhD. Associate Professor of Psychology, Department of Psychology, Sociology & Anthropology, College of Staten Island, City University of New York, Sunnyside Campus, 715 Ocean Terrace, Staten Island, New York, NY 10301, USA.

Louise DeCosta, CSW, BCD. Director, Institute for the Performing Artist, New York. Senior Supervisor (Faculty), Postgraduate Center for Mental Health, 124 East 28th Street, New York, NY 10016, USA.

Robert J. Edelmann, BSc, MPhil, PhD. Lecturer in Clinical Psychology, University of Surrey, Guildford, Surrey, GU2 5XH, England.

Carole H. Field, MA. Marriage, Family & Child Psychotherapist, 13033 Ventura Boulevard, Studio City, California 91604, USA.

David Fontana, BA, MEd, PhD, PGCE, Ad.Dip.Ed, FBPsS, CPsychol. Reader in Educational Psychology, School of Education, University of Wales, Cardiff, Wales.

Dennis C. Gold. North Eastern Pennsylvania Counselling Centre, 676 Wyoming Avenue, Kingston, Pennsylvania 18704, USA.

Jacqueline Hammond, BSc. Research Psychologist, University of Surrey, Guildford, Surrey, GU2 5XH, England.

Elissa C. Haworth, BA. Department of Psychology, University of Manchester, Manchester, M13 9PL, England.

John T. Haworth, BSc, PhD, MLitt. Lecturer, Department of Psychology, University of Manchester, Manchester, M13 9PL, England.

Katharine Hitchcock, BA, MA. Research Psychologist, Department of Psychology, University of Sussex, Falmer, Brighton, Sussex, BN1 9QM, England.

Elly A Konijn, Drs. Research Psychologist, Department of Theatre Studies, State University of Utrecht, Kromme Nieuwe Gracht, 29, 3512 HD Utrecht, The Netherlands.

Sylvia Lindsay, LRAM, ARCM. Director, Council for Music in Hospitals, 340 Lower Road, Little Bookham, Surrey, KT23 4EF.

Martin Lloyd-Elliott, BSc, LISHS. Director, Arts Psychology Consultants Ltd, 38 Earls Court Square, London, SW5 9DQ, England.

Suzanne T. S. MacDonald, MA. Center for Sports Medicine and Dance Medicine, St Francis Hospital, 900 Hyde Street, San Francisco, California 94109, USA.

Glenys McQueen-Fuentes, BA. Assistant Professor, Department of Film Studies, Dramatic & Visual Arts, Brock University, St Catharine's Ontario, L2S 3A1, Canada.

Estelle M. Phillips, BSc, PhD, AFBPsS. Lecturer in Occupational Psychology, Birkbeck College, University of London, Malet Street, London, WC1E 7HX, England.

Barbara Pollack, BA, MA, PhD. Clinical/Consulting Psychologist, Attending Doctor at the Children's Hospital, Denver, 155 So Madison Avenue, Ste. 332, Denver Colorado 80209, USA.

Shelley Reciniello, PhD. Clinical Psychologist, President, SRA Associates, 211 W 56th St, Suite 7M, New York, NY 10019, USA.

Zuleika Robertson. Analytical Psychotherapist, 6 Prospect Park, Exeter, Devon, EX4 6NA, England.

Paul Salmon, PhD. Associate Professor, Department of Psychology, Director of Clinical Research, The Genesis Center, Department of Psychiatry & Behavioral Sciences, University of Louisville, Louisville, Kentucky 40292, USA.

Louise Schuster, MM, MA, PhD. Psychotherapist, 5353 Encino Avenue, Encino, California 91316, USA.

Stephen Snow, PhD. Drama Therapist, Bronx Psychiatric Center, 1500 Waters Place, Bronx, New York 10461, Drama Therapist & Director of Validation Therapy Research, Wartburg Lutheran Home for the Aging, Brooklyn, New York, Instructor in Drama Therapy at The New School for Social Research, New York, USA.

Simone F. Sternberg, EdD. Dean of Training, New York Center for Psychoanalytic Training, Suite 2F, 300 West 72nd Street, New York, NY 10023, USA.

Lucilia Valente, CEPA (Lisbon). PhD student, School of Education, University of Wales, Cardiff, Wales.

Elizabeth R. Valentine, BA, PhD, AFBPsS, CPsychol. Lecturer in Psychology, Royal Holloway and Bedford New College, University of London, Egham Hill, Egham, Surrey, TW20 0EX, England.

Jude Webster, MA, DTR. Project Manager, Monroe Young Family Centre, 33a Daleham Gardens, London, NW3, England.

Daniel T. Wolverton, BA. Trainee Clinical Psychologist, Psychology Department, University of Louisville, Louisville, Kentucky, KY 40292, USA.